Micronutrients in Maternal and Infant Health: Where We Are and Where We Should Go

Micronutrients in Maternal and Infant Health: Where We Are and Where We Should Go

Editor

Yunxian Yu

MDPI • Basel • Beijing • Wuhan • Barcelona • Belgrade • Manchester • Tokyo • Cluj • Tianjin

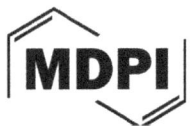

Editor
Yunxian Yu
Zhejiang University School of
Medicine, Hangzhou, China

Editorial Office
MDPI
St. Alban-Anlage 66
4052 Basel, Switzerland

This is a reprint of articles from the Special Issue published online in the open access journal *Nutrients* (ISSN 2072-6643) (available at: https://www.mdpi.com/journal/nutrients/special_issues/micronutrients_maternal_infant).

For citation purposes, cite each article independently as indicated on the article page online and as indicated below:

LastName, A.A.; LastName, B.B.; LastName, C.C. Article Title. *Journal Name* **Year**, *Volume Number*, Page Range.

ISBN 978-3-0365-7272-7 (Hbk)
ISBN 978-3-0365-7273-4 (PDF)

© 2023 by the authors. Articles in this book are Open Access and distributed under the Creative Commons Attribution (CC BY) license, which allows users to download, copy and build upon published articles, as long as the author and publisher are properly credited, which ensures maximum dissemination and a wider impact of our publications.
The book as a whole is distributed by MDPI under the terms and conditions of the Creative Commons license CC BY-NC-ND.

Contents

About the Editor vii

Preface to "Micronutrients in Maternal and Infant Health: Where We Are and Where We Should Go" ix

Yunxian Yu
Association between Plasma Trace Element Concentrations in Early Pregnancy and Gestational Diabetes Mellitus in Shanghai, China
Reprinted from: *Nutrients* **2023**, *15*, 2192, doi:10.3390/nu15092192 1

Ting Wu, Tao Li, Chen Zhang, Hefeng Huang and Yanting Wu
Association between Plasma Trace Element Concentrations in Early Pregnancy and Gestational Diabetes Mellitus in Shanghai, China
Reprinted from: *Nutrients* **2023**, *15*, 115, doi:10.3390/nu15010115 5

Huanmei Zhang, Xiangnan Ren, Zhenyu Yang and Jianqiang Lai
Vitamin A Concentration in Human Milk: A Meta-Analysis
Reprinted from: *Nutrients* **2022**, *14*, 4844, doi:10.3390/nu14224844 19

Hui Wang, Hai-Jun Wang, Mingyuan Jiao, Na Han, Jinhui Xu, Heling Bao, et al.
Associations between Dynamic Vitamin D Level and Thyroid Function during Pregnancy
Reprinted from: *Nutrients* **2022**, *14*, 3780, doi:10.3390/nu14183780 37

Shiqi Lin, Jiajia Li, Yuan Zhang, Xinming Song, Gong Chen and Lijun Pei
Maternal Passive Smoking, Vitamin D Deficiency and Risk of Spontaneous Abortion
Reprinted from: *Nutrients* **2022**, *14*, 3674, doi:10.3390/nu14183674 49

Zhicheng Peng, Shuting Si, Haoyue Cheng, Haibo Zhou, Peihan Chi, Minjia Mo, et al.
The Associations of Maternal Hemoglobin Concentration in Different Time Points and Its Changes during Pregnancy with Birth Weight Outcomes
Reprinted from: *Nutrients* **2022**, *14*, 2542, doi:10.3390/nu14122542 59

Shuting Si, Zhicheng Peng, Haoyue Cheng, Yan Zhuang, Peihan Chi, Xialidan Alifu, et al.
Association of Vitamin D in Different Trimester with Hemoglobin during Pregnancy
Reprinted from: *Nutrients* **2022**, *14*, 2455, doi:10.3390/nu14122455 75

Shuting Si, Minjia Mo, Haoyue Cheng, Zhicheng Peng, Xialidan Alifu, Haibo Zhou, et al.
The Association of Vitamin D and Its Pathway Genes' Polymorphisms with Hypertensive Disorders of Pregnancy: A Prospective Cohort Study
Reprinted from: *Nutrients* **2022**, *14*, 2355, doi:10.3390/nu14112355 87

Huiqing Gang, Hongling Zhang, Tongzhang Zheng, Wei Xia, Shunqing Xu and Yuanyuan Li
Associations between Maternal Selenium Status and Cord Serum Vitamin D Levels: A Birth Cohort Study in Wuhan, China
Reprinted from: *Nutrients* **2022**, *14*, 1715, doi:10.3390/nu14091715 103

Qianling Zhou, Mingyuan Jiao, Na Han, Wangxing Yang, Heling Bao and Zhenghong Ren
The Influence of Maternal Vitamin E Concentrations in Different Trimesters on Gestational Diabetes and Large-for-Gestational-Age: A Retrospective Study in China
Reprinted from: *Nutrients* **2022**, *14*, 1629, doi:10.3390/nu14081629 113

Jiaomei Yang, Yijun Kang, Qianqian Chang, Binyan Zhang, Xin Liu, Lingxia Zeng, et al.
Maternal Zinc, Copper, and Selenium Intakes during Pregnancy and Congenital Heart Defects
Reprinted from: *Nutrients* **2022**, *14*, 1055, doi:10.3390/nu14051055 123

Danmeng Liu, Shanshan Li, Binyan Zhang, Yijun Kang, Yue Cheng, Lingxia Zeng, et al.
Maternal Hemoglobin Concentrations and Birth Weight, Low Birth Weight (LBW), and Small for Gestational Age (SGA): Findings from a Prospective Study in Northwest China
Reprinted from: *Nutrients* **2022**, *14*, 858, doi:10.3390/nu14040858 . . . . **137**

Shanshan Li, Danmeng Liu, Yijun Kang, Pengfei Qu, Baibing Mi, Zhonghai Zhu, et al.
Associations of B Vitamin-Related Dietary Pattern during Pregnancy with Birth Outcomes: A Population-Based Study in Northwest China
Reprinted from: *Nutrients* **2022**, *14*, 600, doi:10.3390/nu14030600 . . . . **153**

Yiming Dai, Jiming Zhang, Xiaojuan Qi, Zheng Wang, Minglan Zheng, Ping Liu, et al.
Cord Blood Manganese Concentrations in Relation to Birth Outcomes and Childhood Physical Growth: A Prospective Birth Cohort Study
Reprinted from: *Nutrients* **2021**, *13*, 4304, doi:10.3390/nu13124304 . . . . **165**

Minjia Mo, Bule Shao, Xing Xin, Wenliang Luo, Shuting Si, Wen Jiang, et al.
The Association of Gene Variants in the Vitamin D Metabolic Pathway and Its Interaction with Vitamin D on Gestational Diabetes Mellitus: A Prospective Cohort Study
Reprinted from: *Nutrients* **2021**, *13*, 4220, doi:10.3390/nu13124220 . . . . **177**

Kai-Lun Hu, Chun-Xi Zhang, Panpan Chen, Dan Zhang and Sarah Hunt
Vitamin D Levels in Early and Middle Pregnancy and Preeclampsia, a Systematic Review and Meta-Analysis
Reprinted from: *Nutrients* **2022**, *14*, 999, doi:10.3390/nu14050999 . . . . **191**

About the Editor

Yunxian Yu

Yunxian Yu is a professor and doctoral supervisor at the Zhejiang University School of Public Health. The main research area of Prof. Yu is the genetic and molecular epidemiology research of pregnancy complications, fetal and child health. More than 110 SCI papers have been published by Prof. Yu and his work contributes significantly to the research on maternal and child nutrition and health, especially in China. Among his research, his studies on Vitamin D during pregnancy and perinatal complications have made remarkable achievements. The recent research found that Vitamin D levels in pregnancy increased with the increase in gestational age, and the variation in Vitamin D pathway genes was an important factor affecting the level of Vitamin D in pregnant women. In addition, Vitamin D deficiency and overweight/obesity during pregnancy significantly increased gestational diabetes, gestational hypertension, anemia and preterm birth. At present, Prof. Yu is still devoting himself to the research of maternal and child health. His main current projects are listed as follows:

(1) National Natural Science Foundation of China: A Mendelian Randomized Study of Vitamin D and preterm prematurely ruptured membranes and its molecular mechanism.

(2) A multi-center randomized controlled study of vitamin D supplementation in pregnant women for prevention of gestational diabetes.

(3) National Key Research and Development Program of the 13th Five-Year Plan: Study on the Epidemiology and Monitoring and early Warning System of Metabolic Diseases of Childhood Obesity.

(4) National Key Research and Development Program of the 14th Five-Year Plan: Demonstration Study on the Pathogenesis and precise Prevention of metabolic diseases of Childhood Obesity.

(5) National Key Research and Development Program of the 14th Five-Year Plan: Construction and comprehensive evaluation of a new multilevel key technology system/demonstration base for the prevention and treatment of embryonic-derived diseases.

Preface to "Micronutrients in Maternal and Infant Health: Where We Are and Where We Should Go"

Maternal and infant nutrition is directly related to perinatal health, and the first 1000 days of life are an important window for disease development throughout the life cycle. Micronutrients are key factors in maintaining pregnancy and fetal growth. As a few of the researchers in the field of maternal and infant health, we are pleased that so many other researchers have joined us. We are delighted to serve as the editors of this book, and we are grateful to all the researchers who have submitted their scientific works for inclusion in this compendium. We also are grateful to the executive editors who helped to us to produce this important work. This book focuses on a variety of micronutrients (including vitamin A, vitamin B, vitamin D and vitamin E, selenium, manganese, copper, zinc and hemoglobin) and explores the associations of micronutrients with various pregnancy complications (including gestational diabetes, gestational hypertension, thyroid function, anemia, abortion, birth outcomes and so on). Another feature of this book is the use of repeated measurements of dynamic micronutrient levels during pregnancy, and micronutrient statuses of mothers and infants are evaluated comprehensively. The works in this book can provide reference for the prevention of related perinatal complications, which has important public health significance. We sincerely hope that you may gain knowledge from these studies or that they may inspire you to undergo further research in related fields, so as to make contributions to maternal and infant health.

Yunxian Yu
Editor

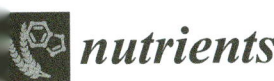 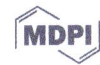

Editorial

Association between Plasma Trace Element Concentrations in Early Pregnancy and Gestational Diabetes Mellitus in Shanghai, China

Yunxian Yu

Department of Epidemiology & Health Statistics, School of Public Health and Medicine, Zhejiang University, Hangzhou 310058, China; yunxianyu@zju.edu.cn

Citation: Yu, Y. Micronutrients in Maternal and Infant Health: Where We Are and Where We Should Go. *Nutrients* **2023**, *15*, 2192. https://doi.org/10.3390/nu15092192

Received: 13 April 2023
Accepted: 21 April 2023
Published: 5 May 2023

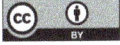

Copyright: © 2022 by the author. Licensee MDPI, Basel, Switzerland. This article is an open access article distributed under the terms and conditions of the Creative Commons Attribution (CC BY) license (https:// creativecommons.org/licenses/by/ 4.0/).

The first 1000 days of life are defined by the World Health Organization as a "window of opportunity" for a person's growth and development, and nutrition is particularly important during this time window [1]. This Special Issue of *Nutrients*, "Micronutrients in Maternal and Infant Health: Where We Are and Where We Should Go", focused on recent research about micronutrients in maternal and infant health. Micronutrients, which play a major role in the metabolism of cellular metabolism and the organ development of the fetus, are important for maintaining pregnancy, fetal growth, and infant health. This issue mainly includes four topics, which are vitamins, race elements, hemoglobin, single nucleotide polymorphisms (SNPs) of genes of the VitD metabolic pathway in maternal and infant health, and the association between micronutrients in maternal or cord blood.

In terms of vitamins, we mainly focused on vitamin D (VitD). VitD deficiency is common during pregnancy. Data from the Chinese Nutrition and Health Survey showed that the prevalence of VitD insufficiency or deficiency in pregnant women in China was about 96.0% [2]. Vitamin D deficiency has been linked to various complications during pregnancy and in infants. Hypertensive disorders of pregnancy (HDP), including gestational hypertension, preeclampsia, eclampsia, pregnancy complicated with chronic hypertension, and chronic hypertension complicated with preeclampsia [3], affect maternal and infant health in the near and long term [4]. Plasma 25(OH)D levels during pregnancy and SNPs in the genes of the VitD metabolic pathway are both important for HDP, as shown by Si et al. [5] In addition, Hu et al. [6] conducted a systematic review and meta-analysis, which indicated that VitD insufficiency or deficiency was associated with an increased risk of preeclampsia. Moreover, maintaining an adequate level of VitD is also beneficial to gestational diabetes (GDM) and thyroid function [7,8]. In addition, Lin et al. [9] suggested that the target group with both VitD deficiency and passive smoking should be paid more attention. Besides VitD, other vitamins are also receiving attention. Vitamin E is a lipid-soluble antioxidant that corrects the oxidative imbalance and protects tissue from damage. Vitamin B is a kind of water-soluble micronutrient, which plays a coenzyme role in many catabolic and anabolic enzyme reactions. Zhou et al. [10] and Li et al. [11] suggested that avoiding excessive vitamin E during pregnancy might be an effective measure to reduce GDM and instances of being large for the gestational age, and adherence to a diet pattern with high vitamin B during pregnancy was associated with higher birth weight and a lower risk of small-for-gestational-age (SGA).

In terms of trace elements, previous studies found that some trace elements participated in regulating and controlling enzyme activity and were involved in the synthesis of many lipids, nucleic acids, and proteins. Recent studies have reported that increased or decreased concentrations of some trace elements were associated with the risk of GDM. Wu et al. [12] also examined the association between maternal exposure to vanadium, chromium, manganese, cobalt, nickel, and selenium in early pregnancy and the risk of GDM, and found that vanadium was positively associated with the risk of GDM, while nickel was negatively associated. Dai et al. [13] reported that prenatal manganese exposure was negatively correlated with childhood physical development, which appeared to be most significant in the early stages. These studies emphasized the importance of detecting the concentrations of trace elements during pregnancy. In addition, dietary and dietary supplements are the main sources of zinc, copper, and selenium in pregnant women. Yang et al. [14] indicated that efforts to promote zinc and selenium intakes during pregnancy needed to be strengthened to reduce the incidence of congenital heart defects in the Chinese population.

Hemoglobin level is also associated with nutritional status and is regarded as a common and economical monitoring indicator for nutritional status assessment during pregnancy. However, the association between hemoglobin levels during pregnancy and the risk of adverse birth outcomes remains controversial. In addition, elevated maternal hemoglobin levels, compared with anemia, are often considered an indicator of good nutritional status and is not always given sufficient clinical attention. However, Liu et al. [15] and Peng et al. [16] evaluated the association between maternal hemoglobin levels and birth weight outcomes and indicated that both severe anemia and high hemoglobin (>130 g/L) should be paid attention to in the practice of maternal and infant health.

Finally, the concentration of micronutrients in human milk and the association between different micronutrients were also explored. Zhang et al. [17] conducted a meta-analysis and found that the level of vitamin A (VitA) in breast milk decreased with the course of breastfeeding, with little difference between China and other countries. These findings provided evidence for the improvement of VitA intake recommendations for exclusively breastfed infants under 6 months of age. In addition, Gang et al. [18] and Si et al. [19] evaluated the association between different micronutrients. Additionally, 25(OH)D levels in cord blood have been linked to diseases in children. Serum selenium and 25(OH)D have been reported in non-pregnant people, and Gang et al. [18] found a positive correlation between maternal urinary selenium levels and cord blood 25(OH)D levels. Si et al. [19] reported that VitD during pregnancy was positive for hemoglobin.

To summarize, micronutrient levels during pregnancy or in infants are essential for programming and the development of complications, which has important public health significance. The studies included in this Special Issue and other related research play important role in future evidence for developing guidelines and management of maternal and infant health through monitoring and supplementing micronutrients, especially for Chinese people. However, the combined effects of various micronutrients on maternal and infant health need to be further studied, and the relevant mechanisms also need to be further explored.

Funding: This research was funded by Chinese National Natural Science Foundation (81973055), the National Key Research and Development Program of China (grant number 2022YFC2703505 and 2021YFC2701901), Major research and development projects of Zhejiang Science and Technology Department (grant number 2018C03010), Key Laboratory of Intelligent Preventive Medicine of Zhejiang Province (grant number 2020E10004), and Leading Innovative and Entrepreneur Team Introduction Pro-gram of Zhejiang (grant number 2019R01007).

Conflicts of Interest: The author declares no conflict of interest.

References

1. Britto, P.R.; Lye, S.J.; Proulx, K.; Yousafzai, A.K.; Matthews, S.G.; Vaivada, T. Nurturing care: Promoting early childhood development. *Lancet* **2017**, *389*, 91–102. [CrossRef] [PubMed]
2. Ramezani Tehrani, F.; Behboudi-Gandevani, S.; Farzadfar, F.; Hosseinpanah, F.; Hadaegh, F.; Khalili, D.; Soleymani-Dodaran, M.; Valizadeh, M.; Abedini, M.; Rahmati, M.; et al. A Cluster Randomized Noninferiority Field Trial of Gestational Diabetes Mellitus Screening. *J. Clin. Endocrinol. Metab.* **2022**, *107*, e2906–e2920. [CrossRef] [PubMed]
3. Hypertension in Pregnancy. Report of the American College of Obstetricians and Gynecologists' Task Force on Hypertension in Pregnancy. *Obstet. Gynecol.* **2013**, *122*, 1122–1131.

4. Theilen, L.H.; Meeks, H.; Fraser, A.; Esplin, M.S.; Smith, K.R.; Varner, M.W. Long-term mortality risk and life expectancy following recurrent hypertensive disease of pregnancy. *Am. J. Obstet. Gynecol.* **2018**, *219*, 107.e1–107.e6. [CrossRef]
5. Si, S.; Mo, M.; Cheng, H.; Peng, Z.; Alifu, X.; Zhou, H.; Chi, P.; Zhuang, Y.; Yu, Y. The Association of Vitamin D and Its Pathway Genes' Polymorphisms with Hypertensive Disorders of Pregnancy: A Prospective Cohort Study. *Nutrients* **2022**, *14*, 2355. [CrossRef] [PubMed]
6. Hu, K.-L.; Zhang, C.-X.; Chen, P.; Zhang, D.; Hunt, S. Vitamin D Levels in Early and Middle Pregnancy and Preeclampsia, a Systematic Review and Meta-Analysis. *Nutrients* **2022**, *14*, 999. [CrossRef] [PubMed]
7. Wang, H.; Wang, H.J.; Jiao, M.; Han, N.; Xu, J.; Bao, H.; Liu, Z.; Ji, Y. Associations between Dynamic Vitamin D Level and Thyroid Function during Pregnancy. *Nutrients* **2022**, *14*, 3780. [CrossRef] [PubMed]
8. Mo, M.; Shao, B.; Xin, X.; Luo, W.; Si, S.; Jiang, W.; Wang, S.; Shen, Y.; Wu, J.; Yu, Y. The Association of Gene Variants in the Vitamin D Metabolic Pathway and Its Interaction with Vitamin D on Gestational Diabetes Mellitus: A Prospective Cohort Study. *Nutrients* **2021**, *13*, 4220. [CrossRef] [PubMed]
9. Lin, S.; Li, J.; Zhang, Y.; Song, X.; Chen, G.; Pei, L. Maternal Passive Smoking, Vitamin D Deficiency and Risk of Spontaneous Abortion. *Nutrients* **2022**, *14*, 3674. [CrossRef] [PubMed]
10. Zhou, Q.; Jiao, M.; Han, N.; Yang, W.; Bao, H.; Ren, Z. The Influence of Maternal Vitamin E Concentrations in Different Trimesters on Gestational Diabetes and Large-for-Gestational-Age: A Retrospective Study in China. *Nutrients* **2022**, *14*, 1629. [CrossRef] [PubMed]
11. Li, S.; Liu, D.; Kang, Y.; Qu, P.; Mi, B.; Zhu, Z.; Han, L.; Zhao, Y.; Chen, F.; Pei, L.; et al. Associations of B Vitamin-Related Dietary Pattern during Pregnancy with Birth Outcomes: A Population-Based Study in Northwest China. *Nutrients* **2022**, *14*, 600. [CrossRef] [PubMed]
12. Wu, T.; Li, T.; Zhang, C.; Huang, H.; Wu, Y. Association between Plasma Trace Element Concentrations in Early Pregnancy and Gestational Diabetes Mellitus in Shanghai, China. *Nutrients* **2022**, *15*, 115. [CrossRef]
13. Dai, Y.; Zhang, J.; Qi, X.; Wang, Z.; Zheng, M.; Liu, P.; Jiang, S.; Guo, J.; Wu, C.; Zhuo, Z. Cord Blood Manganese Concentrations in Relation to Birth Outcomes and Childhood Physical Growth: A Prospective Birth Cohort Study. *Nutrients* **2021**, *13*, 4304. [CrossRef] [PubMed]
14. Yang, J.; Kang, Y.; Chang, Q.; Zhang, B.; Liu, X.; Zeng, L.; Yan, H.; Dang, H. Maternal Zinc, Copper, and Selenium Intakes during Pregnancy and Congenital Heart Defects. *Nutrients* **2022**, *14*, 1055. [CrossRef]
15. Liu, D.; Li, S.; Zhang, B.; Kang, Y.; Cheng, Y.; Zeng, L.; Chen, F.; Mi, B.; Qu, P.; Zhano, D.; et al. Maternal Hemoglobin Concentrations and Birth Weight, Low Birth Weight (LBW), and Small for Gestational Age (SGA): Findings from a Prospective Study in Northwest China. *Nutrients* **2022**, *14*, 858. [CrossRef]
16. Peng, Z.; Si, S.; Cheng, H.; Zhou, H.; Chi, P.; Mo, M.; Zhuang, Y.; Liu, H.; Yu, Y. The Associations of Maternal Hemoglobin Concentration in Different Time Points and Its Changes during Pregnancy with Birth Weight Outcomes. *Nutrients* **2022**, *14*, 2542. [CrossRef] [PubMed]
17. Zhang, H.; Ren, X.; Yang, Z.; Lai, J. Vitamin A Concentration in Human Milk: A Meta-Analysis. *Nutrients* **2022**, *14*, 4844. [CrossRef] [PubMed]
18. Gang, H.; Zhang, H.; Zheng, T.; Xia, W.; Xu, S.; Li, Y. Associations between Maternal Selenium Status and Cord Serum Vitamin D Levels: A Birth Cohort Study in Wuhan, China. *Nutrients* **2022**, *14*, 1715. [CrossRef] [PubMed]
19. Si, S.; Peng, Z.; Cheng, H.; Zhuang, Y.; Chi, P.; Alifu, X.; Zhao, H.; Mo, M.; Yu, Y. Association of Vitamin D in Different Trimester with Hemoglobin during Pregnancy. *Nutrients* **2022**, *14*, 2455. [CrossRef] [PubMed]

Disclaimer/Publisher's Note: The statements, opinions and data contained in all publications are solely those of the individual author(s) and contributor(s) and not of MDPI and/or the editor(s). MDPI and/or the editor(s) disclaim responsibility for any injury to people or property resulting from any ideas, methods, instructions or products referred to in the content.

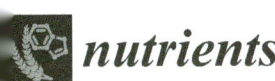

Article

Association between Plasma Trace Element Concentrations in Early Pregnancy and Gestational Diabetes Mellitus in Shanghai, China

Ting Wu [1,2,†], Tao Li [1,2,†], Chen Zhang [1,2], Hefeng Huang [1,2,3,4,5,*] and Yanting Wu [3,4,*]

1. The International Peace Maternity and Child Health Hospital, School of Medicine, Shanghai Jiao Tong University, Shanghai 200030, China
2. Shanghai Key Laboratory of Embryo Original Diseases, Shanghai 200030, China
3. Obstetrics and Gynecology Hospital, Institute of Reproduction and Development, Fudan University, Shanghai 200030, China
4. Research Units of Embryo Original Diseases, Chinese Academy of Medical Sciences, Shanghai 200030, China
5. Women's Hospital, School of Medicine, The Key Laboratory of Reproductive Genetics, Ministry of Education (Zhejiang University), Hangzhou 310058, China
* Correspondence: huanghefg@sjtu.edu.cn (H.H.); yanting_wu@163.com (Y.W.); Tel.: +86-21-6407-0434 (H.H.); +86-21-3318-9900 (Y.W.)
† These authors contributed equally to this work.

Abstract: (1) Background: Trace elements play important roles in gestational diabetes mellitus (GDM), but the results from reported studies are inconsistent. This study aimed to examine the association between maternal exposure to V, Cr, Mn, Co, Ni, and Se in early pregnancy and GDM. (2) Methods: A nested case-control study with 403 GDM patients and 763 controls was conducted. Trace elements were measured using inductively coupled plasma-mass spectrometry in plasma collected from pregnant women in the first trimester of gestation. We used several statistical methods to explore the association between element exposure and GDM risk. (3) Results: Plasma V and Ni were associated with increased and decreased risk of GDM, respectively, in the single-element model. V and Mn were found to be positively, and Ni was found to be negatively associated with GDM risk in the multi-element model. Mn may be the main contributor to GDM risk and Ni the main protective factor against GDM risk in the quantile g computation (QGC). 6.89 µg/L~30.88 µg/L plasma Ni was identified as a safe window for decreased risk of GDM. (4) Conclusions: V was positively associated with GDM risk, while Ni was negatively associated. Ni has dual effects on GDM risk.

Keywords: gestational diabetes mellitus; nickle; trace elements; restricted cubic spline; LASSO regression; quantile g-computation; BKMR models

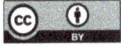

1. Introduction

Gestational diabetes mellitus (GDM), which refers to diabetes diagnosed for the first-time during pregnancy, is one of the most common medical complications of pregnancy [1]. It is associated with substantial short- and long-term adverse complications for both mother and child. The documented prevalence of GDM varies substantially worldwide, ranging from 1% to >30% [2]. The incidence rate of GDM has been increasing worldwide and is approximately 14.8% (95% CI 12.8, 16.7%) in China according to the latest meta-analysis involving 79,064 Chinese participants [3]. In addition to traditional risk factors, such as advanced maternal age, ethnicity, a previous history of gestational diabetes, and a family history of type 2 diabetes mellitus (T2DM), trace elements may play important roles in the development of diabetes [4].

Certain trace elements, such as chromium (Cr), have been suggested to participate in increasing insulin binding and insulin receptor number [5]. Vanadium (V) was found to participate in inhibiting glucose release, improving gluconeogenesis-related enzyme activity, and exerting an insulin-sensitizing effect [6]. Meanwhile, some essential elements, such as manganese (Mn) were found to be associated with a higher risk of hyperglycemia by inhibiting glucose-stimulated insulin secretion and inducing inflammation and oxidative stress [7]. However, not all human studies support the results from laboratory studies. An adult cohort study from Southern Spain suggested that concentrations of certain trace elements (such as Cr) in adipose tissue are associated with the risk of incident T2DM, while V might have a protective effect [8]. A case-control study in China indicated that higher levels of serum selenium (Se) were associated with increased T2DM risk [9].

Some trace elements have recently been suggested to be associated with the risk of GDM in epidemiologic studies. A prospective study demonstrated that increased concentrations of urinary nickel (Ni), Cobalt (Co), and V in early pregnancy are associated with an elevated risk of GDM [10]. In contrast to the results of the above research, two case-control studies indicated an inverse association of V exposure with GDM [11,12], which was reflected by plasma V concentrations and meconium V concentrations. No significant association was found between blood Ni and GDM in the single-metal model in a Chinese birth cohort study [13]. Moreover, a nested case-control study in Xiamen, China, measured Cr concentrations in meconium from newborns delivered by mothers with GDM (137 cases) and without GDM and found a positive association between Cr concentration and GDM prevalence in a dose-dependent manner [14]. One recent meta-analysis showed that the serum Se level of patients with GDM was lower than that in healthy pregnant women. However, no association was found between plasma Se, Cr, and GDM in another nested case-control study [15]. A higher concentration of Mn within a certain range before 24 weeks gestation was demonstrated to impair fasting plasma glucose during pregnancy in a retrospective study [16]. Additionally, a French mother-child cohort study did not find a significant association between blood Mn and the prevalence of GDM [17].

Thus far, the results and conclusions on the relationship between the six trace elements—V, Cr, Mn, Co, Ni, and Se—and GDM are limited and contradictory. In addition, it is essential to study the joint effects of trace elements on GDM risk because elements in the environment exist in the form of co-exposure, and the specific elements included in the analysis individually could be potentially confounded by other elements to which pregnant women are also exposed from the same source. However, when exploring the effects of a multielement mixture in a traditional way, highly unstable results may be obtained if incorporating two or more highly correlated (collinear) elements in a regression model [18]. In recent years, various interdisciplinary methods [19] have been developed to address such issues.

In the present study, we aimed to explore the relationship between these six plasma trace element concentrations before 14 gestational weeks and the risk of GDM. We used least absolute shrinkage and selection operator (LASSO) regression, quantile g computation (QGC), and Bayesian Kernel Machine Regression (BKMR) to screen out independent variables, assess the joint effect of elements on GDM risk and determine the contribution of each element on GDM risk, restricted cubic spline (RCS) was employed to explore the dose-response relationship between elements exposure and GDM risk, with the hope to provide new insights for the prevention of GDM.

2. Materials and Methods

2.1. Study Population

This case-control study was nested in a prospective study initiated in Shanghai, China. From November 2020 to February 2021, pregnant women who visited the International Peace Maternal and Child Hospital (IPMCH) for the first prenatal examination between 8 and 14 gestational weeks and provided enough blood samples were included in the study ($n = 2069$).

The excluded participants were those: (1) who had multiple births ($n = 52$); (2) who were diagnosed with T2DM and other metabolic diseases before pregnancy ($n = 31$); (3) who had serious medical diseases such as cancer ($n = 12$); and (4) who had missing information on birth outcomes ($n = 292$) and missing blood samples ($n = 92$).

Among 1724 finally included pregnant women, 403 pregnant women were diagnosed with GDM and included in the GDM group, and a total of 763 controls were randomly selected from the remaining participants by maternal pre-pregnancy BMI and maternal age (case/control = 1:2 for 360 cases and case/control = 1:1 for 43 cases).

All of the participants in the study signed informed consent forms. This study was approved by the ethics committee of the IPMCH.

2.2. Data Collection

Baseline information was obtained from electronic medical records, including maternal age, ethnic group, pre-pregnancy body mass index (BMI), reproductive history, family and personal disease history, smoking exposure, alcohol consumption, education levels, household income, delivery method, and fetal sex. Maternal BMI was calculated using the formula BMI = weight (kg)/height (m^2). Gestational age was calculated based on the gestational week of delivery and the first day of the last menstrual period. In the present study, smoking exposure was defined as positive if the mother had a smoking history, and alcohol consumption was considered positive if the mother had a drinking history.

2.3. Laboratory Measurements

Plasma concentrations of total cholesterol (CHOL), triglycerides (TG), high-density lipoprotein cholesterol (HDL), low-density lipoprotein cholesterol (LDL), apolipoprotein-A (APO-A), apolipoprotein-B (APO-B) and fasting plasma insulin (FPI) were measured by an automatic chemistry analyzer (BeckmanDXI800, Beckman, Bria, CA, USA). The homeostasis model of assessment-insulin resistance (HOMA-IR) score was obtained according to the following formula: HOMA-IR = FPG (mmol/L) × FPI (μU/mL)/22.5.

Inductively coupled plasma-mass spectrometry (ICP-MS) was used for the determination of the six trace elements. ICP-MS is a quadrupole mass spectrometer, consists of basic components, including the peristaltic pump, nebulizer, spray chamber, ICP torch, interface cones, ion optics, quadrupole, and detector. It has been considered the gold standard analytical method for element measurements in biological samples which meet the interference elimination of the determination of different elements in the sample. We used the NexION 300X device (PerkinElmer, Waltham, MA, USA) and the stander mode for the measurements [20]. Blood was collected between 8 and 14 gestational weeks, and plasma was collected in EDTA tubes after centrifugation at 2000 rpm for 20 min. All plasma samples were frozen at $-80\ °C$ for storage and transferred to a $4\ °C$ refrigerator the night before detection. Several standard curves were prepared by diluting the element standard solution (PerkinElmer, Waltham, MA, USA), and the value of the limit of detection (LOD) of each element was calculated. Plasma (100 μL) was diluted 20 times with sample diluent (1% TMAH1 + % nitric acid) and fully vibrated before detection. See Table S1 for the LOD and detection rate of each element. When the plasma element concentration was below the LOD, LOD/$\sqrt{2}$ was used instead. Standard samples were detected in each batch (30 samples) for quality control purposes.

2.4. Diagnosis of GDM

At 24–28 weeks of gestation, an oral glucose tolerance test (OGTT) was implemented by a 75 g glucose challenge. A diagnosis of GDM was made if fasting plasma glucose was ≥ 5.1 mmol/L (≥ 92 mg/dL), 1-h plasma glucose was ≥ 10.0 mmol/L (≥ 180 mg/dL), or 2-h plasma was ≥ 8.5 mmol/L (≥ 153 mg/dL), according to the recommendations from the Diabetes and Pregnancy Study Group (IADPSG) [21].

2.5. Statistical Analysis

The control group was matched for the GDM group by maternal age and pre-pregnancy BMI using the propensity score matching method (PSM) [22]. Basic demographic characteristics, plasma microelement concentrations, and clinical indicators of the study population were represented using N (%) for categorical variables and median and interquartile range (IQR) for continuous variables. Comparison between case and control groups was determined by the Wilcoxon rank sum test (for continuous variables) or Chi-square (χ^2) test (for categorical variables). The concentrations of trace elements were natural log-transformed [Ln(X)] to normalize their distribution. The pairwise correlations among multiple elements were calculated by Spearman's rank correlation analysis and a correlation-matrix heatmap was plotted. Conditional logistic regression was adopted to evaluate the association between the concentration of trace elements and the risk of GDM by odds ratios (ORs) and 95% confidence intervals (CIs). We chose covariates based on the literature review, stepwise regression, best subset selection, and biological reliability. Potential confounding factors and factors with significant differences between the case and control groups in univariate analysis were included in Model 4, including age (continuous variable), pre-pregnancy BMI (<18.5, 18.5–24, >24), family history of diabetes (yes or no), education level (<10, 10–12, ≥13 years), ethnic groups (Ethnic Han or others), household income level (<0.1 million, 0.2–0.3 million, >0.3 million), TG (continuous variable), CHOL (continuous variable), LDL-cholesterol (continuous variable), HDL-cholesterol (continuous variable) and APOB (continuous variable). Covariates screened by stepwise regression were included in Model 2, including education level, ethnic groups, TG, LDL-cholesterol, HDL-cholesterol, and APOB. Covariates including family history of diabetes, education level, ethnic groups, TG, LDL-cholesterol, and APOB, which were screened by best subset selection, were included in Model 3. The potential nonlinearity of the association of plasma trace elements with odds of GDM, OGTT value, and FPI was further examined using RCS with three knots at the 25th, 50th, and 75th percentiles of Ln (plasma element concentrations) assessed via R version 4.2.0 software ("rms" package).

LASSO regression, QGC, and BKMR models were used to screen out independent variables, assess the joint effect of elements on GDM risk, and determine the contribution of each element to GDM risk. In these analyses, we adjusted for the same variables as in Model 3 of the conditional logistic regression analysis. The 11 covariates and six elements were included in the LASSO regression, and the independent variables with greater influence on the dependent variable were screened when the regression coefficient was compressed to zero. These selected elements were included simultaneously in the multiple-element model adjusted or not adjusted for covariates selected by LASSO (family history of diabetes, education level, ethnic groups, household income level, TG, LDL-cholesterol, HDL-cholesterol, APOB). Quantile g computation, an adaptive adaptation modeling method with weighted quantile sum regression, was used to evaluate the different directions of mixed effects for individual elements and rank important constituents [23]. QGC was conducted using R version 4.2.0 with the "qgcomp" package. BKMR [24] was also used to assess the joint effect of all elements on the risk of GDM and the effect of an individual element as part of the element mixture via the R version 4.2.0 software ("bkmr" package). A PIP (prosterior inclusion probabilities) threshold of 0.5 was considered to be relatively important for individual element exposure to GDM risk.

All statistical analyses were performed using the SPSS 26.0 and R version 4.2.0 software. A p-value (two-tailed) < 0.05 was considered significant.

3. Results

3.1. Characteristics of the Study Population

The characteristics of the study population are presented in Table 1. The median age of the included pregnant women was 32 years. The study population was well-educated, with around 71.78% of educational level reaching university and higher, and the women who developed GDM were less educated than the women in the control group.

Table 1. Characteristics of the study population.

Characteristic	Total (n = 1166)	Non-GDM (n = 763)	GDM (n = 403)	p
Maternal age (years)	32.00 (30.00–34.00)	32.00 (30.00–34.00)	32.00 (30.00–34.00)	0.820
Pre-pregnancy BMI (kg/m^2)				
Underweight (<18.5)	106 (9.10%)	67 (8.80%)	39 (9.70%)	0.056
Normal weight (18.5–23.9)	838 (71.90%)	565 (74.00%)	273 (67.70%)	
Overweight (≥24.0)	222 (19.00%)	131 (17.20%)	91 (22.60%)	
Education level (years)				
High school and lower	89 (7.63%)	55 (7.21%)	34 (8.40%)	0.037 *
Junior or college	240 (20.58%)	141 (18.48%)	99 (24.60%)	
University and higher	837 (71.78%)	567 (74.31%)	270 (67.00%)	
Household income (million Yuan)				
<0.1	88 (7.50%)	64 (8.40%)	24 (5.96%)	0.438
0.2–0.3	739 (63.38%)	483 (63.30%)	256 (63.52%)	
>0.3	339 (29.10%)	216 (28.30%)	123 (30.52%)	
Ethnic groups				
Ethnic Han	1150 (98.60%)	756 (99.10%)	394 (97.80%)	0.060
Others	16 (1.40%)	7 (0.90%)	9 (2.20%)	
Family history of diabetes (Yes)	146 (12.50%)	85 (11.10%)	61 (15.10%)	0.133
Smoking (Yes)	3 (0.30%)	3 (0.40%)	0 (0.00%)	0.277
Drinking (Yes)	6 (0.50%)	4 (0.50%)	2 (0.50%)	0.987
Parity				
Nulliparous	834 (71.53%)	550 (72.08%)	284 (70.47%)	0.728
Multiparous	332 (28.47%)	213 (27.92%)	119 (29.53%)	
Cesarean section (Yes)	554 (51.30%)	358 (50.90%)	196 (52.10%)	0.690
Infant sex				
Male	574 (49.20%)	377 (49.41%)	197 (48.88%)	0.716
Female	506 (43.40%)	327 (42.86%)	179 (44.42%)	
Missing	86 (7.40%)	59 (7.73%)	27 (6.70%)	

GDM, gestational diabetes mellitus; BMI, body mass index; * p < 0.05.

3.2. Levels of Plasma Trace Elements and Glucose and Lipid Metabolism Indices

The exposure levels of the six trace elements in the case and control groups are summarized in Table 2. There were significantly increased levels of plasma V in the GDM group but significantly lower plasma concentrations of Cr and Se. Correlations between trace elements ranged from 0.07–0.82 in Spearman's rank correlation analysis (Figure S1). As shown in Table S2, despite Apo-A, other glucose and lipid metabolism indices were significantly different between the case and control groups, with FPG, OGTT-1h, OGTT-2h, FPI, HOMA-IR, CHOL, TG, LDL-cholesterol, and Apo-B increased significantly and HDL-cholesterol decreased significantly in the GDM group.

Table 2. Profiling of trace elements in maternal plasma of the case-control group.

Element	Total (n = 1166)	Non-GDM (n = 763)	GDM (n = 403)	p
V (μg/L)	6.25 (3.71–9.06)	6.02 (3.32–8.91)	6.60 (4.23–9.18)	0.007 **
Cr (μg/L)	372.40 (250.75–531.44)	391.38 (253.32–535.58)	342.77 (239.58–517.50)	0.021 *
Mn (μg/L)	5.79 (3.51–8.90)	5.61 (3.28–8.88)	5.91 (3.81–9.04)	0.076
Co (μg/L)	56.82 (40.24–81.94)	56.76 (39.66–81.81)	57.02 (41.23–82.13)	0.289
Ni (μg/L)	30.67 (17.34–48.57)	30.84 (18.69–48.89)	30.23 (15.10–48.40)	0.110
Se (μg/L)	87.80 (60.33–120.72)	89.76 (62.16–122.95)	84.30 (58.89–112.91)	0.044 *

GDM, gestational diabetes mellitus; V, Vanadium; Cr, Chromium; Mn, Manganese; Co, Cobalt; Ni, Nickel; Se, Selenium; * p < 0.05, ** p < 0.01.

3.3. Association between Plasma Trace Elements and Risk of GDM

The results of the conditional logistic regression are shown in Table 3. The plasma level of V was positively associated with the risk of GDM, and every unit increase in the natural log of V exposure was associated with 39% (OR = 1.39 (95% CI 1.14, 1.69)) a higher risk of GDM. In contrast, the concentration of plasma Ni was negatively associated with the risk of GDM, and every unit increase in the natural log of Ni exposure was associated with 14% (OR = 0.86 (95% CI 0.77, 0.97)) a lower risk of GDM. Elevated plasma concentrations of Cr, Mn, Co, and Se were not associated with the risk of GDM.

Table 3. Associations between plasma trace element exposure and GDM risk.

Ln-Elements	Single-Element Model OR (95% CI)				Multi-Element Model OR (95% CI)	
	Modle 1	Modle 2	Modle 3	Modle 4	Crude Model	Adjusted Model
V (μg/L)	1.39 (1.14, 1.69) ***	1.47 (1.20, 1.82) ***	1.48 (1.20, 1.82) ***	1.47 (1.20, 1.80) ***	1.27 (1.01, 1.60) *	1.37 (1.07, 1.76) *
Cr (μg/L)	0.81 (0.63, 1.03)	0.79 (0.6, 1.02)	0.77 (0.59, 1.00)	0.78 (0.60, 1.02)	0.82 (0.53, 1.27)	0.75 (0.47, 1.20)
Mn (μg/L)	1.22 (0.99, 1.51)	1.20 (0.96, 1.49)	1.21 (0.97, 1.51)	1.20 (0.96, 1.49)	1.70 (1.22, 2.36) **	1.83 (1.30, 2.59) ***
Co (μg/L)	1.14 (0.91, 1.43)	1.13 (0.89, 1.44)	1.14 (0.89, 1.46)	1.13 (0.89, 1.45)	1.32 (0.95, 1.85)	1.35 (0.94, 1.93)
Ni (μg/L)	0.86 (0.77, 0.97) *	0.82 (0.73, 0.93) **	0.82 (0.72, 0.93) **	0.82 (0.72, 0.93) **	0.72 (0.60, 0.86) ***	0.66 (0.54, 0.80) ***
Se (μg/L)	0.85 (0.67, 1.07)	0.86 (0.67, 1.10)	0.84 (0.66, 1.07)	0.86 (0.67, 1.10)	0.82 (0.57, 1.20)	0.87 (0.59, 1.27)

GDM, gestational diabetes mellitus; OR, odds ratio; CI, confidence interval; * $p < 0.05$, ** $p < 0.01$, *** $p < 0.001$. Model 1 adjusted by education level, ethnic groups, TG, LDL cholesterol, HDL cholesterol, and APOB. Model 2 adjusted by family history of diabetes, education level, ethnic group, TG, LDL cholesterol, HDL cholesterol, and APOB. Model 3 adjusted by age, pre-pregnancy BMI, family history of diabetes, education level, ethnic group, household income level, TG, CHOL, LD, HDL cholesterol, and APOB. Adjusted model adjusted by family history of diabetes, education level, ethnic groups, household income level, TG, LDL cholesterol, HDL cholesterol, and APOB.

3.4. Dose-Response Association of Plasma Trace Element Exposure with GDM Risk, Glucose, and Insulin Level

The potential nonlinearity of the relation between Ln- Ni (p overall < 0.001, p nonlinearity = 0.003) and the risk of GDM was observed in the restricted cubic spline model (Figure 1). In the relatively low levels (<6.89 μg/L) and higher levels (>30.88 μg/L) of plasma Ni, a positive correlation was found between plasma Ni and GDM risk. U-shaped exposure relationships were observed between Ni and FPI ($p = 0.038$), FPG ($p = 0.006$), OGTT-1h ($p < 0.001$), and OGTT-2h ($p = 0.036$) (Figure S2). Additionally, positive dose-response relationships were also observed between V and FPI ($p = 0.005$) and FPG ($p = 0.004$) (Figure S3), Mn and FPI ($p = 0.018$) (Figure S4), and Co and FPI ($p = 0.039$), OGTT-1h ($p = 0.024$) and OGTT-2h ($p = 0.044$) (Figure S5). Nonlinear relationships were not observed between Cr and Se and glucose or insulin levels (Figures S6 and S7).

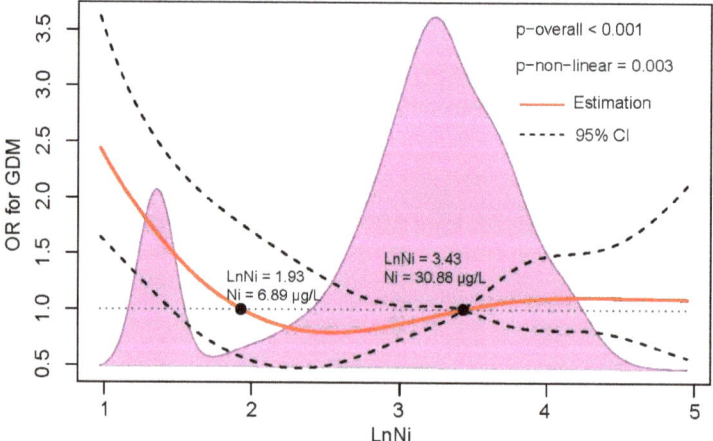

Figure 1. The dose-response relationship of plasma Ni level with GDM risk. RCS regression was used to analyze the dose-response relationship of Ln-Ni with GDM risk after adjusting for family history of diabetes, education level, ethnic groups, TG, LDL-cholesterol, and APO-B. The knots were located at the 25th, 50th, and 75th percentiles. The red line and black dotted line represent the OR value and 95% CI, respectively. The black points represent OR = 1, and the corresponding value of plasma Ni concentration is presented.

3.5. Associations of Metallic Elements Screened by LASSO Regression and Their Coexposure with GDM Risk

The results of LASSO regression showed that all six trace elements had a strong effect on GDM risk (Figure S8). Next, we fitted a logistic regression model and brought all six elements into the model, and additionally adjusted covariates selected by the LASSO regression (Table 3). In this part, increasing Ln-V (OR = 1.27 (95% CI 1.01, 1.60)) and Ln-Ni (OR = 0.72 (95% CI 0.60, 0.86)) were positively and negatively related to the increased risk of GDM, respectively. In addition, increasing Ln-Mn was also observed to be positively associated with an increased risk of GDM (OR = 1.70 (95% CI 1.22, 2.36)).

3.6. Quantile G-Computation Analyses

QGC analysis showed that increasing the Ln-element mixture by one unit was not associated with an increased risk of GDM (OR = 0.97, 95% CI: 0.84, 1.13). The individual weights for each trace element mixture component are shown in Figure 2: Mn (59.1%), Co (31.6%), and V (9.3%) had a positive contribution, and Ni (61.5%), Cr (20.8%) and Se (17.7%) had a negative contribution.

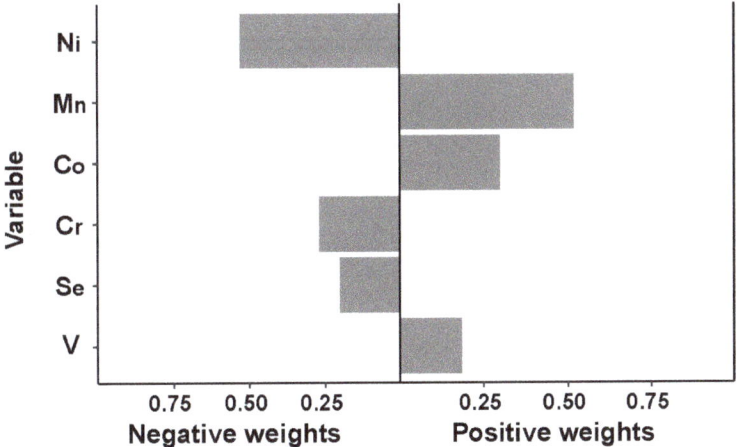

Figure 2. Association between trace element levels and GDM based on quantile g-computation analyses. The estimated weights of each element in the mixture were presented by bootstrapping in either direction.

3.7. Bayesian Kernel Machine Regression Analyses

The PIP of elements varied between 0.7 and 1 (V: 0.8666, Cr: 0.7746, Mn: 1.0000, Co: 0.7742, Se: 1.0000, Ni: 0.8062), and thus, all the elements could be considered important. The univariate relationship between each element and GDM risk is shown in Figure S8. Positive trends were observed between V, Co, and GDM risk (Figure S9a,d), and Cr showed a negative relationship with GDM risk (Figure S9b). A J-shaped relationship between Ni and GDM risk (Figure S9e) and an inverted J-shaped relationship between Mn, Se, and GDM risk (Figure S9c,f) were observed. Considering the comparable positive weight and negative weight of elements on GDM risk, the cumulative effect was not statistically significant, as shown in Figure 3a. Figure 3b illustrates the estimated contribution of individual exposures to the cumulative effect by comparing the GDM risk when a single element was at the 75th percentile compared to when it was at its 25th percentile, where all of the remaining elements were fixed to a particular quantile, such as P25, P50, and P75. When the other element percentiles increased, the higher percentiles of Ni and Mn (P75) presented a more significant negative effect and positive effect on GDM risk compared to their lower concentrations (P25), respectively. The trends of each element in the bivariate exposure-response analysis (Figure S10) were consistent with the univariate relationship analysis, except for the effect of Se on the GDM risk, which was inversely changed when Mn was at a high concentration (P75).

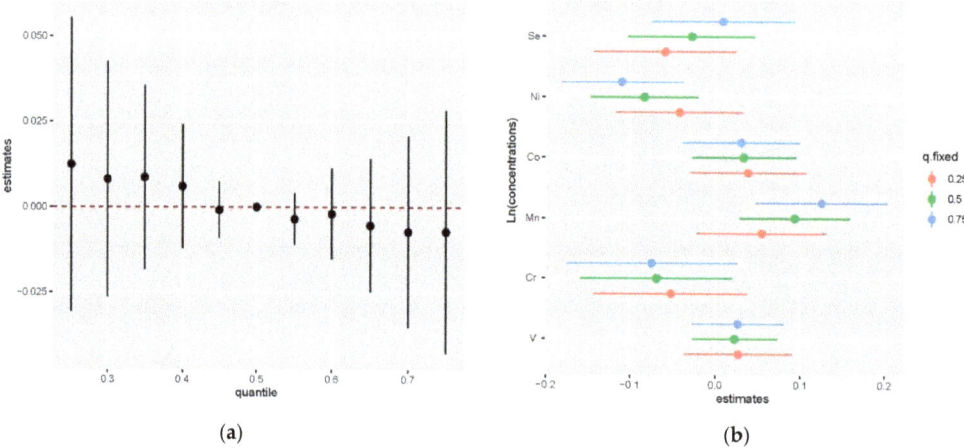

Figure 3. The joint effect of the trace element mixture on GDM by the BKMR model (a) The overall effects of element mixtures (estimates and 95% CI) in elements fixed to different percentiles compared to when they were at their medians (P50). (b) The effects of single exposure when an individual element was at its 75th percentile compared to when that exposure was at its 25th percentile, where all other exposures were fixed to a particular quantile (P25, P50, and P75). The results were adjusted by family history of diabetes, education level, ethnic groups, TG, and LDL-cholesterol.

4. Discussion

In this study, we found that a higher level of plasma V and a lower level of plasma Ni before 14 weeks of pregnancy may be prospectively related to a higher risk of GDM in both single- and multiple-element models. Plasma Mn was found to be positively associated with an increased risk of GDM only in the multiple-element model, and there was no significant relationship between Cr, Co, and Se in the conditional logistic regression. A J-shaped relationship between plasma Ni concentrations and GDM and a U-shaped exposure-response relationship between plasma Ni and OGTT values and FPI were found in RCS analysis. The joint effect of element mixtures on the risk of GDM was not observed in the QGC analysis or the BKMR model. The results from QGC analysis indicate that Mn (59.1%), Co (31.6%), and V (9.3%) had a positive contribution, and Ni (61.5%), Cr (20.8%), and Se (17.7%) had a negative contribution to the risk of GDM. The association of incident GDM with V, Ni, and Mn was consistent in the outcomes of conditional logistic regression, QGC analysis, and BKMR analyses.

V was found to participate in inhibiting glucose release, improving gluconeogenesis-related enzyme activity, and exerting an insulin-sensitizing effect [6]. Two case-control studies showed a positive association between V in plasma [25] and serum [9] with diabetes risk. Two case-control studies based on pregnant women also reported that V exposure, reflected by meconium [12] and plasma V [11] concentrations, respectively, was inversely associated with the odds of GDM. Therefore, we expected that V would reduce the risk for GDM in our study, but the results indicated the opposite. The results from a prospective cohort study conducted in Wuhan, China, were close to those of our study, where there was a significant and positive association between urinary V and GDM based on single-metal models (OR = 1.28, 95% CI: 1.05–1.55) [10]. However, the biological sample of the abovementioned study was inconsistent with our study.

Notably, the median value of plasma V in the present study (6.25 μg/L) was much higher than that in previous studies (plasma V: 0.191 μg/L [25], 0.73 μg/L in GDM cases and 0.80 μg/L in controls [11]), which may account for the inconsistent result. Although V has been found to exert a beneficial effect on the metabolism of carbohydrates, the effective therapeutic dose is difficult to establish, and excess concentrations may lead to several toxic effects [5]. In addition, the health hazards of V, especially when it is at the highest oxidation state (+5), cannot be ignored. V can act as a strong pro-oxidant and pro-apoptotic factor, damage the antioxidant barrier, exacerbate lipid peroxidation (LPO), and lead to programmed cell death (apoptosis) [26]. Therefore, more research is warranted to further explore the effect of V on the risk of GDM and determine the safe exposure range of V.

The epidemiological evidence of Ni in glucose metabolism is limited and inconsistent, although Ni was suggested to adversely affect glucose metabolism by inducing hyperglycemia and glycogenolysis in laboratory studies [27]. Two studies based on Chinese adults and U.S. adults showed that increased urinary Ni concentration is associated with an elevated prevalence of diabetes [28,29]. However, a multisite and multiethnic cohort study of midlife women did not find an association between urinary Ni and an elevated risk of diabetes in midlife women [30]. Another nested case-control study obtained a similar result, and no significant associations were found between plasma Ni and incident diabetes [31]. The evidence of an association between Ni exposure and diabetes in pregnant women was insufficient, and no significant association was found between blood Ni and GDM in the single-metal model in a Chinese birth cohort study [13]. Nevertheless, another Chinese cohort study demonstrated that increased concentrations of urinary Ni in early pregnancy are associated with an elevated risk of GDM [10]. In the present study, a relationship between elevated maternal plasma concentrations of Ni and decreased risk of GDM was observed when evaluated individually or as an element mixture. Additionally, a J-shaped exposure relationship of Ln-Ni with the OR of GDM and U-shaped exposure relationships between Ln-Ni and the three OGTT values and FPI were all observed in the RCS analysis.

When interpreting our study results, the different study biological materials and the much higher concentration of Ni measured in our study should be considered (median (IQR) 30.67 (17.34–48.58) μg/L) when compared to previously published studies (median ranged from 2.48 to 6.484 μg/L [13,31,32]). Urine was a more commonly used biological material in previous studies because of the short half-life period of Ni. Considering that the main exposure source of Ni (from drinking water and food) may be stable in the pregnancy period, our findings may provide new insight into the effect of Ni on glucose metabolism. To the best of our knowledge, this is the first study to demonstrate the dual effect of plasma Ni exposure on the risk of GDM and provide a safety window value of Ni exposure (6.89 μg/L~30.88 μg/L) with potential clinical significance. Interestingly, the cutoff value of 30.88 μg/L was close to the median value of the study population (30.67 μg/L). Thus, we still recommend low levels of Ni exposure in daily life because Ni is potentially essential to the human body, but at high doses is toxic. More research is warranted to further verify our findings and explore the underlying mechanism.

Mn is both an essential nutrient and a potential toxicant, depending on the level of exposure. Mn supplementation may protect mitochondria and islets from ROS by enhancing MnSOD activity and protecting against diabetes [33], but it was also suggested that Mn can inhibit glucose-stimulated insulin secretion in β-cells by impairing mitochondrial function [7]. A cross-sectional study based on coke oven workers indicated that urinary Mn levels were positively associated with hyperglycemia but not with diabetes risk [34]. A U-shaped association between plasma manganese and T2DM was reported by a case-control study [35]. Nevertheless, no significant association was observed between second-trimester blood Mn and GDM in a French mother-child cohort study [17]. A retrospective cohort study from South China demonstrated that serum Mn may prospectively increase the late second trimester OGTT0 but not GDM risk [16].

We measured a relatively low concentration of Mn [median (IQR) 5.79 (3.51–8.90) μg/L] compared with other studies (median ranged from 6.52–21.85 μg/L) [15,17,35]. We found no significant association between Mn and GDM in the single-element model, but interestingly, when we included all the elements in the conditional logistic model, Mn showed a significant positive association with GDM. Additionally, Mn was positively associated with FPI level and was found to be the greatest contributor (59.1%) to GDM in the QGC analysis, which was similar to the results of QGC analysis from a large Japanese study (Mn: 47.4%) [36]. A similar result can also be observed in the BMKR model; when other element percentiles increased, Mn showed a more obvious positive association with GDM. We can speculate that Mn can promote the development of GDM through interactions with other elements such as Se as indicated in the bivariate exposure-response analysis of BKMR models but more evidence is needed to validate the speculation.

Cr, Co, and Se are essential trace elements in the human body. Cr was found to play a significant role in glucose metabolism and have beneficial effects on insulin sensitivity and lipid parameters [37]. Co is an important component of vitamin B12, and Se plays a critical role mainly as a selenoprotein.

Nevertheless, the role of Cr and Co in the development of diabetes mellitus in human studies remains controversial. A positive association was reported between Cr in adipose tissue with T2DM in a 16-year follow-up period prospective adult cohort study [8] and between Co in urine with T2DM in a study based on the National Health and Nutrition Examination Survey (NHANES, 1999–2010) [38]. In a case-control study involving 1471 patients with newly diagnosed T2DM, 682 individuals with newly diagnosed pre-DM indicated that plasma Cr concentrations were inversely associated with T2DM and pre-DM [39]. A negative linear relationship between urinary Co and FPG was found in an ongoing occupational cohort study in China [40]. A large case-control study elucidated a U-shaped relationship between plasma Co concentrations and newly diagnosed T2DM [41].

For pregnant women, Cr in meconium was found to be positively associated with GDM prevalence in a dose-dependent manner in a nested case-control study [14], while data from another two nested case-control studies showed no significant association between Cr levels and the risk of GDM in pregnant women [15,42]. Studies exploring the relationship between Co exposure and GDM are limited; in a prospective cohort study, Co was shown to be significantly and positively associated with GDM [10]. The relationship between Se and GDM has been well established, and most studies support the negative association between Se and the risk of GDM [43]. A recent meta-analysis involving 27 studies showed that the serum Se level of patients with GDM was lower than that in healthy pregnant women [43].

In our present study, although no significant association was observed between Cr, Co, and Se concentrations and GDM in either a single-element or element coexposure logistic regression model. The plasma Cr and Se levels of patients with GDM were lower than those in the control group in our present study. In addition, the positive association between Co and GDM and the negative association between Se and GDM were consistent in the BKMR model and QGC analysis, and Co showed a positive non-linear relationship with FPI, OGTT-1h, and OGTT-2h in RCS analysis.

Our present results showed a much higher concentration of plasma Cr and Co and a comparable concentration of Se than those of previously published studies. Several previous studies showed that the median values varied from 0.2 to 3.97 µg/L for Cr [15,39,44], 1.68–1.9 mg/dL for Co [41,45], and 29.43–94.73 µg/L for Se [15,41,46]. The discrepancies between study populations remain to be elucidated because, aside from Cd, Cr and Co were reported to be the greatest heavy metal pollutant (Cr > Cd > Co > Zn > Ti > Cu) in the surface sediments of the Yangtze River Estuary [47], and there may indeed be a much higher level of metal/element exposure in the Shanghai population. In addition, Cr (III) and Se have been considered to have nutritional or pharmacological effects on the human body [48,49], ranging from antioxidant and anti-inflammatory effects to improving symptoms of insulin resistance, and Se is part of, for instance, Novalac Prenatal pills. The higher plasma level of Se and Cr in pregnant women in the non-GDM group may be the result of their using supplements containing Cr and Se before or during pregnancy. Further well-designed studies should be carried out to explore the role of Cr, Co, and Se in the occurrence, development, and treatment of GDM.

We adopted the BKMR method in our study to determine the joint effects of elements, but the results showed that the increasing percentile of element mixtures was not related to an increased risk of GDM. We speculate that the main explanation is that the contributing effect and protective effect of these six metallic elements on GDM offset each other, as shown in the QGC analysis. Notably, the association between Ni with GDM and Mn with GDM becomes statistically significant along with the increasing percentile of other elements in the BKMR model. There may exist a relatively strong interaction between Ni, Mn, and other elements.

Our study has several strengths. First, we collected blood samples during the first period of pregnancy, which may reflect the causal relationship between element exposure and the risk of GDM. Second, the exposure levels of metallic elements were reflected by a continuous variable (Ln-concentration), which avoids the data loss caused by classification variable conversion. Third, we used several statistical methods to assess the joint effect of all six elements and the independent contribution of each element on the risk of GDM, and the results were stable among these models.

Limitations should also be considered. First, detailed information regarding other potential confounding factors of GDM, such as physical activity and the occupational status during pregnancy, was not well collected. Second, plasma is not the best biological material to reflect body exposure to some elements, such as Ni. Third, we did not take exposure sources such as dietary patterns and residential environment into consideration.

5. Conclusions

In conclusion, our results suggest a positive association between V exposure and a negative association between Ni exposure in early pregnancy with subsequent risk of GDM, regardless of whether they are evaluated individually or as elements mixtures. Plasma Mn was found to be positively associated with an increased risk of GDM in the multiple-element model. In addition, we demonstrate a J-shaped exposure-response relationship between plasma Ni concentrations and GDM and a U-shaped exposure-response relationships between plasma Ni concentrations and FPI, FPG, OGTT-1h, and OGTT-2h. Further studies are warranted to confirm these associations and explore the potential mechanism.

Supplementary Materials: The following supporting information can be downloaded at: https://www.mdpi.com/article/10.3390/nu15010115/s1, Figure S1: Correlations of the plasma concentration of the six trace elements. Spearman's rank correlation was used to analyze the correlations between the Ln-transformed trace elements. Correlation coefficients are presented in the lower left part, and the upper right part is the heatmap of the correlation coefficients between Ln-transformed trace elements. Blue represents a positive correlation, and the darker the color is, the greater the correlation coefficient. * $p < 0.05$, ** $p < 0.01$, *** $p < 0.001$. Figure S2: The dose-response relationships of plasma Ni with FPI and OGTT values. The blue line and gray shadow represent the OR value and 95% CI, respectively. (a) The dose-response relationship of Ln-Ni with FPI. (b) The dose-response relationship of Ln-Ni with FPG. (c) The dose-response relationship of Ln-Ni with OGTT-1h. (d) The dose-response relationship of Ln-Ni with OGTT-2h. Figure S3: The dose-response relationships of plasma V with FPI and OGTT values. The blue line and gray shadow represent the OR value and 95% CI, respectively. (a) The dose-response relationship of Ln-V with FPI. (b) The dose-response relationship of Ln-V with FPG. (c) The dose-response relationship of Ln-V with OGTT-1h. (d) The dose-response relationship of Ln-V with OGTT-2h. Figure S4: The dose-response relationships of plasma Mn with FPI and OGTT values. The blue line and gray shadow represent the OR value and 95% CI, respectively. (a) The dose-response relationship of Ln-Mn with FPI. (b) The dose-response relationship of Ln-Mn with FPG. (c) The dose-response relationship of Ln-Mn with OGTT-1h. (d) The dose-response relationship of Ln-Mn with OGTT-2h. Figure S5: The dose-response relationships of plasma Co with FPI and OGTT values. The blue line and gray shadow represent the OR value and 95% CI, respectively. (a) The dose-response relationship of Ln-Co with FPI. (b) The dose-response relationship of Ln-Co with FPG. (c) The dose-response relationship of Ln-Co with OGTT-1h. (d) The dose-response relationship of

Ln-Co with OGTT-2h. Figure S6: The dose-response relationships of plasma Cr with FPI and OGTT values. The blue line and gray shadow represent the OR value and 95% CI, respectively. (a) The dose-response relationship of Ln-Cr with FPI. (b) The dose-response relationship of Ln-Cr with FPG. (c) The dose-response relationship of Ln-Cr with OGTT-1h. (d) The dose-response relationship of Ln-Cr with OGTT-2h. Figure S7: The dose-response relationships of plasma Se with FPI and OGTT values. The blue line and gray shadow represent the OR value and 95% CI, respectively. (a) The dose-response relationship of Ln-Se with FPI. (b) The dose-response relationship of Ln-Se with FPG. (c) The dose-response relationship of Ln-Se with OGTT-1h. (d) The dose-response relationship of Ln-Se with OGTT-2h. Figure S8: LASSO regression analysis diagram. Maternal age, pre-BMI, ethnic group, educational level, household income level, family history of diabetes, TG, CHOL, LDL, HDL, APO-B, and 6 trace elements were included in the LASSO regression model for analysis. (a) The changing trajectory of misclassification error with the penalty parameter (logλ) (estimates and 95% CI). The dotted line represents the optimal λ value selected after cross-validation. (b) Cross-validation plot for the penalty term. Supplementary Figure S9: Effect of single trace element exposure on GDM by BKMR model Univariate exposure-response functions of each element (95% CI) with others fixed at their medians (P50). The results were adjusted by family history of diabetes, education level, ethnic groups, TG, LDL-cholesterol, and APO-B. Figure S10: Bivariate cross-section effects of trace element exposure on GDM by BKMR model Bivariate cross-section effects of the exposure-response function of a single element where the second element was fixed at P25, P50, and P75. Table S1: Profiling of trace elements in maternal plasma (n = 1166) Table S2: Level of glucose and lipid metabolism indices.

Author Contributions: Conceptualization, T.W. and T.L.; methodology, T.W.; software, T.W.; validation, Y.W. and H.H.; formal analysis, T.W.; investigation, T.L.; resources, T.L.; data curation, T.W.; writing—original draft preparation, T.W.; writing—review and editing, C.Z., H.H. and Y.W.; visualization, T.W. and C.Z.; supervision, H.H. and Y.W; funding acquisition, H.H. and Y.W. All authors have read and agreed to the published version of the manuscript.

Funding: This research was funded by the National Natural Science Foundation of China (82088102), CAMS Innovation Fund for Medical Sciences (2019-I2M-5-064), Collaborative Innovation Program of Shanghai Municipal Health Commission (2020CXJQ01), Clinical Research Plan of SHDC (SHDC2020CR1008A) and Shanghai Frontiers Science Research Base of Reproduction and Development.

Institutional Review Board Statement: The study was conducted in accordance with the Declaration of Helsinnki and approved by the Ethics Committee of the International Peace Maternal and Child Hospital (IPMCH)((GKLW) 2019-51).

Informed Consent Statement: Informed consent was obtained from all subjects involved in the study.

Data Availability Statement: The data presented in this study are available on reasonable request from the corresponding author.

Acknowledgments: We would like to thank the participants and the medical staff of the International Peace Maternal and Child Hospital (IPMCH). We would like to acknowledge the School of Public Health, Fudan University, for providing the detection platform. We would like to thank Yiming Dai, Qiang Liu, and Zhijun Zhou. We thank them for the instrument maintenance during element detection. We would like to thank Chun Xia, a graduate student from Tongji University, for helping us test the samples and process the raw data.

Conflicts of Interest: The authors declare no conflict of interest. The funders had no role in the design of the study; in the collection, analyses, or interpretation of data; in the writing of the manuscript; or in the decision to publish the results.

References

1. Guariguata, L.; Linnenkamp, U.; Beagley, J.; Whiting, D.R.; Cho, N.H. Global estimates of the prevalence of hyperglycaemia in pregnancy. *Diabetes Res. Clin. Pract.* **2014**, *103*, 176–185. [CrossRef] [PubMed]
2. McIntyre, H.D.; Catalano, P.; Zhang, C.; Desoye, G.; Mathiesen, E.R.; Damm, P. Gestational diabetes mellitus. *Nat. Rev. Dis. Prim.* **2019**, *5*, 47. [CrossRef] [PubMed]
3. Gao, C.; Sun, X.; Lu, L.; Liu, F.; Yuan, J. Prevalence of gestational diabetes mellitus in mainland China: A systematic review and meta-analysis. *J. Diabetes Investig.* **2019**, *10*, 154–162. [CrossRef] [PubMed]
4. Zhang, Y.; Chen, T.; Zhang, Y.; Hu, Q.; Wang, X.; Chang, H.; Mao, J.-H.; Snijders, A.M.; Xia, Y. Contribution of trace element exposure to gestational diabetes mellitus through disturbing the gut microbiome. *Environ. Int.* **2021**, *153*, 106520. [CrossRef]

1. Dubey, P.; Thakur, V.; Chattopadhyay, M. Role of Minerals and Trace Elements in Diabetes and Insulin Resistance. *Nutrients* **2020**, *12*, 1864. [CrossRef]
2. Gruzewska, K.; Michno, A.; Pawelczyk, T.; Bielarczyk, H. Essentiality and toxicity of vanadium supplements in health and pathology. *J. Physiol. Pharmacol. Off. J. Pol. Physiol. Soc.* **2014**, *65*, 603–611.
3. Dover, E.N.; Patel, N.; Stýblo, M. Impact of in vitro heavy metal exposure on pancreatic β-cell function. *Toxicol. Lett.* **2018**, *299*, 137–144. [CrossRef]
4. Rodríguez-Pérez, C.; Gómez-Peña, C.; Pérez-Carrascosa, F.M.; Vrhovnik, P.; Echeverría, R.; Salcedo-Bellido, I.; Mustieles, V.; Željka, F.; Arrebola, J.P. Trace elements concentration in adipose tissue and the risk of incident type 2 diabetes in a prospective adult cohort. *Environ. Pollut.* **2021**, *286*, 117496. [CrossRef]
5. Lv, Y.; Xie, L.; Dong, C.; Yang, R.; Long, T.; Yang, H.; Chen, L.; Zhang, L.; Chen, X.; Luo, X.; et al. Co-exposure of serum calcium, selenium and vanadium is nonlinearly associated with increased risk of type 2 diabetes mellitus in a Chinese population. *Chemosphere* **2021**, *263*, 128021. [CrossRef]
6. Wang, X.; Gao, D.; Zhang, G.; Zhang, X.; Li, Q.; Gao, Q.; Chen, R.; Xu, S.; Huang, L.; Zhang, Y.; et al. Exposure to multiple metals in early pregnancy and gestational diabetes mellitus: A prospective cohort study. *Environ. Int.* **2020**, *135*, 105370. [CrossRef]
7. Li, X.; Zhu, Y.; Yin, J.; Li, B.; Li, P.; Cao, B.; Wang, Q.; Xu, J.; Liu, L. Inverse Association of Plasma Vanadium Concentrations with Gestational Diabetes Mellitus. *Nutrients* **2022**, *14*, 1415. [CrossRef] [PubMed]
8. Wu, Y.; Zhang, J.; Peng, S.; Wang, X.; Luo, L.; Liu, L.; Huang, Q.; Tian, M.; Zhang, X.; Shen, H. Multiple elements related to metabolic markers in the context of gestational diabetes mellitus in meconium. *Environ. Int.* **2018**, *121 Pt 2*, 1227–1234. [CrossRef]
9. Wang, Y.; Zhang, P.; Chen, X.; Wu, W.; Feng, Y.; Yang, H.; Li, M.; Xie, B.; Guo, P.; Warren, J.L.; et al. Multiple metal concentrations and gestational diabetes mellitus in Taiyuan, China. *Chemosphere* **2019**, *237*, 124412. [CrossRef] [PubMed]
10. Peng, S.; Liu, L.; Zhang, X.; Heinrich, J.; Zhang, J.; Schramm, K.-W.; Huang, Q.; Tian, M.; Eqani, S.; Shen, H. A nested case-control study indicating heavy metal residues in meconium associate with maternal gestational diabetes mellitus risk. *Environ. Health A Glob. Access Sci. Source* **2015**, *14*, 19. [CrossRef] [PubMed]
11. Zhu, G.; Zheng, T.; Xia, C.; Qi, L.; Papandonatos, G.D.; Ming, Y.; Zeng, Z.; Zhang, X.; Zhang, H.; Li, Y. Plasma levels of trace element status in early pregnancy and the risk of gestational diabetes mellitus: A nested case-control study. *J. Trace Elem. Med. Biol. Organ Soc. Miner. Trace Elem.* **2021**, *68*, 126829. [CrossRef] [PubMed]
12. Zhou, Z.; Chen, G.; Li, P.; Rao, J.; Wang, L.; Yu, D.; Lin, D.; Fan, D.; Ye, S.; Wu, S.; et al. Prospective association of metal levels with gestational diabetes mellitus and glucose: A retrospective cohort study from South China. *Ecotoxicol. Environ. Saf.* **2021**, *210*, 111854. [CrossRef]
13. Soomro, M.H.; Baiz, N.; Huel, G.; Yazbeck, C.; Botton, J.; Heude, B.; Bornehag, C.-G.; Annesi-Maesano, I. Exposure to heavy metals during pregnancy related to gestational diabetes mellitus in diabetes-free mothers. *Sci. Total Environ.* **2019**, *656*, 870–876. [CrossRef]
14. Ranganathan, P.; Pramesh, C.S.; Aggarwal, R. Common pitfalls in statistical analysis: Logistic regression. *Perspect. Clin. Res.* **2017**, *8*, 148–151.
15. Yu, L.; Liu, W.; Wang, X.; Ye, Z.; Tan, Q.; Qiu, W.; Nie, X.; Li, M.; Wang, B.; Chen, W. A review of practical statistical methods used in epidemiological studies to estimate the health effects of multi-pollutant mixture. *Environ. Pollut.* **2022**, *306*, 119356. [CrossRef]
16. Yang, H.S.; LaFrance, D.; Hao, Y. Elemental Testing Using Inductively Coupled Plasma Mass Spectrometry in Clinical Laboratories. *Am. J. Clin. Pathol.* **2021**, *156*, 167–175. [CrossRef]
17. American Diabetes Association. Classification and Diagnosis of Diabetes. *Diabetes Care* **2018**, *41* (Suppl. 1), S22–S24.
18. Austin, P.C. An Introduction to Propensity Score Methods for Reducing the Effects of Confounding in Observational Studies. *Multivar. Behav. Res.* **2011**, *46*, 399–424. [CrossRef] [PubMed]
19. Keil, A.P.; Buckley, J.P.; O'Brien, K.M.; Ferguson, K.K.; Zhao, S.; White, A.J. A Quantile-Based g-Computation Approach to Addressing the Effects of Exposure Mixtures. *Environ. Health Perspect.* **2020**, *128*, 47004. [CrossRef]
20. Bobb, J.F.; Claus Henn, B.; Valeri, L.; Coull, B.A. Statistical software for analyzing the health effects of multiple concurrent exposures via Bayesian kernel machine regression. *Environ. Health A Glob. Access Sci. Source* **2018**, *17*, 67. [CrossRef] [PubMed]
21. Li, X.T.; Yu, P.F.; Gao, Y.; Guo, W.H.; Wang, J.; Liu, X.; Gu, A.H.; Ji, G.X.; Dong, Q.; Wang, B.S.; et al. Association between Plasma Metal Levels and Diabetes Risk: A Case-control Study in China. *Biomed. Environ. Sci. BES* **2017**, *30*, 482–491. [PubMed]
22. Ścibior, A.; Pietrzyk, Ł.; Plewa, Z.; Skiba, A. Vanadium: Risks and possible benefits in the light of a comprehensive overview of its pharmacotoxicological mechanisms and multi-applications with a summary of further research trends. *J. Trace Elem. Med. Biol. Organ Soc. Miner. Trace Elem.* **2020**, *61*, 126508. [CrossRef]
23. Kubrak, O.I.; Rovenko, B.M.; Husak, V.V.; Storey, J.M.; Storey, K.B.; Lushchak, V.I. Nickel induces hyperglycemia and glycogenolysis and affects the antioxidant system in liver and white muscle of goldfish *Carassius auratus* L. *Ecotoxicol. Environ. Saf.* **2012**, *80*, 231–237. [CrossRef]
24. Liu, G.; Sun, L.; Pan, A.; Zhu, M.; Li, Z.; ZhenzhenWang, Z.; Liu, X.; Ye, X.; Li, H.; Zheng, H.; et al. Nickel exposure is associated with the prevalence of type 2 diabetes in Chinese adults. *Int. J. Epidemiol.* **2015**, *44*, 240–248. [CrossRef]
25. Titcomb, T.J.; Liu, B.; Lehmler, H.-J.; Snetselaar, L.G.; Bao, W. Environmental Nickel Exposure and Diabetes in a Nationally Representative Sample of US Adults. *Expo. Health* **2021**, *13*, 697–704. [CrossRef]
26. Wang, X.; Karvonen-Gutierrez, C.A.; Herman, W.H.; Mukherjee, B.; Harlow, S.D.; Park, S.K. Urinary metals and incident diabetes in midlife women: Study of Women's Health Across the Nation (SWAN). *BMJ Open Diabetes Res. Care* **2020**, *8*.

31. Yuan, Y.; Xiao, Y.; Yu, Y.; Liu, Y.; Feng, W.; Qiu, G.; Wang, H.; Liu, B.; Wang, J.; Zhou, L.; et al. Associations of multiple plasma metals with incident type 2 diabetes in Chinese adults: The Dongfeng-Tongji Cohort. *Environ. Pollut.* **2018**, *237*, 917–925. [CrossRef] [PubMed]
32. Li, Z.; Long, T.; Wang, R.; Feng, Y.; Hu, H.; Xu, Y.; Wei, Y.; Wang, F.; Guo, H.; Zhang, X.; et al. Plasma metals and cancer incidence in patients with type 2 diabetes. *Sci. Total Environ.* **2021**, *758*, 143616. [CrossRef] [PubMed]
33. Burlet, E.; Jain, S. Manganese supplementation reduces high glucose-induced monocyte adhesion to endothelial cells and endothelial dysfunction in Zucker diabetic fatty rats. *J. Biol. Chem.* **2013**, *288*, 6409–6416. [CrossRef] [PubMed]
34. Liu, B.; Feng, W.; Wang, J.; Li, Y.; Han, X.; Hu, H.; Guo, H.; Zhang, X.; He, M. Association of urinary metals levels with type 2 diabetes risk in coke oven workers. *Environ. Pollut.* **2016**, *210*, 1–8. [CrossRef] [PubMed]
35. Shan, Z.; Chen, S.; Sun, T.; Luo, C.; Guo, Y.; Yu, X.; Yang, W.; Hu, F.B.; Liu, L. U-Shaped Association between Plasma Manganese Levels and Type 2 Diabetes. *Environ. Health Perspect.* **2016**, *124*, 1876–1881. [CrossRef]
36. Tatsuta, N.; Iwai-Shimada, M.; Nakayama, S.F.; Iwama, N.; Metoki, H.; Arima, T.; Sakurai, K.; Anai, A.; Asato, K.; Kuriyama, S.; et al. Association between whole blood metallic elements concentrations and gestational diabetes mellitus in Japanese women: The Japan environment and Children's study. *Environ. Res.* **2022**, *212 (Pt B)*, 113231. [CrossRef]
37. White, P.E.; Król, E.; Szwengiel, A.; Tubacka, M.; Szczepankiewicz, D.; Staniek, H.; Vincent, J.B.; Krejpcio, Z. Effects of Bitter Melon and a Chromium Propionate Complex on Symptoms of Insulin Resistance and Type 2 Diabetes in Rat Models. *Biol. Trace Elem. Res.* **2021**, *199*, 1013–1026. [CrossRef]
38. Menke, A.; Guallar, E.; Cowie, C. Metals in Urine and Diabetes in U.S. Adults. *Diabetes* **2016**, *65*, 164–171. [CrossRef]
39. Chen, S.; Jin, X.; Shan, Z.; Li, S.; Yin, J.; Sun, T.; Luo, C.; Yang, W.; Yao, P.; Yu, K.; et al. Inverse Association of Plasma Chromium Levels with Newly Diagnosed Type 2 Diabetes: A Case-Control Study. *Nutrients* **2017**, *9*, 294. [CrossRef]
40. Yang, A.; Liu, S.; Cheng, Z.; Pu, H.; Cheng, N.; Ding, J.; Li, J.; Li, H.; Hu, X.; Ren, X.; et al. Dose-response analysis of environmental exposure to multiple metals and their joint effects with fasting plasma glucose among occupational workers. *Chemosphere* **2017**, *186*, 314–321. [CrossRef]
41. Cao, B.; Fang, C.; Peng, X.; Li, X.; Hu, X.; Xiang, P.; Zhou, L.; Liu, H.; Huang, Y.; Zhang, Q.; et al. U-shaped association between plasma cobalt levels and type 2 diabetes. *Chemosphere* **2021**, *267*, 129224. [CrossRef]
42. Onat, T.; Demir Caltekin, M.; Turksoy, V.A.; Baser, E.; Aydogan Kirmizi, D.; Kara, M.; Yalvac, E.S. The Relationship Between Heavy Metal Exposure, Trace Element Level, and Monocyte to HDL Cholesterol Ratio with Gestational Diabetes Mellitus. *Biol. Trace Elem. Res.* **2021**, *199*, 1306–1315. [CrossRef]
43. Xu, W.; Tang, Y.; Ji, Y.; Yu, H.; Li, Y.; Piao, C.; Xie, L. The association between serum selenium level and gestational diabetes mellitus: A systematic review and meta-analysis. *Diabetes/Metab. Res. Rev.* **2022**, *38*, e3522. [CrossRef] [PubMed]
44. Lin, C.-C.; Tsweng, G.-J.; Lee, C.-F.; Chen, B.-H.; Huang, Y.-L. Magnesium, zinc, and chromium levels in children, adolescents, and young adults with type 1 diabetes. *Clin. Nutr.* **2016**, *35*, 880–884. [CrossRef] [PubMed]
45. Alimonti, A.; Bocca, B.; Mannella, E.; Petrucci, F.; Zennaro, F.; Cotichini, R.; D'Ippolito, C.; Agresti, A.; Caimi, S.; Forte, G. Assessment of reference values for selected elements in a healthy urban population. *Ann. Dell'Istituto Super. Sanita* **2005**, *41*, 181–187.
46. Liu, P.J.; Yao, A.; Ma, L.; Chen, X.Y.; Yu, S.L.; Liu, Y.; Hou, Y.X. Associations of Serum Selenium Levels in the First Trimester of Pregnancy with the Risk of Gestational Diabetes Mellitus and Preterm Birth: A Preliminary Cohort Study. *Biol. Trace Elem. Res.* **2021**, *199*, 527–534. [CrossRef]
47. Zhuang, W.; Zhou, F. Distribution, source and pollution assessment of heavy metals in the surface sediments of the Yangtze River Estuary and its adjacent East China Sea. *Mar. Pollut. Bull.* **2021**, *164*, 112002. [CrossRef]
48. Vincent, J.B. Effects of chromium supplementation on body composition, human and animal health, and insulin and glucose metabolism. *Curr. Opin. Clin. Nutr. Metab. Care* **2019**, *22*, 483–489. [CrossRef]
49. Rayman, M.P. Selenium and human health. *Lancet* **2012**, *379*, 1256–1268. [CrossRef]

Disclaimer/Publisher's Note: The statements, opinions and data contained in all publications are solely those of the individual author(s) and contributor(s) and not of MDPI and/or the editor(s). MDPI and/or the editor(s) disclaim responsibility for any injury to people or property resulting from any ideas, methods, instructions or products referred to in the content.

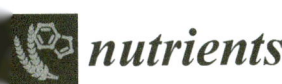

Article

Vitamin A Concentration in Human Milk: A Meta-Analysis

Huanmei Zhang [1,2], Xiangnan Ren [1,2], Zhenyu Yang [1,2] and Jianqiang Lai [2,3,*]

1. Department of Maternal and Child Nutrition, National Institute for Nutrition and Health, Chinese Center for Disease Control and Prevention, Beijing 100050, China
2. China-DRIs Expert Committee on Human Milk Composition, Chinese Nutrition Society, Beijing 100050, China
3. National Institute for Nutrition and Health, Chinese Center for Disease Control and Prevention, Beijing 100050, China
* Correspondence: laijq@ninh.chinacdc.cn

Abstract: Humans require vitamin A (VA). However, pooled VA data in human milk is uncommon internationally and offers little support for dietary reference intake (DRIs) revision of infants under 6 months. As a result, we conducted a literature review and a meta-analysis to study VA concentration in breast milk throughout lactation across seven databases by August 2021. Observational or intervention studies involving nursing mothers between the ages of 18 and 45, with no recognized health concerns and who had full-term infants under 48 months were included. Studies in which retinol concentration was expressed as a mass concentration on a volume basis and determined using high-, ultra-, or ultra-fast performance liquid chromatography (HPLC, UPLC, or UFLC) were chosen. Finally, 76 papers involving 9171 samples published between 1985 and 2021 qualified for quantitative synthesis. Results from the random-effects model showed that the VA concentration of healthy term human milk decreased significantly as lactation progressed. VA (μg/L) with 95% CI at the colostrum, transitional, early mature and late mature stages being 920.7 (744.5, 1095.8), 523.7 (313.7, 733.6), 402.4 (342.5, 462.3) and 254.7 (223.7, 285.7), respectively (X^2 = 71.36, $p < 0.01$). Subgroup analysis revealed no significant differences identified in VA concentration (μg/L) between Chinese and non-Chinese samples at each stage, being 1039.1 vs. 895.8 (p = 0.64), 505.7 vs. 542.2(p = 0.88), 408.4 vs. 401.2 (p = 0.92), 240.0 vs. 259.3 (p = 0.41). The findings have significant implications for the revision of DRIs for infants under six months.

Keywords: vitamin A; retinol; human milk; full-term infant; lactation stage

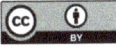

1. Introduction

VA involves various physiological processes including retinal vision, gene expression, immune strength, reproduction, embryonic development, and growth [1,2]. Latest research shows that VA may have protective effects on outcomes of some viral infections such as HPV and measles [3]. Breastfed infants, particularly exclusively breastfed infants, acquire VA through human milk to achieve such needs. Breast-milk VA is a good indication of infants and lactating mothers' VA status, according to the World Health Organization (WHO) [4,5]. The WHO, European Food Safety Authority (EFSA), and other competent scientific organizations have established dietary reference VA values for infants and lactating women [2,6,7]. However, such recommendations by the WHO or EFSA were based on hypotheses, carried out with limited research and few subjects [8]. There have been quite a few publications about human milk VA concentrations worldwide; however, there is a wide range as shown in publications [9–11]. Meta-analysis methodology has been viewed as a beneficial method for statistically combining and summarizing the results from various studies, so as to obtain pooled data or estimates that may better represent what is true in the population [12]. However, relatively few systematic reviews and meta-analyses have been undertaken to synthesize VA concentration in human milk using international data [13,14], resulting in scarcity of updated and solid breast milk VA levels. Such data is critical for establishing dietary reference intakes (DRIs) for groups, particularly newborns and breastfeeding mothers [8].

To inform DRI revision for the group of healthy full-term infants aged 0 to 6 months, we conducted a meta-analysis study to analyze human milk's VA concentration on volume base, determined by advanced methods (HPLC, UPLC, or UFLC), and to explore the influence of potential confounders using meta-regression.

2. Materials and Methods

2.1. Literature Search

Articles in English were searched through PubMed, Web of Science, Embase and Cochrane Central Register of Controlled Trials employing matching keywords "vitamin A" or "retinol" with "human * milk", "woman * milk", "mother * milk", "breast * milk", "lactation" or "lactating". Articles in Chinese were searched through the China National Knowledge Internet (CNKI), Wan Fang Database, or China Science and Technology Journal Database (CSTJ) utilizing matching Chinese keywords covering "human milk" and "vitamin A", the former keyword including "human milk", "breast milk", or "lactating mother" and the latter including "vitamins", "vitamin A", "retinol", "nutrients" or "nutritional composition". Articles published by 21 August 2021 were taken into account.

2.2. Study Selection and Screening

Studies were considered if they matched the following criteria: (1) intervention or observational studies that reported the level of VA in human milk; (2) mothers were aged between 18 to 45 years; (3) healthy lactating mothers free of degenerative or metabolic illnesses; (4) full-term infants aged 0 to 48 months; and (5) high-, ultra-, or ultra-fast performance liquid chromatography (HPLC, UPLC or UFLC) determination method. Criteria for exclusion: (1) VA supplementation or particular diet intervention was used; (2) studies were presented as a review, case report, conference abstract, or proceedings without full-text articles, communication letters, texts described in language other than English or Chinese, duplicate publications, or full-text inaccessible; (3) preterm milk studies or data derived from a blend of preterm and term breast milk; (4) research with identical samples, or concentration data not in volume unit, inconsistent data, or unusual data; (5) no clear identification of lactation stage. EndNote version 20.3 (Clarivate Analytics (UK) Limited, London, UK) was used to screen and choose studies.

Data of Orhon et al. [15] at the colostrum stage, Vaisman et al. [16] at the transitional phase and Redeuil et al. [9] at the transitional and late mature stages were removed due to unusual data distribution. That of Eagle-Stone et al. [17] was omitted because participants in some regions likely took high-dose VA supplements three months before the survey. The supplementing effect on raised VA levels of human milk was considered durable within 6 months [4].

2.3. Data Extraction

Papers were chosen in the order of title, abstract and entire contents based on the inclusion and exclusion criteria stated above. Four detectives extracted and double-checked the data. A fifth investigator was consulted for assistance if there was any doubt throughout the selection process. First author, publication year, study design, study location, analysis methods, participant characteristics (sample size, mother age, lactation stage) and VA concentration of human milk sample were all extracted.

Data from various lactating stages were retrieved and included in cohort studies. A median point was chosen if more than one human milk sample subgroup was tested within the same lactation stage. In intervention studies, baseline data from the intervention and control groups were retrieved, and follow-up data from the control group were treated similarly to cohort research. When both full breast-milk samples and random samples were used in the same study, data of the former was extracted. All extracted data was recorded using Excel.

2.4. Data Analysis

The VA concentration data were given as mean± standard deviation of retinol. If retinyl palmitate levels were also given, they were converted in proportion. If provided as geometric mean and 95% CI, geometric mean was deemed identical to arithmetic mean values, and 95% CI was regarded arithmetic mean values. Zhang et al. [18] were consulted on the data transformation. The transformation of VA concentration in human milk from mass base to volume was multiplied by a factor of 1.032. Individual sample size formation was used in the computation when many samples were used in a single study, and weighted mean and standard deviation were required. The following are the relevant functions:

$$\text{Mean} = (n1 \times M1 + n2 \times M2 + n3 \times M3 + \ldots + ni \times Mi)/(n1 + n2 + n3 + \ldots + ni) \quad (1)$$

$$A_i = S_i^2 (n_i - 1) + M_i^2 \times n_i \quad (2)$$

$$SD = \sqrt{\frac{\sum A_i - \frac{[\sum (M_i n_i)]^2}{N}}{N - 1}} \quad (3)$$

The individual mean value, sample size and standard deviation of personal research are represented by Mi, ni and Si, respectively.

A weighted mean and standard deviation were determined for a common lactation stage. If the VA result of an individual study exceeded the range of Mean ± 2SD, the data was considered an outlier and was excluded. The other studies were then incorporated and integrated using meta-analysis with a random-effects model because there are differences between studies in both population and performance. Subgroup analysis at each lactation stage was conducted by countries: Chinese and non-Chinese studies.

The I^2 test with a significance level of $\alpha = 0.05$ was used to visually analyze heterogeneity among studies regarding the human milk VA level and to quantify the magnitude of heterogeneity. Individual trials were examined using sensitivity analysis at each stage of breastfeeding. Sources of heterogeneity were assessed using meta-regression analysis, which included research design, publication year, mother's age, country, sampling time, sampling volume, and whether the breast was empty after sampled. R packages version 4.1.3 (10 March 2022) were used for meta-analysis and meta-regression.

3. Results

3.1. Study Identification

Database searching yielded 12,887 entries, including 11,089 abstracts in English and 1798 in Chinese (Figure 1). After all duplicates were removed, 9558 records were tested against the title and abstract. In addition, three articles were included during the paper-chasing procedure [18–20]. To establish eligibility for inclusion in the review, we evaluated 118 full-text studies. Finally, 76 studies from 33 countries met the inclusion and exclusion criteria. They were assessed for data review, with seventy-one full-texts in English [9–11,16,20–87], four in Chinese [88–91], and one in Spanish but with abstract in English [74].

3.2. Study Characteristics

There was one human milk bank study, forty cross-sectional studies, sixteen randomized-control studies, four cohort studies, eleven intervention studies, one cross-sectional study in parallel to one intervention study, and three longitudinal studies (Table 1), with six studies involving Chinese participants, sixty-nine studies involving non-Chinese participants and one study involving multinational participants. A total of 9171 human milk samples were included, with VA concentrations in colostrum, transitional and mature human milk determined in 2170, 719 and 6282 models, respectively. There were 4082 and 950 samples included as early mature and late mature human milk, respectively, yet 999 specimens with no clear indication whether they were early or late mature. There were 2053 Chinese and 5602 non-Chinese participants. These studies were published between Year 1985–2021.

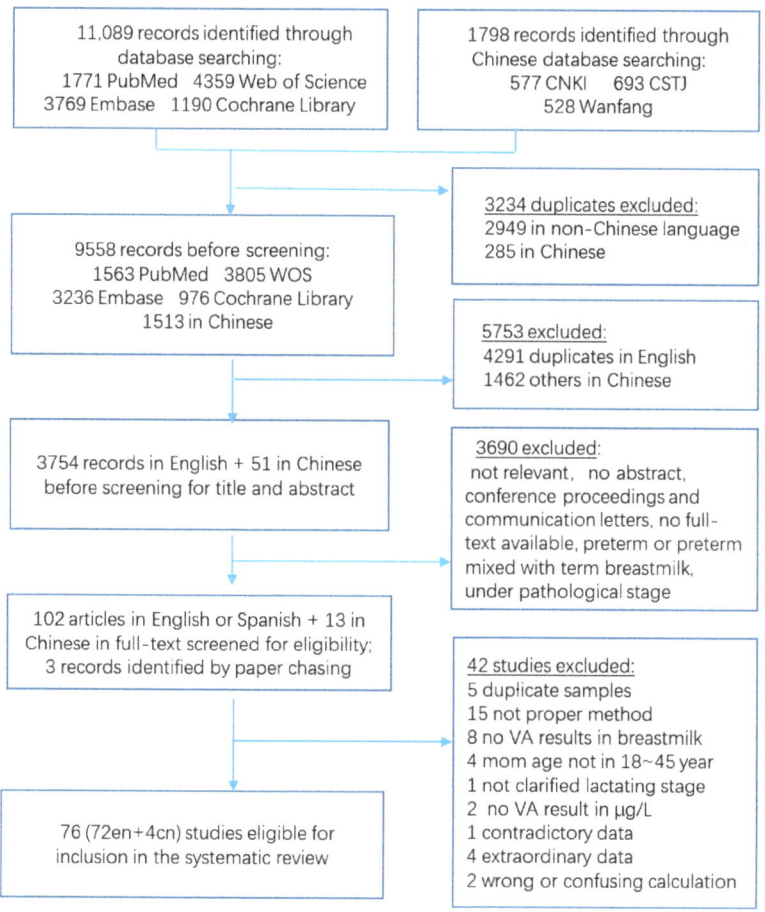

Figure 1. Flow diagram of literature review.

3.3. VA Concentration in Human Milk

The VA concentration (µg/L) with 95% CI of human milk at colostrum, transitional, early and late mature stages was 920.7 (744.5, 1096.8), 523.7 (313.7, 733.6), 402.4 (342.5, 462.3) and 254.7 (223.7, 285.7) for all samples, respectively (Table 2). The VA concentration with 95% CI of mature human milk was 385.3 (339.4, 431.3) µg/L. Subgroup analysis by lactation stage showed there were significant difference between the colostrum, transitional and mature stages ($X^2 = 170.02$, $p < 0.01$) (Figure S1) and between the colostrum, transitional, early and late mature stages ($X^2 = 71.36$, $p < 0.01$) (Figure S2).

At the colostrum stage, which is within 7 days following delivery, there were five studies performed on 429 Chinese participants and twenty-two studies completed on 1741 non-Chinese subjects (Figure 2). The VA content with 95% CI was 1039.1 (470.3, 1607.8) µg/L in Chinese specimens and 895.75 (714.1, 1077.4) in non-Chinese. There was no statistically significant variance between the two population groups ($X^2 = 0.22$, $p = 0.64$).

Table 1. Summary Characteristics of included studies.

First Author and Publication Year	Country	Study Design	Postpartum Days	Lactation Stage	Age of Mothers (y)	Subjects	Sample Size	Empty Breast or Not	Sampling Time #
Abebe 2019 [22]	Ethiopia	CSS	180	3	23.0–33.6	110	110	No	AM
Agne-Djigo 2012 [23]	Senegalese	IS	156–198	3 + 4	20.9–35.3	59	59	Yes	AM
Ahmed 2004 [10]	Bangladesh	CSS	2	1	18.7–27.5	105	105	No	NS
Alam 2010 [24]	Bangladesh	RCT	61–89	3	21–33	251	251	No	AM + PM
Atalhi 2020 [25]	Morocco	IS	15	3	19–40	68	68	No	AM
Ayah 2007 [26]	Kenya	RCT	92–98	3	18.0–30.8	201	201	NS	NS
Barua 1997 [27]	Bangladesh	CSS	45–780	3	18–32	61	61	No	AM
Bezerra 2010 [11]	Brazil	IS	1	1	19.2–29.8	143	143	No	AM
Bezerra 2020 [28]	Brazil	CSS	1	1	19.4–30.2	65	65	No	AM
Canfield 1997 [21]	China	IS	75–277	3 + 4 *	24.8–32.6	6	6	Yes	PM
Canfield 1998 [20]	China	IS	30–298	3 + 4	20.8–35.6	3	3	Yes	PM
Canfield 1999 [31]	Honduras	IS	30–365	3 + 4	17.3–30.1	36	36	Yes	AM
Canfield 2001 [30]	Honduras	IS	90–330	3 + 4	19.5–32.5	79	79	no	AM
Canfield 2003 [29]	Multination &	CSS	25–193	3, 3 + 4	24.6–30.4	471	471	Yes	PM
Chappell 1985 [32]	Canada	CS	1–25	1, 3	NA	12	24	Yes	AM
da Silva 2019 [33]	Brazil	CS	25–134	3	20.4–35.2	42	42	No	NS
da Silva 2010 [34]	Brazil	CSS	1	1	19.6–31.2	86	86	Yes	AM
Daniels 2019 [35]	Indonesia	CSS	14	2	19.7–31.9	113	113	Yes	AM
de Lira 2013 [36]	Brazil	CSS	1–3	1	17–31	103	103	no	AM
de Pee 1995 [37]	Indonesia	RCT	150–384	3 + 4	17–40	175	175	yes	AM
de Pee 1997 [38]	Indonesia	CSS+ IS	90–180, 181–548	3, 4	17–40	168	168	Yes	AM
Deminice 2018 [39]	Brazil	CSS	2–6	1	20.3–31.4	154	154	No	NS
Denic 2019 [40]	Serbia	CSS	1–30	1, 3	18–40	43	86	Yes	AM
Dimenstein 2003 [41]	Brazil	CSS	1–2	1	18–39	42	42	No	AM + PM
Ding 2021 [42]	China	RCT	30–45	3	26.0–34.9	294	294	No	AM
Duan 2021 [43]	South Korea	CSS	NA	3 + 4	NA	34	34	NS	NS
Duda 2009 [44]	Poland	CSS	30–360	3 + 4	25.7–31.7	30	30	NS	NS

Table 1. Cont.

First Author and Publication Year	Country	Study Design	Postpartum Days	Lactation Stage	Age of Mothers (y)	Subjects	Sample Size	Empty Breast or Not	Sampling Time #
Ettyang 2004 [45]	Kenya	CSS	14~450	3 + 4	23–35	62	62	No	random
Fang 2014 [88]	China	CSS	3–30	1,3	NA	70	70	NS	NS
Garcia-Guerra 2009 [46]	Mexico	LS	30	3	18–28.8	122	122	Yes	AM + PM
Gibson 2020 [47]	Indonesia	LS	60–150	2	22–34.8	193	193	Yes	AM
Goes 2002 [48]	Brazil	CSS	30–180	3	NA	60	60	NS	NS
Grilo 2015 [49]	Brazil	RCT	1	1	18–35	33	33	No	AM
Grilo 2016 [50]	Brazil	RCT	1–30	1,3	16–31	88	132	No	AM
Gross 1998 [51]	Indonesia	CSS	30–114	3	20.2–30.6	81	81	Yes	AM
Gurgel 2018 [52]	Brazil	CSS	1–2	1	24.8–34.0	424	424	No	AM
Hampel 2017 [53]	Bangladesh	LS	60–120	3	18–22	17	17	Yes	AM
Haskell 2021 [54]	Malawi	RCT	180	3	19–31	103	103	No	NS
Jiang 2016 [55]	China	CS	1–42	1, 2, 3	20–35	102	306	No	AM
Khan 2007 [56]	Vietnam	RCT	174–342	4	21.2–31.2	268	268	NS	AM
Kim 1990 [58]	USA	CSS	30–210	3 + 4	NA	54	54	NS	AM
Kim 2017 [57]	South Korea	CSS	30–330	3, 4	28.6–34.8	334	334	Yes	random
Klevor 2016 [59]	Ghana	RCT	180	3	21.1–32.1	243	243	No	NS
Lira 2018 [60]	Brazil	CSS	2	1	18.3–35.5	134	134	No	AM
Liu 2016 [90]	China	CSS	3–180	1, 3	NA	43	43	NS	NS
Liyanage 2008 [61]	Sri Lanka	CSS	60–270	3 + 4	21.0–33.2	88	88	NS	NS
Lopez-Teros 2017 [62]	Mexico	CSS	30–150	3	22–32	56	56	No	AM
Machado 2019 [63]	Brazil	LS	85–105	3	20–40	19	19	No	AM
Martin 2010 [64]	Brazil	RCT	20–30	3	19.3–30.7	61	61	NS	AM
Matamoros 2018 [65]	Argentina	CSS	30–90	3	18–33	79	79	Yes	AM
Mello-Neto 2009 [66]	Brazil	CSS	20–60	3	16–44	136	136	NS	random
Meneses 2005 [67]	Brazil	CSS	28–83	3	20.3–32.9	49	49	Yes	AM
Muslimatun 2001 [68]	Indonesia	RCT	4–7	1	17–35	31	31	Yes	AM
Olafsdottir 2001 [69]	Iceland	CSS	60–120	3	27–35	77	77	No	NS

Table 1. Cont.

First Author and Publication Year	Country	Study Design	Postpartum Days	Lactation Stage	Age of Mothers (y)	Subjects	Sample Size	Empty Breast or Not	Sampling Time #
Ortega 1997 [70]	Spain	IS	13–40	2,3	24.2–31.6	57	114	No	AM
Palmer 2016 [71]	Zambia	RCT	120–360	3 + 4	18–30	140	140	Yes	AM
Palmer 2021 [72]	Zambia	RCT	270	4	21–34	216	216	Yes	AM
Panpanich 2002 [73]	Thailand	CSS	120–360	3, 4	19.2–31.6	226	226	No	NS
Redeuil 2021 [9]	Switzerland	CS	1–308	1, 3	27.0–35.4	49	102	Yes	AM
Ribeiro 2007 [74]	Brazil	CSS	1	1	18–40	24	24	No	NS
Rice 2000 [75]	Bangladesh	RCT	90	3	20.9–32.3	35	35	Yes	NS
Samano 2017 [76]	Mexico	CSS	30–60	3	19.0–35.0	32	32	Yes	AM
Sânzio Gurgel 2016 [77]	Brazil	CSS	1–7	1	24.6–32.6	25	25	No	AM
Schulz 2007 [78]	Germany	CSS	2	1	24.9–32.9	29	29	No	NS
Schweigert 2004 [79]	Germany	CSS	2–21	1, 3	24–36	21	42	Yes	NS
Souza 2015 [80]	Brazil	CSS	30	3	22.4–35.0	80	80	No	AM
Szlagatys-Sidorkiewicz 2012 [81]	Poland	LS	30–32	3	23.0–29.2	25	25	Yes	AM
Szlagatys-Sidorkiewicx 2012 [82]	Poland	CSS	3–32	1, 3	22.0–32.6	49	98	Yes	AM
Tijerina-Saenz 2009 [83]	Canada	CSS	30	3	20–40	60	60	No	NS
Tokusoglu 2008 [84]	Turkey	CSS	60–90	3	20–40	92	92	No	AM
Tomiya 2017 [85]	Brazil	RCT	1	1	18–31	101	101	NS	NS
Turner 2013 [86]	Bangladesh	RCT	78–267	3 + 4	20–26	135	135	Yes	NS
Vaisman 1985 [16]	Israel	CSS	7–28	1, 3	NA	7	14	Yes	random
Whitefield 2020 [87]	Cambodian	IS	21–187	3	21.4–30.7	68	68	Yes	NS
Zhang 2001 [89]	China	CSS	1–90	1, 2, 3	21–31	365	365	No	NS
Zhang 2021 [91]	China	CSS	1–330	1, 2, 3, 4	22.2–30.4	923	923	Yes	AM

Note: study design: CSS-Cross Sectional Study; CS- Cohort Study; IS-Intervention study; LS- Longitudinal study; RCT-Randomized Control Test. Lactating stage: 1 colostrum; 2 transitional human milk; 3 early mature human milk; 4 late mature human milk. * 3 + 4 Denotes there was no precise specification of mature human milk. & Multination included AU, CA, CL, CHN, JPN, MEX, PH, UK and USA. # AM: Morning. PM: afternoon or evening; NS: not specified; Random: single sampling and specified daytime but not clarify exact sampling hours.

Table 2. Summary of findings for the comparison between Chinese and non-Chinese human milk samples.

Lactation Stage	Studies Enrolling Chinese Participants				Studies Enrolling Non-Chinese Participants				X^2	p	Total Studies			
	No.	Sample Size	Mean	95% CI	No.	Sample Size	Mean	95% CI			No.	Sample Size	Mean	95% CI
Colostrum	5	429	1039.1	470.3, 1607.8	22	1741	895.8	714.1, 1077.4	0.22	0.64	27	2170	920.7	744.5, 1096.8
Transitional	3	356	505.7	118.0, 893.4	3	363	542.2	278.9, 805.6	0.02	0.88	6	719	523.7	313.7, 733.6
Mature	7	1268	386.4	270.6, 502.3	53	5014	385.2	335.1, 435.3	0.00	0.98	59	6282	385.4	339.4, 431.3
Early	7	1112	408.4	282.6, 534.1	38	3221	401.2	333.6, 468.6	0.01	0.92	44	4333	402.4	342.5, 462.3
Late	1	156	240.0	214.9, 265.1	5	794	259.3	220.8, 297.8	0.68	0.41	6	950	254.7	223.7, 285.7

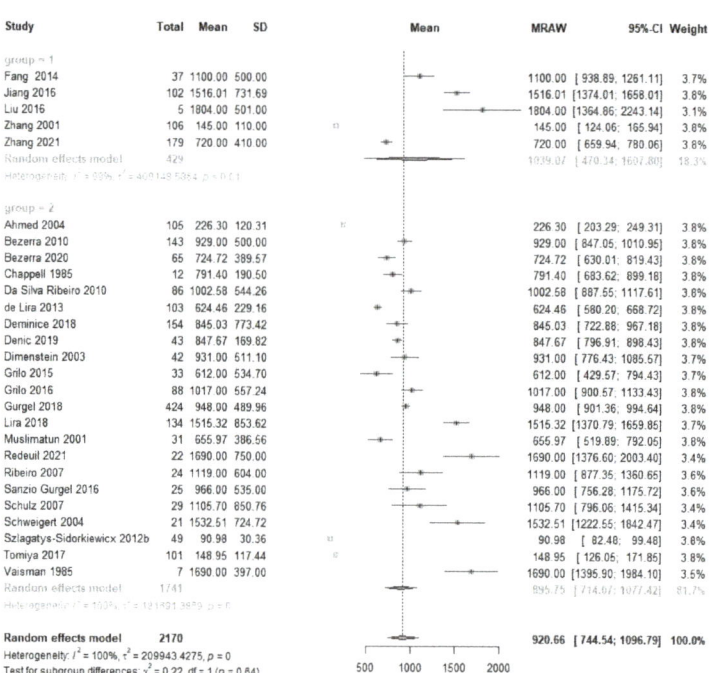

Figure 2. Forest plot of colostrum VA concentration and subgroup analysis between Chinese and non-Chinese samples.

At the transitional stage, which is postpartum 8–14 days, there were three studies carried out among 356 Chinese subjects and three studies among 363 non-Chinese subjects (Figure 3). The VA concentration with 95% CI was 505.7 (118.0, 893.4) μg/L for Chinese and 542.2 (278.9, 805.6) for non-Chinese samples, respectively. There was no significant difference between the two populations (X^2 = 0.02, p = 0.88).

There were seven studies conducted among 1268 Chinese subjects and fifty-three studies among 5014 non-Chinese participants at the mature human milk stage (Figure S3), covering seven studies with 1112 Chinese and thirty-eight studies with 3221 non-Chinese at early mature stage (Figure 4), one study with 156 Chinese and five studies with 794 non-Chinese subjects at late mature stage (Figure 5). The VA concentration with 95% CI between Chinese and non-Chinese participants was 386.4 (270.6, 502.3) μg/L vs. 385.2 (335.1, 435.3) μg/L at the mature stage (X^2 = 0.00, p = 0.98), 408.4 (282.6, 534.1) μg/L vs. 401.2 (333.6, 468.8) μg/L at the early mature stage ($X^2 = 0.01$, $p = 0.92$) and 240.0 (214.9, 265.1) µg/L vs. 259.3 (220.8, 297.8) µg/L at the late mature stage ($X^2 = 0.68$, $p = 0.41$). There was no significant difference when comparing population subgroups at the mature, early mature or late mature lactation stage.

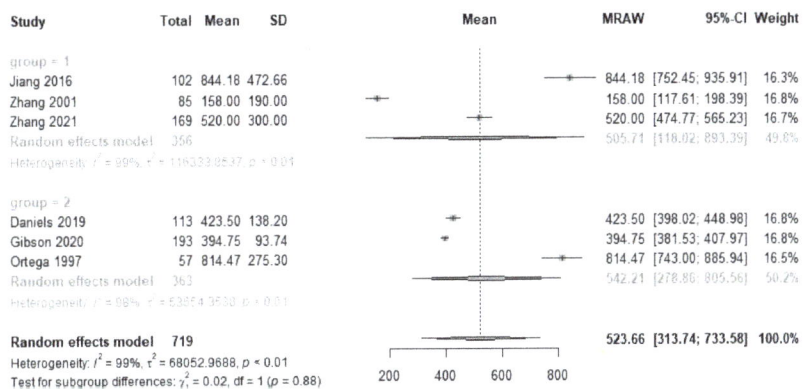

Figure 3. Forest plot of transitional human milk VA concentration and subgroup analysis between Chinese and non-Chinese samples.

3.4. Heterogeneity and Sensitivity Analysis

All analyses revealed substantial heterogeneity (I^2 in 85~100%). Following sensitivity testing, no significant change in the combined effect of VA levels was seen at each lactation stage, indicating that all respective synthesized results was stable.

3.5. Meta-Regression

The results of the univariate meta-regression analysis revealed that none of the following, i.e., publication year, sampling time, whether emptying breast or not after sampling, whether Chinese or not, or study design type at each lactation stage, were significantly associated with heterogeneity between studies (all $p > 0.05$) except maternal age (≥ 30 years vs. <30 years) and nationality (Table A1). The explained heterogeneity of country changed very little following correction for maternal age, i.e., 54.58% to 54.20% at early mature human milk stage (both $p < 0.0001$), but the effect of maternal age changed from significant to insignificant, i.e., its p value being increased from 0.025 to 0.051. Equally, at the colostrum stage, the explained heterogeneity of country after correction resulted in a minute change, i.e., 21.56% to 25.94% but with the p value decreasing from 0.34 to 0.044, whereas the impact of maternal age changed from significant to insignificant again, with the p value increasing from 0.041 to 0.48. The results of the multivariate meta-regression study results suggested that country was a source of heterogeneity, while maternal age was not.

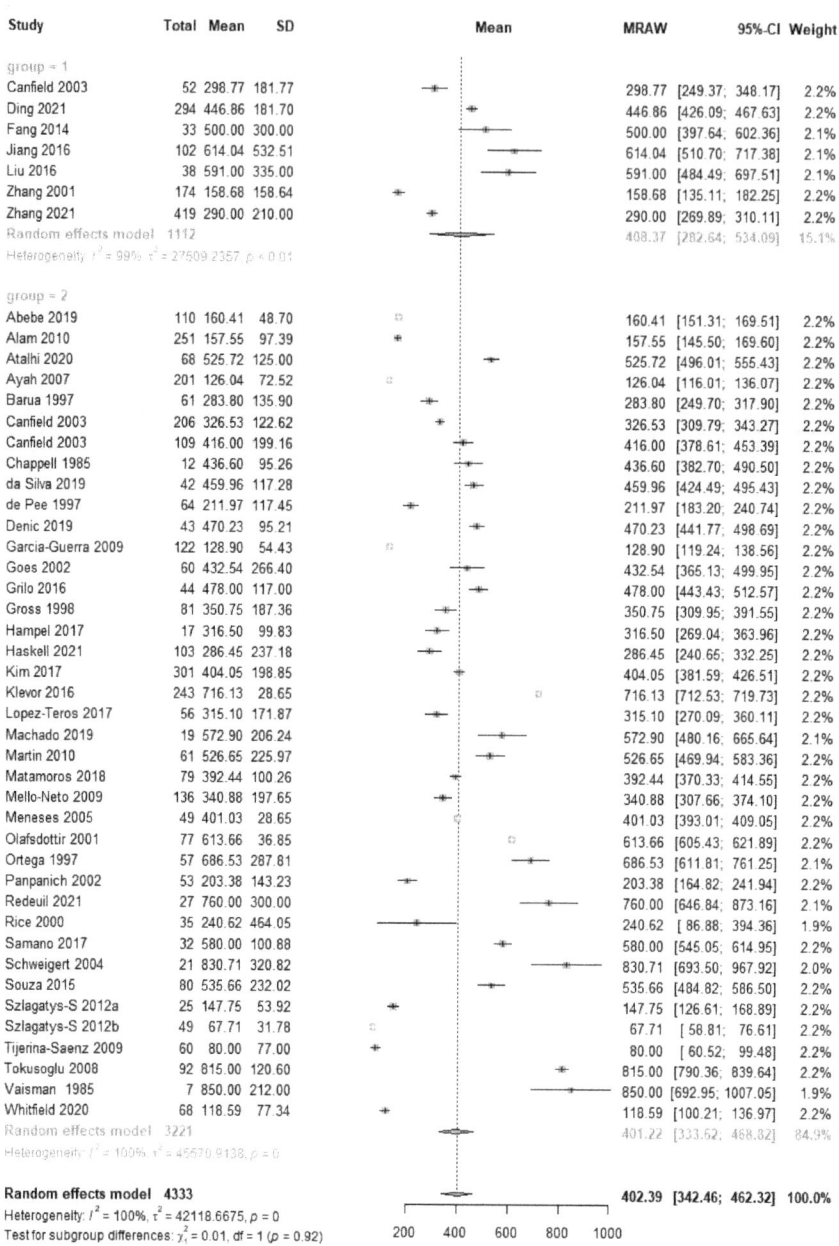

Figure 4. Forest plot of early mature human milk VA concentration and subgroup analysis between Chinese and non-Chinese samples.

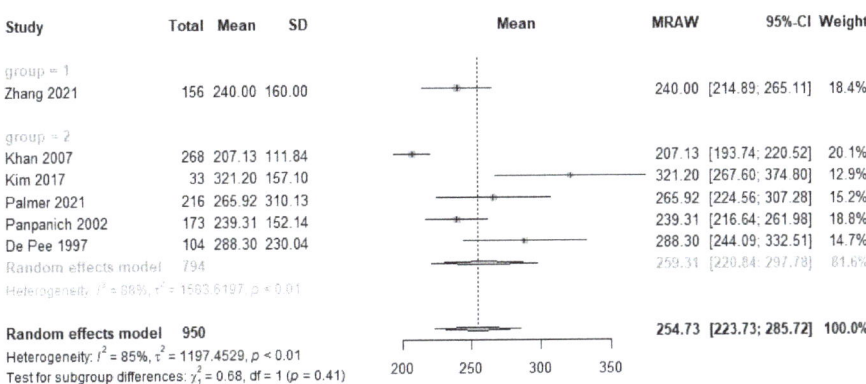

Figure 5. Forest plot of late mature human milk VA concentration and subgroup analysis between Chinese and non-Chinese samples.

4. Discussion

In this study, we compiled previously published data on retinol concentrations in term human milk at each step of the four lactation stages and compared them between Chinese and non-Chinese studies. Our research comprised 76 articles, including 9171 participants from 33 countries from 1985 to 2021, for calculating human milk VA levels determined by HPLC, UPLC, or UFLC. At the colostrum, transitional, early mature and late mature stages of human milk, the VA levels were 920.7 µg/L (3.21 µmol/L), 523.7 µg/L (1.83 µmol/L), 402.4 µg/L (1.40 µmol/L), and 254.7 µg/L (0.89 µmol/L), respectively. There was no significant difference in the VA levels between Chinese and non-Chinese human milk at each lactation stage. This research has crucial implications for DRIs VA modification.

4.1. Data Interpretation

Our findings were compatible with previous meta-analysis findings on VA levels in human milk and the declining tendency with the lactation stage. Dror et al. [14] examined retinol levels in colostrum in four included studies and the mature stage in twenty-four studies (21~365-day lactation). The systematic approach chose the retinol-to-fat ratio (µmol/g fat) as the primary outcome measure which led to nearly two-thirds of the relevant literature being excluded for the meta-analysis. Despite this, the outcomes of our research at the two segmental stages were similar to those of Dror et al., namely 920.7 µg/L vs. 999.7 µg/L, 385.4 µg/L vs. 383.8 µg/L. de Vries et al. [13] conducted a systematic review of 11 studies on the relationship between colostrum VA and maternal serum (plasma) vitamin concentration but did not carry out a meta-analysis. As a result, our findings have greater precision and comprehensiveness.

The respective wide data distribution could explain the similar VA level of human milk at between Chinese and non-Chinese individuals at each lactation stage. Typically, the samples by Zhang et al. [91] were from 20 counties in 11 provinces across China, including urban and rural locations. In contrast, the non-Chinese samples came from 32 nations, comprising both developed, developing, and under-developed ones. Our multivariate meta-regression results, on the other hand, showed that the country factor explained more than 50% of the heterogeneity, implying that the remaining variation between studies could be due to factors such as VA intake, maternal status or sampling protocol rather than the insignificant factors such as study design, publication year, and so on that we analyzed here. Previous research has shown that inadequate dietary VA consumption, maternal VA status during pregnancy and lactation all contribute to clinical heterogeneity, while breast milk sampling protocol accounts for methodological heterogeneity [53,63,66,70,92].

4.2. Implications of Our Results for DRIs Revision

Two studies reported mean liver VA concentration of perinatal normal-weight newborns [93,94], one being 17.3 ± 17.4 µg/g liver in Thai fetuses in gestational age of 37–40 week ($n = 10$), the other being 22 ± 26 µg/g liver in USA infants aged 0–6 days ($n = 22$). Assuming that the liver represents 4.3% of body weight and the liver VA concentration is 20 µg/g, a 3.2-kg full-term newborn has stores of 2.8 mg VA. In contrast, an exclusively breast-fed infant consumes approximately 54.3 mg of VA from mother's milk (402.4 µg/L × 0.75 L/day × 180 days). About 19.4 times more VA is transferred from a mother to a baby during the 6 months of lactation than is accumulated by the fetus during 9 months of gestation. Obviously, the VA in breast milk is of paramount importance for maintaining adequate VA status in early postnatal life of infants as compared to accumulation of VA in the liver prenatally.

A proper estimation of human milk VA level is critical for reference setting in terms of dietary adequate intake requirement for the population of exclusively breastfed infants under six months of age to guarantee optimal growth and development of the newborns. Accurate VA adequacy information for newborns and nursing mothers is desperately needed [8]. As a result, we proposed that the VA content in early mature human milk expressed as a mean with a 95% CI of 402.4 (342.5, 462.3) µg/L or 1.40 (1.20, 1.61) µmol/L, could be used as data support for the purpose. First, a VA level in human milk greater than >1.05 µmol/L may prevent clinical VA deficiency during the first six months of infancy [5]. Second, in this investigation, the synthesis result of VA level at the early mature stage showed less variance than colostrum and transitional phase and had a greater level than at later mature stage, indicating a better representative of human milk VA level. Third, an equilibrium of VA secretion appeared to be obtained in early mature human milk for human beings, as evidenced by the relatively comparable levels of VA in both Chinese and non-Chinese participants at this stage. It is worth noting that 923 mother-infant dyad participants in the Zhang 2021 [91] study had generally adequate nutrition and health status. The comparable VA concentration in early mature human milk is 0.25 mg/L (0.87 µmol/L). This threshold is far lower than the level proposed here. Fourth, past values presented by authoritative groups might have been overstated. The current acceptable intake level of VA for infants aged 0 to 6 months established by EFSA or IOM was based on the average amount of VA consumed in humans [1,2]. However, if the figures are derived from a small number of articles, there is a risk of overestimating the average demand for this group. The EFSA limit of 530 µg/L, chosen as the midpoint of a range of averages (229–831) µg/L, was based on five studies conducted in western countries that did not differentiate between early mature and later-stage human milk. Based on four investigations [19–21,32], the IOM established 485 µg/L (1.70 µmol/L) as the VA level in human milk in 2001 and adopted the level from one of the studies, which was undertaken among three healthy, well-nourished mothers within 75~277 days postpartum [21]. Our data analysis included these four research studies, whereas one study [19] was omitted due to outdated methodology. According to EFSA [7], the average levels of total VA concentration in western countries have generally been estimated to be between 450 and 600 µg/L. Nevertheless, we proposed a reference concentration range of VA in human milk of 402.4 (95% CI: 342.5, 462.3) µg/L for DRIs VA modification for infants ≤ 6 months of age. The range could also be helpful to nursing women and to optimizing the VA level of infant formula.

4.3. Study Limitations

Since the availability of the individual studies limited our meta-analysis of studies at the transitional and later mature lactation stages, the influence of country variability on human milk VA level at transitional stage may be weak, and it was not possible to assess it at the later mature stage. As a result, the meta-regression results for these two stages should be interpreted with caution.

5. Conclusions

The current study found that synthesized human milk VA levels decreased as breastfeeding progressed and that there was no significant difference in human milk VA levels between China and other countries, even though country played a vital role in the variation. Our findings have important implications for DRIs VA revision for the population of exclusively breastfed infants under six months.

Supplementary Materials: The following supporting information can be downloaded at: https://www.mdpi.com/article/10.3390/nu14224844/s1, Figure S1: Forest plot of VA in human milk by 3 lactation stages; Figure S2: Forest plot of VA in human milk by 4 lactation stages; Figure S3: Forest plot of VA in mature human milk by population.

Author Contributions: H.Z. worked on the study design, data extraction, analysis, interpretation and manuscript writing. X.R. contributed to the study design, data extraction, data check and editing. Z.Y. contributes the study design, data check, data analysis, data interpretation and manuscript review. J.L. contributed to funding acquisition, study design and manuscript review. All authors have read and agreed to the published version of the manuscript.

Funding: CNS Research Fund for DRIs.

Institutional Review Board Statement: Not applicable.

Informed Consent Statement: Not applicable.

Data Availability Statement: The data presented in this study are available in the inserted articles.

Acknowledgments: We are thankful for the assistance by Ai Zhao and Yuandi Xi on data extraction.

Conflicts of Interest: The authors declare no conflict of interest.

Appendix A

Table A1. Univariate Meta-regression of enrolled studies for heterogeneity source.

	Stage 1		Stage 2		Stage 3		Stage 4	
	p	R^2	p	R^2	p	R^2	p	R^2
Country	0.066	21.56%	0.49	0.00%	<0.0001	54.58%	-&	-
Population (Chinese vs. Non-Chinese)	0.59	0.00%	0.81	0.00%	0.97	0.00%	0.68	0.00%
Publication year	0.94	0.00%	0.91	0.00%	0.88	0.00%	0.82	0.00%
Sampling time	0.24	3.39%	0.06	33.90%	0.29	1.88%	0.11	45.00%
Study design	0.15	6.59%	0.052	49.13%	0.53	0.00%	0.295	1.62%
Whether emptying breast or not	0.23	2.18%	0.49	0.00%	0.37	0.00%	0.12	36.45%
Maternal age (<30 years vs. ≥30 years)	0.019	17.65%	-$	-	0.025	9.50%	0.015	66.48%

Note: Lactating stage: 1 colostrum; 2 transitional human milk; 3 early mature human milk; 4 late mature human milk. R^2: Accounted for amount of heterogeneity. & Unable to make analysis due to limited number of studies. $ Unable to make analysis due to same age stratification.

References

1. Institute of Medicine. *Dietary Reference Intakes for Vitamin A, Vitamin K, Arsenic, Boron, Chromium, Copper, Iodine, Iron, Manganese, Molybdenum, Nickel, Silicon, Vanadium and Zinc*; National Academy Press: Washington, DC, USA, 2001.
2. EFSA NDA Panel (EFSA Panel on Dietetic Products, Nutrition, and Allergies (NDA). Scientific opinion on Dietary Reference Values for vitamin A. *EFSA J.* **2015**, *13*, 4028. [CrossRef]
3. Sinopoli, A.; Caminada, S.; Isonne, C.; Santoro, M.M.; Baccolini, V. What Are the Effects of Vitamin A Oral Supplementation in the Prevention and Management of Viral Infections? A Systematic Review of Randomized Clinical Trials. *Nutrients* **2022**, *14*, 4081. [CrossRef] [PubMed]
4. Underwood, B.A. Maternal vitamin A status and its importance in infancy and early childhood. *Am. J. Clin. Nutr.* **1994**, *59*, 517S–522S. [CrossRef] [PubMed]

5. Stoltzfus, R.J.; Underwood, B.A. Breast-milk vitamin A as an indicator of the vitamin A status of women and infants. *Bull. World Health Organ.* **1995**, *73*, 703–711. [PubMed]
6. Joint FAO/WHO Expert Consultation on Human Vitamin and Mineral Requirements. *Vitamin and Mineral Requirements in Human Nutrition: Report of a Joint FAO/WHO Expert Consultation*; WHO: Geneva, Switzerland, 1998; p. 341.
7. EFSA NDA Panel (EFSA Panel on Dietetic Products, Nutrition, and Allergies (NDA). Nutrient requirements and dietary intakes of infants and young children in the EU. *EFSA J.* **2013**, *11*, 3408–3510.
8. Ross, A.C.; Moran, N.E. Our Current Dietary Reference Intakes for Vitamin A-Now 20 Years Old. *Curr. Dev. Nutr.* **2020**, *4*, nzaa096. [CrossRef]
9. Redeuil, K.; Lévêques, A.; Oberson, J.M.; Bénet, S.; Tissot, E.; Longet, K.; de Castro, A.; Romagny, C.; Beauport, L.; Fischer Fumeaux, C.J.; et al. Vitamins and carotenoids in human milk delivering preterm and term infants: Implications for preterm nutrient requirements and human milk fortification strategies. *Clin. Nutr.* **2021**, *40*, 222–228. [CrossRef]
10. Ahmed, L.; Nazrul Islam, S.; Khan, M.N.; Huque, S.; Ahsan, M. Antioxidant micronutrient profile (vitamin E, C, A, copper, zinc, iron) of colostrum: Association with maternal characteristics. *J. Trop. Pediatr.* **2004**, *50*, 357–358. [CrossRef]
11. Bezerra, D.S.; de Araújo, K.F.; Azevêdo, G.M.; Dimenstein, R. A randomized trial evaluating the effect of 2 regimens of maternal vitamin a supplementation on breast milk retinol levels. *J. Hum. Lact.* **2010**, *26*, 148–156. [CrossRef]
12. Andrade, C. Understanding the Basics of Meta-Analysis and How to Read a Forest Plot: As Simple as It Gets. *J. Clin. Psychiatry* **2020**, *81*, 20f13698. [CrossRef]
13. de Vries, Y.; Pundir, S.; McKenzie, E.; Keijer, J.; Kussmann, M. Maternal Circulating Vitamin Status and Colostrum Vitamin Composition in Healthy Lactating Women—A Systematic Approach. *Nutrients* **2018**, *10*, 687. [CrossRef] [PubMed]
14. Dror, D.K.; Allen, L.H. Retinol-to-Fat Ratio and Retinol Concentration in Human Milk Show Similar Time Trends and Associations with Maternal Factors at the Population Level: A Systematic Review and Meta-Analysis. *Adv. Nutr.* **2018**, *9*, 332s–346s. [CrossRef]
15. Orhon, F.S.; Ulukol, B.; Kahya, D.; Cengiz, B.; Başkan, S.; Tezcan, S. The influence of maternal smoking on maternal and newborn oxidant and antioxidant status. *Eur. J. Pediatr.* **2009**, *168*, 975–981. [CrossRef] [PubMed]
16. Vaisman, N.; Mogilner, B.M.; Sklan, D. Vitamin A and E content of preterm and term milk. *Nutr. Res.* **1985**, *5*, 931–935. [CrossRef]
17. Engle-Stone, R.; Haskell, M.J.; Nankap, M.; Ndjebayi, A.O.; Brown, K.H. Breast milk retinol and plasma retinol-binding protein concentrations provide similar estimates of vitamin A deficiency prevalence and identify similar risk groups among women in Cameroon but breast milk retinol underestimates the prevalence of deficiency among young children. *J. Nutr.* **2014**, *144*, 209–217. [CrossRef]
18. Zhang, Z.; Wang, Y.; Yang, X.; Chen, Y.; Zhang, H.; Xu, X.; Zhou, J.; Chen, H.; Su, M.; Yang, Y.; et al. Human Milk Lipid Profiles Around the World: A Systematic Review and Meta-Analysis. *Adv. Nutr.* **2022**, 1–18. [CrossRef]
19. Butte, N.F.; Calloway, D.H. Evaluation of lactational performance of Navajo women. *Am. J. Clin. Nutr.* **1981**, *34*, 2210–2215. [CrossRef]
20. Canfield, L.M.; Giuliano, A.R.; Neilson, E.M.; Blashil, B.M.; Graver, E.J.; Yap, H.H. Kinetics of the response of milk and serum beta-carotene to daily beta-carotene supplementation in healthy, lactating women. *Am. J. Clin. Nutr.* **1998**, *67*, 276–283. [CrossRef]
21. Canfield, L.M.; Giuliano, A.R.; Neilson, E.M.; Yap, H.H.; Graver, E.J.; Cui, H.A.; Blashill, B.M. beta-Carotene in breast milk and serum is increased after a single beta-carotene dose. *Am. J. Clin. Nutr.* **1997**, *66*, 52–61. [CrossRef]
22. Abebe, Z.; Haki, G.D.; Schweigert, F.J.; Henkel, I.M.; Baye, K. Low human milk vitamin A concentration is prevalent in rural Ethiopia. *Eur. J. Clin. Nutr.* **2019**, *73*, 1110–1116. [CrossRef]
23. Agne-Djigo, A.; Idohou-Dossou, N.; Kwadjode, K.M.; Tanumihardjo, S.A.; Wade, S. High prevalence of vitamin A deficiency is detected by the modified relative dose-response test in six-month-old Senegalese breast-fed infants. *J. Nutr.* **2012**, *142*, 1991–1996. [CrossRef] [PubMed]
24. Alam, D.S.; van Raaij, J.M.; Hautvast, J.G.; Yunus, M.; Wahed, M.A.; Fuchs, G.J. Effect of dietary fat supplementation during late pregnancy and first six months of lactation on maternal and infant vitamin A status in rural Bangladesh. *J. Health Popul. Nutr.* **2010**, *28*, 333–342. [CrossRef] [PubMed]
25. Atalhi, N.; El Hamdouchi, A.; Barkat, A.; Elkari, K.; Hamrani, A.; El Mzibri, M.; Haskell, M.J.; Mokhtar, N.; Aguenaou, H. Combined consumption of a single high-dose vitamin A supplement with provision of vitamin A fortified oil to households maintains adequate milk retinol concentrations for 6 months in lactating Moroccan women. *Appl. Physiol. Nutr. Metab.* **2020**, *45*, 275–282. [CrossRef]
26. Ayah, R.A.; Mwaniki, D.L.; Magnussen, P.; Tedstone, A.E.; Marshall, T.; Alusala, D.; Luoba, A.; Kaestel, P.; Michaelsen, K.F.; Friis, H. The effects of maternal and infant vitamin A supplementation on vitamin A status: A randomised trial in Kenya. *Br. J. Nutr.* **2007**, *98*, 422–430. [CrossRef] [PubMed]
27. Barua, S.; Tarannum, S.; Nahar, L.; Mohiduzzaman, M. Retinol and alpha-tocopherol content in breast milk of Bangladeshi mothers under low socio-economic status. *Int. J. Food Sci. Nutr.* **1997**, *48*, 13–18. [CrossRef] [PubMed]
28. Bezerra, D.S.; Ribeiro, K.D.S.; Lima, M.S.R.; Pires Medeiros, J.F.; da Silva, A.; Dimenstein, R.; Osório, M.M. Retinol status and associated factors in mother-newborn pairs. *J. Hum. Nutr. Diet.* **2020**, *33*, 222–231. [CrossRef]
29. Canfield, L.M.; Clandinin, M.T.; Davies, D.P.; Fernandez, M.C.; Jackson, J.; Hawkes, J.; Goldman, W.J.; Pramuk, K.; Reyes, H.; Sablan, B.; et al. Multinational study of major breast milk carotenoids of healthy mothers. *Eur. J. Nutr.* **2003**, *42*, 133–141. [CrossRef]

30. Canfield, L.M.; Kaminsky, R.G.; Taren, D.L.; Shaw, E.; Sander, J.K. Red palm oil in the maternal diet increases provitamin A carotenoids in human milk and serum of the mother-infant dyad. *Eur. J. Nutr.* **2001**, *40*, 30–38. [CrossRef]
31. Canfield, L.M.; Taren, D.L.; Kaminsky, R.G.; Mahal, Z. Short-term β-carotene supplementation of lactating mothers consuming diets low in vitamin A. *J. Nutr. Biochem.* **1999**, *10*, 532–538. [CrossRef]
32. Chappell, J.E.; Francis, T.; Clandinin, M.T. Vitamin A and E content of human milk at early stages of lactation. *Early Hum. Dev.* **1985**, *11*, 157–167. [CrossRef]
33. da Silva, A.G.C.L.; de Sousa Rebouças, A.; Mendonça, B.M.A.; Silva, D.C.N.E.; Dimenstein, R.; Ribeiro, K.D.D.S. Relationship between the dietary intake, serum, and breast milk concentrations of vitamin A and vitamin E in a cohort of women over the course of lactation. *Mater. Child Nutr.* **2019**, *15*, e12772. [CrossRef] [PubMed]
34. da Silva Ribeiro, K.D.; de Araújo, K.F.; de Souza, H.H.; Soares, F.B.; da Costa Pereira, M.; Dimenstein, R. Nutritional vitamin A status in northeast Brazilian lactating mothers. *J. Hum. Nutr. Diet.* **2010**, *23*, 154–161. [CrossRef] [PubMed]
35. Daniels, L.; Gibson, R.S.; Diana, A.; Haszard, J.J.; Rahmannia, S.; Luftimas, D.E.; Hampel, D.; Shahab-Ferdows, S.; Reid, M.; Melo, L.; et al. Micronutrient intakes of lactating mothers and their association with breast milk concentrations and micronutrient adequacy of exclusively breastfed Indonesian infants. *Am. J. Clin. Nutr.* **2019**, *110*, 391–400. [CrossRef] [PubMed]
36. de Lira, L.Q.; Lima, M.S.R.; de Medeiros, J.M.S.; da Silva, I.F.; Dimenstein, R. Correlation of vitamin A nutritional status on alpha-tocopherol in the colostrum of lactating women. *Mater. Child Nutr.* **2013**, *9*, 31–40. [CrossRef]
37. De Pee, S.; West, C.E.; Muhilal; Karyadi, D.; Hautvast, J.G.A.J. Lack of improvement in vitamin A status with increased consumption of dark-green leafy vegetables. *Lancet* **1995**, *346*, 75–81. [CrossRef]
38. De Pee, S.; Yuniar, Y.; West, C.E.; Muhilal. Evaluation of biochemical indicators of vitamin A status in breast- feeding and non-breast-feeding Indonesian women. *Am. J. Clin. Nutr.* **1997**, *66*, 160–167. [CrossRef]
39. Deminice, T.M.M.; Ferraz, I.S.; Monteiro, J.P.; Jordão, A.A.; Ambrósio, L.M.C.S.; Nogueira-de-Almeida, C.A. Vitamin A intake of Brazilian mothers and retinol concentrations in maternal blood, human milk, and the umbilical cord. *J. Int. Med. Res.* **2018**, *46*, 1555–1569. [CrossRef]
40. Denić, M.; Sunarić, S.; Genčić, M.; Živković, J.; Jovanović, T.; Kocić, G.; Jonović, M. Maternal age has more pronounced effect on breast milk retinol and β-carotene content than maternal dietary pattern. *Nutrition* **2019**, *65*, 120–125. [CrossRef]
41. Dimenstein, R.; Simplício, J.L.; Ribeiro, K.D.S.; Melo, I.L.P. Retinol levels in human colostrum: Influence of child, maternal and socioeconomic variables. *J. Pediatr.* **2003**, *79*, 513–518. [CrossRef]
42. Ding, Y.; Hu, P.; Yang, Y.; Xu, F.; Li, F.; Lu, X.; Xie, Z.; Wang, Z. Impact of maternal daily oral low-dose vitamin a supplementation on the mother–infant pair: A randomised placebo-controlled trial in China. *Nutrients* **2021**, *13*, 2370. [CrossRef]
43. Duan, B.B.; So, H.J.; Shin, J.A.; Qin, Y.; Yang, J.; Lee, K.T. Different content of cholesterol, retinol, and tocopherols in human milk according to its fat content. *Eur. Food Res. Technol.* **2021**, *247*, 1307–1318. [CrossRef]
44. Duda, G.; Nogala-Kalucka, M.; Karwowska, W.; Kupczyk, B.; Lampart-Szczapa, E. Influence of the lactating women diet on the concentration of the lipophilic vitamins in human milk. *Pak. J. Nutr.* **2009**, *8*, 629–634. [CrossRef]
45. Ettyang, G.A.; Oloo, A.; van Marken Lichtenbelt, W.; Saris, W. Consumption of vitamin A by breastfeeding children in rural Kenya. *Food Nutr. Bull.* **2004**, *25*, 256–263. [CrossRef]
46. García-Guerra, A.; Neufeld, L.M.; Hernández-Cordero, S.; Rivera, J.; Martorell, R.; Ramakrishnan, U. Prenatal multiple micronutrient supplementation impact on biochemical indicators during pregnancy and postpartum. *Salud Publica M.* **2009**, *51*, 327–335. [CrossRef]
47. Gibson, R.S.; Rahmannia, S.; Diana, A.; Leong, C.; Haszard, J.J.; Hampel, D.; Reid, M.; Erhardt, J.; Suryanto, A.H.; Sofiah, W.N.; et al. Association of maternal diet, micronutrient status, and milk volume with milk micronutrient concentrations in Indonesian mothers at 2 and 5 months postpartum. *Am. J. Clin. Nutr.* **2020**, *112*, 1039–1050. [CrossRef]
48. Góes, H.C.A.; Torres, A.G.; Donangelo, C.M.; Trugo, N.M.F. Nutrient composition of banked human milk in Brazil and influence of processing on zinc distribution in milk fractions. *Nutrition* **2002**, *18*, 590–594. [CrossRef]
49. Grilo, E.C.; Lima, M.S.R.; Cunha, L.R.F.; Gurgel, C.S.S.; Clemente, H.A.; Dimenstein, R. Effect of maternal vitamin A supplementation on retinol concentration in colostrum. *J. Pediatr.* **2015**, *91*, 81–86. [CrossRef]
50. Grilo, E.C.; Medeiros, W.F.; Silva, A.G.; Gurgel, C.S.; Ramalho, H.M.; Dimenstein, R. Maternal supplementation with a megadose of vitamin A reduces colostrum level of α-tocopherol: A randomised controlled trial. *J. Hum. Nutr. Diet.* **2016**, *29*, 652–661. [CrossRef]
51. Gross, R.; Hänsel, H.; Schultink, W.; Shrimpton, R.; Matulessi, P.; Gross, G.; Tagliaferri, E.; Sastroamdijojo, S. Moderate zinc and vitamin A deficiency in breast milk of mothers from East-Jakarta. *Eur. J. Clin. Nutr.* **1998**, *52*, 884–890. [CrossRef]
52. Gurgel, C.S.S.; Grilo, E.C.; Lira, L.Q.; Assunção, D.G.F.; Oliveira, P.G.; Melo, L.R.M.d.; de Medeiros, S.V.; Pessanha, L.C.; Dimenstein, R.; Lyra, C.O. Vitamin A nutritional status in high- and low-income postpartum women and its effect on colostrum and the requirements of the term newborn. *J. Pediatr.* **2018**, *94*, 207–215. [CrossRef]
53. Hampel, D.; Shahab-Ferdows, S.; Islam, M.M.; Peerson, J.M.; Allen, L.H. Vitamin Concentrations in Human Milk Vary with Time within Feed, Circadian Rhythm, and Single-Dose Supplementation. *J. Nutr.* **2017**, *147*, 603–611. [CrossRef] [PubMed]
54. Haskell, M.J.; Young, M.; Adu-Afarwuah, S.; Lartey, A.; Okronipa, H.E.T.; Maleta, K.; Ashorn, U.; Jorgensen, J.M.; Fan, Y.M.; Arnold, C.D.; et al. Small-Quantity Lipid-Based Nutrient Supplements Do Not Affect Plasma or Milk Retinol Concentrations Among Malawian Mothers, or Plasma Retinol Concentrations among Young Malawian or Ghanaian Children in Two Randomized Trials. *J. Nutr.* **2021**, *151*, 1029–1037. [CrossRef] [PubMed]

55. Jiang, J.; Xiao, H.; Wu, K.; Yu, Z.; Ren, Y.; Zhao, Y.; Li, K.; Li, J.; Li, D. Retinol and α-tocopherol in human milk and their relationship with dietary intake during lactation. *Food Funct.* **2016**, *7*, 1985–1991. [CrossRef] [PubMed]
56. Khan, N.C.; West, C.E.; de Pee, S.; Bosch, D.; Phuong, H.D.; Hulshof, P.J.; Khoi, H.H.; Verhoef, H.; Hautvast, J.G. The contribution of plant foods to the vitamin A supply of lactating women in Vietnam: A randomized controlled trial. *Am. J. Clin. Nutr.* **2007**, *85*, 1112–1120. [CrossRef] [PubMed]
57. Kim, H.; Jung, B.M.; Lee, B.N.; Kim, Y.J.; Jung, J.A.; Chang, N. Retinol, α-tocopherol, and selected minerals in breast milk of lactating women with full-term infants in South Korea. *Nutr. Res. Pract.* **2017**, *11*, 64–69. [CrossRef]
58. Kim, Y.; English, C.; Reich, P.; Gerber, L.E.; Simpson, K.L. VITAMIN-A AND CAROTENOIDS IN HUMAN-MILK. *J. Agric. Food Chem.* **1990**, *38*, 1930–1933. [CrossRef]
59. Klevor, M.K.; Haskell, M.J.; Lartey, A.; Adu-Afarwuah, S.; Zeilani, M.; Dewey, K.G. Lipid-Based Nutrient Supplements Providing Approximately the Recommended Daily Intake of Vitamin A Do Not Increase Breast Milk Retinol Concentrations among Ghanaian Women. *J. Nutr.* **2016**, *146*, 335–342. [CrossRef]
60. Lira, L.Q.; de Souza, A.F.; Amâncio, A.M.; Bezerra, C.G.; Pimentel, J.B.; Moia, M.N.; Dimenstein, R. Retinol and Betacarotene Status in Mother-Infant Dyads and Associations between Them. *Ann. Nutr. Metab.* **2018**, *72*, 50–56. [CrossRef]
61. Liyanage, C.; Hettiarachchi, M.; Mangalajeewa, P.; Malawipathirana, S. Adequacy of vitamin A and fat in the breast milk of lactating women in south Sri Lanka. *Public Health Nutr.* **2008**, *11*, 747–750. [CrossRef]
62. Lopez-Teros, V.; Limon-Miro, A.T.; Astiazaran-Garcia, H.; Tanumihardjo, S.A.; Tortoledo-Ortiz, O.; Valencia, M.E. 'Dose-to-Mother' Deuterium Oxide Dilution Technique: An Accurate Strategy to Measure Vitamin A Intake in Breastfed Infants. *Nutrients* **2017**, *9*, 169. [CrossRef]
63. Machado, M.R.; Kamp, F.; Nunes, J.C.; El-Bacha, T.; Torres, A.G. Breast Milk Content of Vitamin A and E from Early- to Mid-Lactation Is Affected by Inadequate Dietary Intake in Brazilian Adult Women. *Nutrients* **2019**, *11*, 2025. [CrossRef] [PubMed]
64. Martins, T.M.; Ferraz, I.S.; Daneluzzi, J.C.; Martinelli, C.E.; Del Ciampo, L.A.; Ricco, R.G.; Jordo, A.A.; Patta, M.C.; Vannucchi, H. Impact of maternal vitamin A supplementation on the mother-Infant pair in Brazil. *Eur. J. Clin. Nutr.* **2010**, *64*, 1302–1307. [CrossRef] [PubMed]
65. Matamoros, N.; Visentin, S.; Ferrari, G.; Falivene, M.; Fasano, V.; González, H.F. Vitamin A content in mature breast milk and its adequacy to the nutritional recommendations for infants. *Arch. Argent Pediatr.* **2018**, *116*, 146–148. [CrossRef] [PubMed]
66. Mello-Neto, J.; Rondó, P.H.C.; Oshiiwa, M.; Morgano, M.A.; Zacari, C.Z.; Domingues, S. The influence of maternal factors on the concentration of vitamin A in mature breast milk. *Clin. Nutr.* **2009**, *28*, 178–181. [CrossRef] [PubMed]
67. Meneses, F.; Trugo, N.M.F. Retinol, β-carotene, and lutein + zeaxanthin in the milk of Brazilian nursing women: Associations with plasma concentrations and influences of maternal characteristics. *Nutr. Res.* **2005**, *25*, 443–451. [CrossRef]
68. Muslimatun, S.; Schmidt, M.K.; West, C.E.; Schultink, W.; Hautvast, J.G.A.J.; Karyadi, D. Weekly vitamin A and iron supplementation during pregnancy increases vitamin A concentration of breast milk but not iron status in indonesian lactating women. *J. Nutr.* **2001**, *131*, 2664–2669. [CrossRef]
69. Olafsdottir, A.S.; Wagner, K.H.; Thorsdottir, I.; Elmadfa, I. Fat-soluble vitamins in the maternal diet, influence of cod liver oil supplementation and impact of the maternal diet on human milk composition. *Ann. Nutr. Metab.* **2001**, *45*, 265–272. [CrossRef]
70. Ortega, R.M.; Andrés, P.; Martínez, R.M.; López-Sobaler, A.M. Vitamin A status during the third trimester of pregnancy in Spanish women: Influence on concentrations of vitamin A in breast milk. *Am. J. Clin. Nutr.* **1997**, *66*, 564–568. [CrossRef]
71. Palmer, A.C.; Chileshe, J.; Hall, A.G.; Barffour, M.A.; Molobeka, N.; West, K.P.; Haskell, M.J. Short-term daily consumption of provitamin a carotenoid-biofortified maize has limited impact on breast milk retinol concentrations in Zambian women enrolled in a randomized controlled feeding trial. *J. Nutr.* **2016**, *146*, 1783–1792. [CrossRef]
72. Palmer, A.C.; Jobarteh, M.L.; Chipili, M.; Greene, M.D.; Oxley, A.; Lietz, G.; Mwanza, R.; Haskell, M.J. Biofortified and fortified maize consumption reduces prevalence of low milk retinol, but does not increase vitamin A stores of breastfeeding Zambian infants with adequate reserves: A randomized controlled trial. *Am. J. Clin. Nutr.* **2021**, *113*, 1209–1220. [CrossRef]
73. Panpanich, R.; Vitsupakorn, K.; Harper, G.; Brabin, B. Serum and breast-milk vitamin A in women during lactation in rural Chiang Mai, Thailand. *Ann. Trop. Paediatr.* **2002**, *22*, 321–324. [CrossRef]
74. Ribeiro, K.D.; Araújo, K.F.; Pereira, M.C.; Dimenstein, R. Evaluation of retinol levels in human colostrum in two samples collected at an interval of 24 hours. *J. Pediatr.* **2007**, *83*, 377–380. [CrossRef]
75. Rice, A.L.; Stoltzfus, R.J.; De Francisco, A.; Kjolhede, C.L. Evaluation of serum retinol, the modified-relative-dose-response ratio, and breast-milk vitamin A as indicators of response to postpartum maternal vitamin A supplementation. *Am. J. Clin. Nutr.* **2000**, *71*, 799–806. [CrossRef]
76. Samano, R.; Martinez-Rojano, H.; Hernandez, R.M.; Ramirez, C.; Quijano, M.E.F.; Espindola-Polis, J.M.; Veruete, D. Retinol and alpha-Tocopherol in the Breast Milk of Women after a High-Risk Pregnancy. *Nutrients* **2017**, *9*, 14. [CrossRef]
77. Sânzio Gurgel, C.S.; Alves de Araújo Pereira, L.; de Assis Costa, A.; Adja da Silva Souza, M.; Araújo de Brito, P.; Miranda de Melo, L.R.; Dimenstein, R. Effect of routine prenatal supplementation on vitamin concentrations in maternal serum and breast milk. *Nutrition* **2017**, *33*, 261–265. [CrossRef]
78. Schulz, C.; Engel, U.; Kreienberg, R.; Biesalski, H.K. Vitamin A and β-carotene supply of women with gemini or short birth intervals: A pilot study. *Eur. J. Nutr.* **2007**, *46*, 12–20. [CrossRef]
79. Schweigert, F.J.; Bathe, K.; Chen, F.; Büscher, U.; Dudenhausen, J.W. Effect of the stage of lactation in humans on carotenoid levels in milk, blood plasma and plasma lipoprotein fractions. *Eur. J. Nutr.* **2004**, *43*, 39–44. [CrossRef]

80. Souza, G.; Dolinsky, M.; Matos, A.; Chagas, C.; Ramalho, A. Vitamin A concentration in human milk and its relationship with liver reserve formation and compliance with the recommended daily intake of vitamin A in pre-term and term infants in exclusive breastfeeding. *Arch. Gynecol. Obstet.* **2015**, *291*, 319–325. [CrossRef]
81. Szlagatys-Sidorkiewicz, A.; Zagierski, M.; Jankowska, A.; Łuczak, G.; Macur, K.; Baogonekczek, T.; Korzon, M.; Krzykowski, G.; Martysiak-Zurowska, D.; Kamińska, B. Longitudinal study of vitamins A, E and lipid oxidative damage in human milk throughout lactation. *Early Hum. Dev.* **2012**, *88*, 421–424. [CrossRef]
82. Szlagatys-Sidorkiewicz, A.; Zagierski, M.; Łuczak, G.; MacUr, K.; Bączek, T.; Kamińska, B. Maternal smoking does not influence vitamin A and e concentrations in mature human milk. *Breastfeed. Med.* **2012**, *7*, 285–289. [CrossRef]
83. Tijerina-Sáenz, A.; Innis, S.M.; Kitts, D.D. Antioxidant capacity of human milk and its association with vitamins A and E and fatty acid composition. *Acta Paediatr.* **2009**, *98*, 1793–1798. [CrossRef]
84. Tokuşoğlu, Ö.; Tansuğ, N.; Akşit, S.; Dinç, G.; Kasirga, E.; Özcan, C. Retinol and α-tocopherol concentrations in breast milk of Turkish lactating mothers under different socio-economic status. *Int. J. Food Sci. Nutr.* **2008**, *59*, 166–174. [CrossRef]
85. Tomiya, M.T.O.; de Arruda, I.K.G.; da Silva Diniz, A.; Santana, R.A.; da Silveira, K.C.; Andreto, L.M. The effect of vitamin A supplementation with 400 000 IU vs 200 000 IU on retinol concentrations in the breast milk: A randomized clinical trial. *Clin. Nutr.* **2017**, *36*, 100–106. [CrossRef]
86. Turner, T.; Burri, B.J.; Jamil, K.M.; Jamil, M. The effects of daily consumption of β-cryptoxanthin-rich tangerines and β-carotene-rich sweet potatoes on vitamin A and carotenoid concentrations in plasma and breast milk of Bangladeshi women with low vitamin A status in a randomized controlled trial. *Am. J. Clin. Nutr.* **2013**, *98*, 1200–1208. [CrossRef]
87. Whitfield, K.C.; Shahab-Ferdows, S.; Kroeun, H.; Sophonneary, P.; Green, T.J.; Allen, L.H.; Hampel, D. Macro- and Micronutrients in Milk from Healthy Cambodian Mothers: Status and Interrelations. *J. Nutr.* **2020**, *150*, 1461–1469. [CrossRef]
88. Fang, F.; Li, T.; Liu, Y.; Liu, B.; Ye, W. vestigation of the Contents of the Fat-Soluble Vitamins A, D and E in Human Milk from Hohho. *J. Dairy Sci. Technol.* **2014**, *37*, 5–7.
89. Zhang, L.; Bao, J.; Chen, H. Determination of vitamin A of human milk from Zhoushan islands from Zhejiang Province. *J. Hygiene Res.* **2001**, *30*, 234–236. [CrossRef]
90. Liu, J. Study on the Vitamin Contents of Human Milk in Huhhot. *Food Res. Dev.* **2016**, *37*, 20–22.
91. Zhang, H.; Wan, R.; Chen, B.; Wang, J.; Yang, Z.; Yin, S. Concentrations of vitamin A and vitamin E in breast milk at different lactation stages from urban and rural china. *Acta Nutr. Sin.* **2021**, *43*, 347–351+357. [CrossRef]
92. Fares, S.; Sethom, M.M.; Kacem, S.; Ksibi, I.; Feki, M.; Jebnoun, S.; Kaabachi, N. Retinol and Alpha-tocopherol in the Colostrum of Lactating Tunisian Women Delivering Prematurely: Associations with Maternal Characteristics. *Pediatr. Neonatol.* **2016**, *57*, 120–126. [CrossRef]
93. Montreewasuwat, N.; Olson, J.A. Serum and liver concentrations of vitamin A in Thai fetuses as a function of gestational age. *Am. J. Clin. Nutr.* **1979**, *32*, 601–606. [CrossRef]
94. Olson, J.A.; Gunning, D.B.; Tilton, R.A. Liver concentrations of vitamin A and carotenoids, as a function of age and other parameters, of American children who died of various causes. *Am. J. Clin. Nutr.* **1984**, *39*, 903–910. [CrossRef]

Associations between Dynamic Vitamin D Level and Thyroid Function during Pregnancy

Hui Wang [1], Hai-Jun Wang [1], Mingyuan Jiao [2], Na Han [2], Jinhui Xu [1], Heling Bao [1], Zheng Liu [1] and Yuelong Ji [1,*]

[1] Department of Maternal and Child Health, School of Public Health, Peking University, Beijing 100191, China
[2] Maternal and Child Health Care Hospital of Tongzhou District, Beijing 100191, China
* Correspondence: yuelong.ji@pku.edu.cn; Tel./Fax: +86-010-82801222

Abstract: Optimal Vitamin D (VitD) status and thyroid function are essential for pregnant women. This study aimed to explore associations between dynamic VitD status and thyroid function parameters in each trimester and throughout the pregnancy period. Information on all 8828 eligible participants was extracted from the Peking University Retrospective Birth Cohort in Tongzhou. Dynamic VitD status was represented as a combination of deficiency/sufficiency in the first and second trimesters. Thyroid function was assessed in three trimesters. The associations between VitD and thyroid function were assessed by multiple linear regression and generalized estimating equation models in each trimester and throughout the pregnancy period, respectively. The results indicated that both free thyroxine (fT4; $\beta = 0.004$; 95%CI: 0.003, 0.006; $p < 0.001$) and free triiodothyronine (fT3; $\beta = 0.009$; 95%CI: 0.004, 0.015; $p = 0.001$) had positive associations with VitD status in the first trimester. A VitD status that was sufficient in the first trimester and deficient in the second trimester had a lower TSH ($\beta = -0.370$; 95%CI: -0.710, -0.031; $p = 0.033$) compared with the group with sufficient VitD for both first and second trimesters. In conclusion, the associations between VitD and thyroid parameters existed throughout the pregnancy. Maintaining an adequate concentration of VitD is critical to support optimal thyroid function during pregnancy.

Keywords: Vitamin D; deficiency; thyroid-stimulating hormone; free thyroxine; free triiodothyronine

1. Introduction

Thyroid hormones are crucial for the maintenance of many fundamental functions in both adults and children [1]. During pregnancy, adequate thyroid hormone levels are essential for normal pregnancy and optimal fetal growth and development [2]. Maternal thyroid hormone is needed to support the development of placental and fetal hormones over the first half of pregnancy [3]. Since the fetal thyroid gland matures only after 18–20 weeks of gestation, before that, all thyroid hormones depend on maternal thyroxin (T4) transferred through the placenta [2]. Additionally, serum levels of thyroid-binding globulin (TBG) increase during pregnancy; this is consequently combined with free T4 (fT4) and free triiodothyronine (fT3) and then results in a slight decrease (10–15%) of these two hormones when pregnant women live in an area with sufficient iodine [4]. Meanwhile, increased urinary iodide clearance, thyroid hormone degradation, and human chorionic gonadotropin (hCG), which is a weak agonist of the thyroid-stimulating hormone receptor (TSH), all trigger higher thyroid hormone demand [5]. The total concentration of thyroxine should increase by around 20–50% to reach a euthyroid level during pregnancy [6]. Overall, pregnancy has a critical impact on the thyroid gland and its function.

Vitamin D (VitD) plays a pleiotropic role in the physiological and biological processes of the human body, such as cell growth, differentiation, maturation, anticarcinogenic effects, and anti-autoimmune activities, due to the wide expression of the VitD receptor (VDR) [7,8]. Recent studies have indicated that VitD deficiency is associated with thyroid disease since VDR is expressed in thyrocytes [9]. Vitamin deficiency has been associated with autoimmune thyroid disease (AITD), such as Grave's disease (GD) and Hashimoto's thyroiditis

(HT) [10,11]. Studies have indicated that VitD deficiency is prevalent in China [12,13] and the prevalence of VitD deficiency in pregnant women is around 70% [14]. Furthermore, VitD deficiency or thyroid disorder during pregnancy has a similarly adverse impact on the pregnant woman and fetus, for example, preeclampsia, gestational diabetes, premature birth, and abnormal fetal mental development.

All the aforementioned phenomena indicate a potential association between VitD and thyroid function. Some studies have investigated the associations between VitD status and thyroid function during pregnancy; their general weakness was that they investigated the associations in the first or second trimester or in three trimesters with different participants [15–17]. Only one study explored the dynamic association between VitD status and thyroid function parameters across three trimesters among 50 pregnant women, which had relatively low statistical power [18]. Three out of four studies did not find associations between VitD and thyroid function, and only one study detected a positive association between VitD concentration and TSH in the second trimester. Therefore, the present study aimed to fill this research gap by using a relatively larger sample size to capture the dynamic associations between VitD status and thyroid function in the Peking University Retrospective Birth Cohort in Tongzhou.

2. Participants and Methods

2.1. Study Population

The present study is a retrospective cohort study. Information on all eligible participants was extracted from the Peking University Retrospective Birth Cohort in Tongzhou (39° N latitude) based on the hospital information system of Beijing [19]. The inclusion criteria were (1) singleton pregnancy; (2) maternal age between 18 and 49 years old; (3) the initial thyroid function test was performed in the first trimester; (4) without assisted reproduction; (5) without heart disease, hypertension, diabetes mellitus, kidney disease, and autoimmunity disease before pregnancy; (6) without family or personal history of thyroid disease; (7) information on the first pregnancy was retained if more than one pregnancy was detected for the same woman; and (8) verified last menstrual period between 28 October 2015 and 29 May 2019. Exclusion criteria were (1) levothyroxine (LT4) intake during pregnancy ($n = 901$); (2) no Vitamin D test for the first and second trimesters ($n = 9290$); and (3) absence of important covariables ($n = 56$). Finally, information on 8828 pregnant women who visited and delivered in the Tongzhou Maternal and Children Health Hospital and had vitamin tests twice was collected. Among them, 1552 pregnant women were tested for thyroid function in the first and second trimesters; 562 for thyroid function in the first and third trimesters; and 212 for the first, second, and third trimesters (Figure S1).

2.2. Data Collection

2.2.1. Assessment of VitD Deficiency and Thyroid Function

Serum 25-hydroxyVitamin D [25(OH)D] was measured in the first (median 9.5 weeks of gestation) and second trimester (median 26.8 week of gestation) as the combination of 25(OH)D2 and 25(OH)D3 using the high-performance liquid chromatography mass spectrometry method. Thus, the combined value of 25(OH)D2 and 25(OH)D3 was used to represent the level of 25(OH)D. When $25(OH)D \leq 20.0$ ng/mL, then the corresponding participant was defined as having maternal VitD deficiency. We classified VitD status into four groups: deficient in the first trimester and sufficient in the second trimester (D1S2), deficient in the second trimester and sufficient in the first trimester (S1D2), sufficient in both trimesters (S1S2), and deficient in both trimesters (D1D2). This classification method could better reflect the dynamic VitD status in the first two trimesters. Furthermore, we categorized the first trimester VitD status into quartiles (quartile 1: median 10.3 nmol/L (full range 2.4–13.1); quartile 2: median 15.8 nmol/L (full range 3.1–18.3); quartile 3: median 21.3 nmol/L (full range 18.3–24.3); quartile 4: median 28.3 nmol/L (full range 24.3–92.9).

The thyroid function was assessed primarily during the first trimester of pregnancy. A small fraction of the pregnant women had three thyroid function tests during the pregnancy period. Fasting blood samples were taken from all participants between 8:00 a.m. and 10:00 a.m. Then, serum was used for testing TSH, free T4 (fT4), free T3 (fT3), and TPOAb via electrochemiluminescence immunoassays (ARCHITECT i2000, Abbott Core Laboratory, Abbott Park, IL, USA). According to the reference range provided by the manufacturer, TPOAb > 5.6 IU/mL was considered positive. All the reagents were matched with ARCHITECT i2000 and supplied by the same company. The intra and inter-assay coefficients of variation for the above-mentioned three indicators were all smaller than 10%.

2.2.2. Assessment of Covariates

The following relevant sociodemographic and clinical variables were considered as covariates: maternal age, maternal educational level (high school or below, college, and university or above), employment status (yes, no), race (Han, other), parity history (primipara, multipara), folate supplementation status (yes, no), and VitD supplementation status (yes, no). Based on the data of the present study, 91% of pregnant women took VitD as a supplement. All demographic and medical information was collected by trained health professionals when the pregnant women initialized the perinatal files in the first trimester, including birth date, race, educational attainment, occupation, pregnancy history, disease history, and LMP. Body mass index (BMI) was calculated by using weight (kg) divided by the square of height (m^2) with the first antenatal visit data and participants were classified as underweight (BMI < 18.5 kg/m^2), normal weight (18.5 ≤ BMI < 24.0 kg/m^2), obese (24.0 ≤ BMI < 28.0 kg/m^2), or overweight (BMI > 28.0 kg/m^2) according to the criteria issued by the Working Group on Obesity in China (WGOC) [20]. Since VitD is influenced by sunlight, we categorized the conception period (last menstrual period) into spring (February–May), summer (June–July), autumn (August–October) and winter (November–January) to generally represent the fluctuation of VitD concentrations.

2.3. Approval of Ethics

The study was approved by the Ethics Committee of the Peking University Health Science Center (IRB00001052-21023).

2.4. Statistical Analyses

Continuous variables were checked for normal distribution using the Kolmogorov–Smirnov test and were presented as mean (standard deviation, SD) for normally distributed data and as median (IQR) for skewed data. Continuous variables were compared by using one-way ANOVA test or Kruskal–Wallis rank sum test among the four subgroups. Categorical variables were presented as frequency (percentage), and compared using the Chi-square test or Fisher's exact test among the four subgroups. Multiple linear regression was applied to assess associations of VitD status with thyroid function parameters at each trimester. Generalized estimation equation (GEE) analysis was applied to assess the associations of VitD status with thyroid function parameters throughout the pregnancy using identity link function and exchangeable correlation structure. The crude model was built without adjusting for any covariates, whereas the adjusted model was adjusted for all the covariates (maternal age, maternal educational levels, maternal employment status, parity, pre-pregnancy BMI class, Vitamin D supplement during pregnancy, gestational diabetes, and gestational hypertension disorder). The data analyses were performed using R software (version 4.1.1). A two-tailed p-value < 0.05 was considered statistically significant.

3. Results

3.1. Characteristics of the Study Population

The median value of maternal VitD (25(OH)D) was 18.3 ng/mL in the first trimester and 30.5 ng/mL in the second trimester (Table 1). The proportion of VitD deficiency reduced from 57.1% in the first trimester to 19.8% in the second trimester among total participants. In the present study, the prevalence of gestational diabetes mellitus was 28.6% and the gestational hypertensive disorder was 2.1%.

Table 1. Characteristics of participants in three different trimesters.

Characteristic	First Trimester, $n = 8828$	Second Trimester [1], $n = 1396$	Third Trimester [2], $n = 562$	p [4]
Maternal age	29.40 (5.10) [3]	29.20 (4.82)	29.75 (5.38)	0.033
Maternal education				0.894
Low (high school or below)	1308 (14.8)	197 (14.1)	77 (13.7)	
Middle (college)	3828 (43.4)	607 (43.5)	251 (44.7)	
High (university or above)	3692 (41.8)	592 (42.4)	234 (41.6)	
Maternal employment				0.194
Unemployed	980 (11.1)	140 (10.0)	72 (12.8)	
Employed	7848 (88.9)	1256 (90.0)	490 (87.2)	
Race/ethnicity				0.960
Han	8305 (94.1)	1316 (94.3)	529 (94.1)	
Other	523 (5.9)	80 (5.7)	33 (5.9)	
Parity				0.143
Primiparous	5049 (57.2)	785 (56.2)	343 (61.0)	
Multiparous	3779 (42.8)	611 (43.8)	219 (39.0)	
Maternal BMI class				0.130
Underweight	840 (9.5)	151 (10.8)	43 (7.7)	
Normal	5823 (66.0)	940 (67.3)	380 (67.6)	
Overweight	1716 (19.4)	247 (17.7)	106 (18.9)	
Obese	449 (5.1)	58 (4.2)	33 (5.9)	
Folate supplement				0.462
No	760 (8.6)	107 (7.7)	45 (8.0)	
Yes	8068 (91.4)	1289 (92.3)	517 (92.0)	
Multivitamin supplement				0.765
No	4290 (48.6)	671 (48.1)	265 (47.2)	
Yes	4538 (51.4)	725 (51.9)	297 (52.8)	
Season of conception				0.011
Spring	1974 (22.4)	301 (21.6)	134 (23.8)	
Summer	1631 (18.5)	257 (18.4)	133 (23.7)	
Autumn	2614 (29.6)	436 (31.2)	163 (29.0)	
Winter	2609 (29.6)	402 (28.8)	132 (23.5)	
Vitamin D (0–13 weeks), ng/mL	18.30 (11.20)	18.20 (11.70)	19.20 (10.67)	0.312
Vitamin D deficiency (0–13 weeks)				0.410
No	3783 (42.9)	600 (43.0)	257 (45.7)	
Yes	5045 (57.1)	796 (57.0)	305 (54.3)	
Vitamin D (14–28 weeks), ng/mL	30.50 (16.20)	30.55 (16.32)	30.50 (14.85)	0.905
Vitamin D deficiency (14–28 weeks)				0.124
No	7081 (80.2)	1106 (79.2)	468 (83.3)	
Yes	1747 (19.8)	290 (20.8)	94 (16.7)	
Vitamin D supplement				0.264
No	810 (9.2)	113 (8.1)	44 (7.8)	
Yes	8018 (90.8)	1283 (91.9)	518 (92.2)	
TPOAb positive (0–13 weeks)	993 (11.2)	234 (16.8)	105 (18.7)	<0.001
Gestational hypertensive disorder	185 (2.1)	26 (1.9)	27 (4.8)	<0.001
Gestational diabetes mellitus	2492 (28.2)	382 (27.4)	227 (40.4)	<0.001

[1] Second-trimester participants should have both first- and second-trimester thyroid function tests irrespective of the third trimester thyroid function test. [2] Third-trimester participants should have both first- and third-trimester thyroid function tests irrespective of the second trimester thyroid function test. [3] Values are n (%) for categorical variables and median (IQR) for a continuous variable with a skewed distribution. Vitamin D concentration was measured with 25-hydroxyVitamin D in the serum. [4] Continuous variables were compared by using one-way ANOVA test for normal distribution data or Kruskal–Wallis rank sum test for skew distribution data among the four subgroups.

3.2. Characteristics of Thyroid Function with Different VitD Status

From the quartile analysis based on the first trimester, only fT3 increased steadily with higher VitD concentration in the first trimester ($p < 0.001$, Table S1). Within the group of participants with two VitD measurements, the number of participants was the lowest in the S1D2 group (Table 2). In the first trimester, levels of fT3 and fT4 were different among those four groups (both $p < 0.05$). The highest median levels of fT3 and fT4 were detected in the S1D2 group. In the third trimester, the TSH levels were different among the four groups ($p < 0.001$), and the S1D2 group had the highest TSH level among these four groups.

Table 2. Parameters of thyroid function with different VitD status in three trimesters.

Characteristic	S1S2 [1]	D1S2	S1D2	D1D2	p [3]
First trimester (n = 8828)	n = 3324	n = 3757	n = 459	n = 1288	
TPOAb (IU/mL)	0.37 (0.66) [2]	0.33 (0.59)	0.37 (0.67)	0.33 (0.53)	0.983
TSH (μIU/mL)	0.92 (0.91)	0.90 (0.97)	0.93 (1.01)	0.88 (0.97)	0.513
fT3 (pmol/L)	4.26 (0.62)	4.19 (0.61)	4.27 (0.64)	4.16 (0.64)	0.002
fT4 (pmol/L)	13.35 (2.05)	13.20 (2.08)	13.51 (2.03)	13.25 (2.04)	0.024
Second trimester (n = 1396)	n = 515	n = 591	n = 85	n = 205	
TSH (μIU/mL)	0.85 (0.82)	0.90 (0.81)	0.74 (0.90)	0.86 (0.87)	0.379
fT3 (pmol/L)	4.06 (0.60)	4.10 (0.60)	3.97 (0.49)	4.05 (0.59)	0.052
fT4 (pmol/L)	11.21 (1.70)	11.25 (1.76)	11.43 (1.91)	11.05 (1.86)	0.928
Third trimester (n = 562)	n = 225	n = 243	n = 32	n = 62	
TSH (μIU/mL)	1.27 (1.03)	1.31 (1.08)	1.69 (1.53)	1.25 (1.20)	<0.001
fT3 (pmol/L)	3.80 (0.66)	3.84 (0.66)	3.78 (0.52)	3.89 (0.60)	0.597
fT4 (pmol/L)	9.91 (1.78)	9.96 (1.74)	9.66 (1.46)	9.91 (1.85)	0.619

[1] S1S2 means that VitD was sufficient in both the first and second trimester; D1S2 means that VitD was deficient in the first trimester and sufficient in the second trimester; S1D2 means that VitD was sufficient in the first trimester and deficient in the second trimester; D1D2 means that VitD was deficient in both the first and second trimesters. [2] Values are median (IQR) for a continuous variable with a skewed distribution. Vitamin D concentration was measured with 25-hydroxyVitamin D in the serum. [3] Continuous variables were compared by using one-way ANOVA test for normal distribution data or Kruskal–Wallis rank sum test for skew distribution data among the four subgroups.

3.3. Associations between VitD Status and Thyroid Function in Each Trimester Separately

In the first trimester, the contemporaneous VitD status was positively associated with fT3 and fT4 levels both in the continuous analysis ($\beta = 0.004$; 95%CI: 0.003, 0.006; $p < 0.001$ and $\beta = 0.009$; 95%CI: 0.004, 0.015; $P = 0.001$) and categorical analysis ($\beta = -0.056$; 95%CI: $-0.097, -0.016$; $p = 0.007$ and $\beta = -0.196$; 95%CI: $-0.331, -0.060$; $p = 0.001$), respectively (Table 3). In the second trimester, the contemporaneous VitD status was positively associated with fT3 ($\beta = 0.003$; 95%CI: 0.001, 0.006; $p = 0.014$). In the third trimester, the VitD status of the second trimester had a positive association with the fT4 level in the third trimester ($\beta = 0.011$; 95%CI: 0.001, 0.022; $p = 0.030$). However, the association between VitD status and TSH was more complex. The VitD level in the second trimester seems to have had a negative association with TSH level in the third trimester in the continuous analysis ($\beta = -0.009$; 95%CI: $-0.016, -0.001$; $p = 0.024$).

3.4. Associations between VitD Status and Thyroid Function across Three Trimesters

To further portray the associations between VitD and thyroid function throughout three trimesters, GEE analyses were conducted in 212 pregnant women who had thyroid parameters measured at each trimester (Table 4). S1D2 of VitD status had positive association with TSH ($\beta = -0.370$; 95%CI: $-0.710, -0.031$; $p = 0.033$), that is, compared with VitD that was sufficient in both the first and second trimester, the status of deficiency could reduce TSH. Since the sample size shrank substantially, therefore, further characteristics comparisons were performed between 212 pregnant women and the rest of the total population (Table S2). It indicated that there is higher prevalence of TPOAb positivity (10.7% vs. 31.6%), GHD (2.0% vs. 4.2%), and GDM (28.0% vs. 37.7%) in the population who had three thyroid function tests (Table S2).

Table 3. Associations between VitD status and thyroid function parameter in each trimester [1].

Indicators	Vitamin D Status	First Trimester (n = 8828)			Second Trimester (n = 1396)			Third Trimester (n = 562)		
		β	95%CI	p	β	95%CI	p	β	95%CI	p
TSH	VitD level in 1st trimester	0.001	−0.001, 0.003	0.311	−0.001	−0.006, 0.003	0.547	−0.001	−0.011, 0.010	0.884
	VitD level in 2nd trimester				0.002	−0.001, 0.006	0.188	−0.009	−0.016, −0.001	0.024
	Vit D deficiency classification									
	D1S2	−0.016	−0.049, 0.018	0.365	−0.029	−0.116, 0.058	0.511	0.178	−0.011, 0.367	0.066
	S1D2	0.001	−0.040, 0.041	0.980	0.019	−0.081, 0.120	0.707	−0.378	−0.587, −0.169	<0.001
	D1D2	0.001	−0.045, 0.048	0.953	0.075	−0.037, 0.188	0.190	−0.455	−0.690, −0.221	<0.001
fT3	VitD level in 1st trimester	0.004	0.003, 0.006	<0.001	−0.001	−0.005, 0.002	0.512	−0.004	−0.010, 0.003	0.262
	VitD level in 2nd trimester				0.003	0.001, 0.006	0.014	−0.0001	−0.005, 0.005	0.962
	Vit D deficiency classification									
	D1S2	−0.027	−0.056, 0.003	0.076	−0.074	−0.138, −0.009	0.025	0.018	−0.099, 0.136	0.762
	S1D2	−0.014	−0.049, 0.021	0.436	0.001	−0.072, 0.075	0.972	0.055	−0.075, 0.184	0.410
	D1D2	−0.056	−0.097, −0.016	0.007	0.078	−0.004, 0.161	0.064	0.083	−0.063, 0.228	0.265
fT4	VitD level in 1st trimester	0.009	0.004, 0.015	0.001	0.009	−0.002, 0.020	0.106	0.001	−0.013, 0.016	0.842
	VitD level in 2nd trimester				0.001	−0.007, 0.009	0.849	0.011	0.001, 0.022	0.030
	Vit D deficiency classification									
	D1S2	0.077	−0.023, 0.176	0.130	−0.046	−0.241, 0.148	0.640	−0.090	−0.350, 0.170	0.498
	S1D2	−0.050	−0.168, 0.069	0.411	0.049	−0.175, 0.273	0.669	0.113	−0.175, 0.400	0.442
	D1D2	−0.196	−0.331, −0.060	0.005	0.013	−0.238, 0.264	0.921	0.146	−0.176, 0.469	0.374

[1] Multiple linear regression was applied to assess the associations of the Vitamin D status with thyroid function parameters at each trimester. Adjusted for maternal age, maternal educational levels, maternal employment status, parity, prenatal BMI class, Vitamin D supplement, folate and multivitamin supplementation, GHD, GDM, TPOAb positivity during pregnancy, and seasons of conception.

Table 4. Associations between VitD status and thyroid function parameter across three trimesters [1] (n = 212).

Indicator	VitD Status	Unadjusted Analysis			Adjusted Analysis [2]		
		Beta	95%CI	p	Beta	95%CI	p
TSH	VitD level in 1st trimester	0.001	−0.012, 0.014	0.855	0.004	−0.009, 0.018	0.519
	VitD level in 2nd trimester	0.002	−0.008, 0.012	0.696	0.001	−0.008, 0.011	0.786
	VitD deficiency classification						
	D1S2	−0.155	−0.367, 0.057	0.152	−0.133	−0.358, 0.091	0.245
	S1D2	−0.283	−0.586, 0.020	0.067	−0.370	−0.710, −0.031	0.033
	D1D2	−0.050	−0.422, 0.323	0.794	−0.215	−0.632, 0.202	0.312
FT3	VitD level in 1st trimester	−0.012	−0.025, 0.002	0.089	−0.015	−0.030, 0.000	0.053
	VitD level in 2nd trimester	−0.002	−0.011, 0.008	0.716	−0.002	−0.014, 0.009	0.695
	VitD deficiency classification						
	D1S2	0.010	−0.232, 0.252	0.935	0.072	−0.201, 0.344	0.605
	S1D2	−0.010	−0.238, 0.218	0.933	−0.054	−0.309, 0.201	0.678
	D1D2	0.193	−0.020, 0.407	0.076	0.181	−0.084, 0.445	0.181
FT4	VitD level in 1st trimester	−0.021	−0.054, 0.013	0.222	−0.030	−0.067, 0.008	0.121
	VitD level in 2nd trimester	0.000	−0.0278, 0.0287	0.975	−0.004	−0.034, 0.027	0.819
	VitD deficiency classification						
	D1S2	0.546	−0.413, 1.504	0.265	0.755	−0.167, 1.678	0.109
	S1D2	0.781	−0.066, 1.627	0.071	0.853	−0.009, 1.715	0.052
	D1D2	0.760	0.043, 1.477	0.038	0.799	−0.023, 1.622	0.057

[1] Generalized estimation equation (GEE) analysis was applied to assess associations of the Vitamin D status with thyroid function parameters throughout pregnancy using identity link function and exchangeable correlation structure. [2] Adjusted for maternal age, maternal educational levels, maternal employment status, parity, pre-pregnancy BMI class, Vitamin D supplement, folate and multivitamin supplementation, positivity for GHD, GDM, TPOAb during pregnancy, and seasons of conception.

4. Discussion

In the current study, we delineated the complex associations between VitD and thyroid function parameters in each trimester with the birth cohort data. The results indicated that fT4 and fT3 both had positive associations with VitD status in the first trimester. A VitD status that was sufficient in the first trimester and deficient in the second trimester had a lower TSH, compared with the group with sufficient VitD for both first and second trimesters. Previous research indicated that VitD status was negatively associated with GHD, GDM, and TPOAb positivity [21–23], and these diseases or syndromes were also associated with thyroid functions [24]. Therefore, we adjusted these factors rather than directly censoring them from the data.

The VitD levels during pregnancy showed large variation across nations and regions. Additionally, due to the different VitD supplementation recommendations within and between jurisdictions during pregnancy, the supplementation also varies among pregnant women. VitD deficiency is common in pregnant women, and the worldwide prevalence of VitD deficiency was 54% in pregnant women [25]. A study based on China Nutrition and Health Surveillance (CNHS) indicated that the prevalence of VitD deficiency (<20 ng/mL) was higher in 2015–2017 (87.43%) compared with 2010–2012 (73.4%) among pregnant women, regardless of VitD supplementation [26]. The prevalence of VitD deficiency was 30.57% in the Shanghai birth cohort in the first trimester, which was less than our current study (57.1%) [27]. A plausible reason might be that the altitude is higher in Beijing in comparison with Shanghai.

The natural process of pregnancy might also influence the levels of VitD. One study focusing on pregnant women who did not have VitD supplementation showed that the deficiency rate could reach 96% in the first trimester. Interestingly, the prevalence decreased to 78% and 76% in the second and third trimesters individually [18]. Therefore, it might indicate that there is a physiological increase in VitD during pregnancy, the lowest concentration of VitD was in the first trimester. In addition, this result was confirmed with a larger sample size in the Shanghai birth cohort in both the VitD-supplemented group and the non-supplemented group [27], and Indian pregnant women [28]. Although VitD concentration was substantially influenced by seasons, concentration trends were similar in different trimesters [28].

In the aspects of thyroid function parameters, the physiological changes of TSH, fT4, and fT3 are non-linear and intricate [2]. During the first 8–10 weeks of gestation, hCG concentration reaches the highest level and the α subunit of hCG is structurally similar to TSH, which increases the serum concentration of thyroxine, particularly in T4, and this in turn reduces the level of TSH *per se* through negative feedback via the hypothalamic–pituitary–thyroid axis [29]. Generally, for every 10,000 IU/L increasing in hCG, TSH decreases by 0.1 mU/L; TSH value drops to the valley at the gestation age of 10–12 weeks [30]. Therefore, during pregnancy, women normally have lower serum TSH concentrations than before pregnancy. After a first trimester, with the reduced concentration of hCG, the TSH concentration slowly increases and maintains at the plateau around 25 weeks of gestation. However, there are 10% and 5% fractions of women with a suppressed TSH in the second and the third trimester, respectively [29]. In contrast, the level of fT4 peaks around gestation age of 10–12 weeks and shifts downwards after this until birth [2]. To date, there have been only a few studies measuring fT3 through three trimesters with the gold standard measurement LC-MS/MS. According to the published data, the levels of fT3 synchronize with fT4 in late pregnancy [31,32]. Overall, the TSH, fT3, and fT4 levels should be dissected based on the different trimesters. Therefore, we drew a theoretical schematic diagram for VitD and thyroid parameter (Figure S2) for a better understanding.

In the present study, positive associations were detected between VitD concentration and fT3 and fT4 levels in the first trimester, individually. These results were logical and corresponded to physiological changes among pregnant women based on the aforementioned findings (Figure S2). In contrast, no association between VitD and thyroid functional parameters was detected in Zhao's study with 50 Chinese women [18]. The plausible differences could be attributed two major aspects. First, the number of participants was only 50 in Zhao's study, which generated relatively low R^2 values in the multiple linear regression. Second, all participants did not supplement with VitD before or during pregnancy, which resulted in a generally low serum VitD level. Musa's study was conducted with 132 Sudanese women in the first trimester and also did not find relationship between VitD level and thyroid parameters [16]. Both Zhao's and Musa's studies included participants who did not use VitD supplementation, although the non-supplementation period was different. The period of no supplementation of VitD in Musa's study only accounted for the last six months before recruitment [16], while Zhao's study recruited participants who did not use VitD or calcium supplementation before or during pregnancy. Nonetheless, the prevalence of VitD deficiency was significantly high in both Zhao's (98%) and Musa's (99.2%) cohorts.

Ahi et al. conducted correlation analyses between maternal VitD and thyroid function analysis with 66 Iranian pregnant women without VitD supplementation. The participants were approximately divided into three trimesters, and each trimester included 22 pregnant women. However, no statistical association was detected and the prevalence of VitD deficiency was 45.46% [15]. All of these results indicated that associations can only be detected with a certain amount of VitD. Intriguingly, Nizar carried out a study with sufficient levels of VitD (>30 ng/mL) in Ammaman-Jordan women and detected a negative association between VitD and TSH ($r = -0.51$, $p < 0.005$) [33]. However, Nizar did not indicate which trimester those participants were in when they conducted the study. We hypothesize that this scenario fits into the theoretical relationship between VitD and TSH in the first trimester (Figure S2). In the present study, we detect a positive association between VitD and TSH in the third-trimester model and the GEE model. These results indicated that the TSH level started to increase in the second trimester and mainly bounced up in the third trimester. Then, the overall average effect of VitD on TSH was positive during the entire pregnancy period. In addition, Pan et al. performed an association analysis with

277 pregnant women (without any thyroid-antibody positivity) in the second trimester; they revealed a positive association between TSH and VitD and negative associations between fT3/fT4 and VitD, respectively. In our present study, we revealed a positive association between fT3/fT4 and VitD in the first trimester. Overall, all those results fitted into the theoretical model in the first trimester (our present study) and second trimester (Pan's study) individually (Figure S2).

Until now, the regulations between VitD and thyroid parameters have not been fully illustrated. The majority of studies have examined VitD deficiency and autoimmune thyroid disease (AITD) [9]. Since 1,25(OH)2D can suppress the adaptive immune system, it improves immune tolerance and represents a beneficial effect on a number of autoimmune diseases [34]. Additionally, animal studies have indicated that 1,25(OH)2D combined with cyclosporine could result in a synergistic effect to prevent the induction of experimental autoimmune thyroiditis (EAT) in CBA mice [35,36]. Furthermore, BALB/C mice could develop persistent hyperthyroidism after immunization with the TSH receptor only in VitD-deficient mice [37]. In rat experiments, researchers found that 1,25(OH)D3 could bind to the thyroid hormone receptors at the pituitary levels and modulated the secretion of TSH [38]. Kano et al. demonstrated that VitD concentration could be elevated after increasing T3, T4, and TSH in rats [39]. More related experiments should be conducted to further elucidate the mechanism of VitD and thyroid hormone interactions. Nonetheless, both adequate VitD level and euthyroidism are vital for fetal development. Therefore, VitD supplementation seems more important in the first trimester.

Several merits of the current study should be mentioned. It was the first study to reveal the associations between VitD and thyroid parameters across three trimesters with a relatively moderate population size, with the birth cohort data. Furthermore, we also dynamically considered Vitamin D concentration during the first two trimesters in terms of the high supplementation rate, which strengthened our findings. However, the present study also encountered limitations. Most pregnant women were only measured for their thyroid function in the first trimester routinely. Those participants who had more than one measurement of their thyroid functions had a high prevalence of gestational complications, such as GDM and GHD, which may mean the associations between VitD and thyroid function parameters were underestimated. Second, most participants did not have a VitD measurement in the third trimester, which made it difficult to portray the full view of VitD and thyroid function in our own dataset. Finally, it was an observational study in which causal inference ability was also limited.

In conclusion, the associations between VitD and thyroid parameters are dynamic. fT3 and fT4 were positively associated with VitD in the first trimester. TSH was positively associated with VitD, particularly in the third trimester. It is important to maintain an adequate level of VitD to support normal thyroid function from a nutritional point of view.

Supplementary Materials: The following supporting information can be downloaded at: https://www.mdpi.com/article/10.3390/nu14183780/s1, Figure S1: Flowchart of selection of participants; Figure S2: Schematic diagram of theoretically physiological changes of Vitamin D and thyroid parameters. (Modified from thyroid disease in pregnancy: new insights in diagnosis and clinical management). Table S1: hyroid function in the quartile of VitD level 1 quartile in each trimester; Table S2: Comparison of characteristics between the population of the total population and the GEE population.

Author Contributions: Conceptualization, H.W., M.J. and Y.J.; methodology, N.H. and Y.J.; data collection and cleaning, M.J., N.H., H.B. and J.X.; data analysis, Y.J., J.X. and Z.L.; draft preparation, H.W. and Y.J.; comprehensive review and editing, H.-J.W.; funding acquisition, H.-J.W. and Y.J. All authors have read and agreed to the published version of the manuscript.

Funding: The present research was funded by Peking University Medicine Fund for the world's leading discipline or discipline cluster development (BMU2022XY030), the National Natural Science Foundation of China (81973053), and Peking University Medicine Fund of Fostering Young Scholars' Scientific & Technological Innovation (BMU2022PY018).

Institutional Review Board Statement: The study was approved by the Ethics Committee of the Peking University Health Science Center (IRB00001052-21023).

Informed Consent Statement: Written informed consent was obtained from all subjects involved in the study.

Data Availability Statement: The data presented in this study are available on request from the corresponding author.

Acknowledgments: We sincerely thank the research group of the Peking University Retrospective Birth Cohort in Tongzhou based on the hospital information system. We appreciate the health professionals in the Tongzhou Maternal and Child Health Care Hospital of Beijing for data collection and management.

Conflicts of Interest: All authors declare no conflict of interest.

References

1. Springer, D.; Jiskra, J.; Limanova, Z.; Zima, T.; Potlukova, E. Thyroid in pregnancy: From physiology to screening. *Crit. Rev. Clin. Lab. Sci.* **2017**, *54*, 102–116. [CrossRef] [PubMed]
2. Korevaar, T.I.M.; Medici, M.; Visser, T.J.; Peeters, R.P. Thyroid disease in pregnancy: New insights in diagnosis and clinical management. *Nat. Rev. Endocrinol.* **2017**, *13*, 610–622. [CrossRef] [PubMed]
3. Glinoer, D. What happens to the normal thyroid during pregnancy? *Thyroid* **1999**, *9*, 631–635. [CrossRef] [PubMed]
4. Krassas, G.E.; Poppe, K.; Glinoer, D. Thyroid function and human reproductive health. *Endocr. Rev.* **2010**, *31*, 702–755. [CrossRef] [PubMed]
5. Lee, S.Y.; Pearce, E.N. Assessment and treatment of thyroid disorders in pregnancy and the postpartum period. *Nat. Rev. Endocrinol.* **2022**, *18*, 158–171. [CrossRef] [PubMed]
6. Alexander, E.K.; Pearce, E.N.; Brent, G.A.; Brown, R.S.; Chen, H.; Dosiou, C.; Grobman, W.A.; Laurberg, P.; Lazarus, J.H.; Mandel, S.J.; et al. 2017 Guidelines of the American Thyroid Association for the Diagnosis and Management of Thyroid Disease During Pregnancy and the Postpartum. *Thyroid* **2017**, *27*, 315–389. [CrossRef]
7. Shirvani, S.S.; Nouri, M.; Sakhinia, E.; Babaloo, Z.; Mohammadzaeh, A.; Alipour, S.; Jadideslam, G.; Khabbazi, A. The molecular and clinical evidence of Vitamin D signaling as a modulator of the immune system: Role in Behcet's disease. *Immunol. Lett.* **2019**, *210*, 10–19. [CrossRef]
8. Brown, A.J.; Dusso, A.; Slatopolsky, E. Vitamin D. *Am. J. Physiol.* **1999**, *277*, F157–F175. [CrossRef]
9. Kim, D. The Role of Vitamin D in Thyroid Diseases. *Int. J. Mol. Sci.* **2017**, *18*, 1949. [CrossRef]
10. Muscogiuri, G.; Tirabassi, G.; Bizzaro, G.; Orio, F.; Paschou, S.A.; Vryonidou, A.; Balercia, G.; Shoenfeld, Y.; Colao, A. Vitamin D and thyroid disease: To D or not to D? *Eur. J. Clin. Nutr.* **2015**, *69*, 291–296. [CrossRef]
11. Taheriniya, S.; Arab, A.; Hadi, A.; Fadel, A.; Askari, G. Vitamin d and thyroid disorders: A systematic review and meta-analysis of observational studies. *BMC Endocr. Disord.* **2021**, *21*, 171. [CrossRef] [PubMed]
12. Ning, Z.; Song, S.; Miao, L.; Zhang, P.; Wang, X.; Liu, J.; Hu, Y.; Xu, Y.; Zhao, T.; Liang, Y.; et al. High prevalence of Vitamin D deficiency in urban health checkup population. *Clin. Nutr.* **2016**, *35*, 859–863. [CrossRef] [PubMed]
13. Jiang, W.; Wu, D.B.; Xiao, G.B.; Ding, B.; Chen, E.Q. An epidemiology survey of Vitamin D deficiency and its influencing factors. *Med. Clin.* **2020**, *154*, 7–12. [CrossRef] [PubMed]
14. Yang, C.; Jing, W.; Ge, S.; Sun, W. Vitamin D status and Vitamin D deficiency risk factors among pregnancy of Shanghai in China. *BMC Pregnancy Childbirth* **2021**, *21*, 431. [CrossRef]
15. Ahi, S.; Adelpour, M.; Fereydooni, I.; Hatami, N. Correlation between Maternal Vitamin D and Thyroid Function in Pregnancy with Maternal and Neonatal Outcomes: A Cross-Sectional Study. *Int. J. Endocrinol.* **2022**, *2022*, 6295775. [CrossRef]
16. Musa, I.R.; Rayis, D.A.; Ahmed, M.A.; Khamis, A.H.; Nasr, A.M.; Adam, I. Thyroid Function and 25 (OH) Vitamin D Level among Sudanese Women in Early Pregnancy. *Open Access Maced. J. Med. Sci.* **2018**, *6*, 488–492. [CrossRef]
17. Pan, Y.; Zhong, S.; Liu, Q.; Wang, C.B.; Zhu, W.H.; Shen, X.A.; Lu, B.; Shen, L.W.; Zeng, Y. Investigating the relationship between 25-hydroxyVitamin D and thyroid function in second-trimester pregnant women. *Gynecol. Endocrinol.* **2018**, *34*, 345–348. [CrossRef]
18. Zhao, Y.; Miao, W.; Li, C.; Yu, X.; Shan, Z.; Guan, H.; Teng, W. Dynamic changes in serum 25-hydroxyVitamin D during pregnancy and lack of effect on thyroid parameters. *PLoS ONE* **2014**, *9*, e90161. [CrossRef]
19. Liu, Z.; Meng, T.; Liu, J.; Xu, X.; Luo, S.; Jin, C.; Han, N.; Wang, H.J. The individual and joint effects of maternal 25(OH)D deficiency and gestational diabetes on infant birth size. *Nutr. Metab. Cardiovasc. Dis.* **2020**, *30*, 2398–2405. [CrossRef]
20. National Health and Family Planning Commission of People's Replulic of China. *Criteria of Weight for Adults*; Standards Press of China: Beijing, China, 2013.
21. Fogacci, S.; Fogacci, F.; Banach, M.; Michos, E.D.; Hernandez, A.V.; Lip, G.Y.H.; Blaha, M.J.; Toth, P.P.; Borghi, C.; Cicero, A.F.G.; et al. Vitamin D supplementation and incident preeclampsia: A systematic review and meta-analysis of randomized clinical trials. *Clin. Nutr.* **2020**, *39*, 1742–1752. [CrossRef]

22. Burris, H.H.; Rifas-Shiman, S.L.; Kleinman, K.; Litonjua, A.A.; Huh, S.Y.; Rich-Edwards, J.W.; Camargo, C.A., Jr.; Gillman, M.W. Vitamin D deficiency in pregnancy and gestational diabetes mellitus. *Am. J. Obstet Gynecol.* **2012**, *207*, 182.e1–182.e8. [CrossRef] [PubMed]
23. Zhao, R.; Zhang, W.; Ma, C.; Zhao, Y.; Xiong, R.; Wang, H.; Chen, W.; Zheng, S.G. Immunomodulatory Function of Vitamin D and Its Role in Autoimmune Thyroid Disease. *Front. Immunol.* **2021**, *12*, 574967. [CrossRef] [PubMed]
24. Wang, J.; Gong, X.H.; Peng, T.; Wu, J.N. Association of Thyroid Function During Pregnancy With the Risk of Pre-eclampsia and Gestational Diabetes Mellitus. *Endocr. Pract.* **2021**, *27*, 819–825. [CrossRef]
25. Kiely, M.E.; Wagner, C.L.; Roth, D.E. Vitamin D in pregnancy: Where we are and where we should go. *J. Steroid Biochem. Mol. Biol.* **2020**, *201*, 105669. [CrossRef] [PubMed]
26. Hu, Y.; Wang, R.; Mao, D.; Chen, J.; Li, M.; Li, W.; Yang, Y.; Zhao, L.; Zhang, J.; Piao, J.; et al. Vitamin D Nutritional Status of Chinese Pregnant Women, Comparing the Chinese National Nutrition Surveillance (CNHS) 2015–2017 with CNHS 2010–2012. *Nutrients* **2021**, *13*, 2237. [CrossRef]
27. Wang, X.; Jiao, X.; Tian, Y.; Zhang, J.; Zhang, Y.; Li, J.; Yang, F.; Xu, M.; Yu, X.; for the Shanghai Birth Cohort Study. Associations between maternal Vitamin D status during three trimesters and cord blood 25(OH)D concentrations in newborns: A prospective Shanghai birth cohort study. *Eur. J. Nutr.* **2021**, *60*, 3473–3483. [CrossRef]
28. Marwaha, R.K.; Tandon, N.; Chopra, S.; Agarwal, N.; Garg, M.K.; Sharma, B.; Kanwar, R.S.; Bhadra, K.; Singh, S.; Mani, K.; et al. Vitamin D status in pregnant Indian women across trimesters and different seasons and its correlation with neonatal serum 25-hydroxyVitamin D levels. *Br. J. Nutr.* **2011**, *106*, 1383–1389. [CrossRef]
29. Glinoer, D. The regulation of thyroid function in pregnancy: Pathways of endocrine adaptation from physiology to pathology. *Endocr. Rev.* **1997**, *18*, 404–433. [CrossRef]
30. Negro, R. *Significance and Management of Low TSH in Pregnancy*; Georg Thieme Verlag: New York, NY, USA, 2009; pp. 84–95.
31. Weeke, J.; Dybkjaer, L.; Granlie, K.; Eskjaer Jensen, S.; Kjaerulff, E.; Laurberg, P.; Magnusson, B. A longitudinal study of serum TSH, and total and free iodothyronines during normal pregnancy. *Acta Endocrinol.* **1982**, *101*, 531–537. [CrossRef]
32. Berghout, A.; Wiersinga, W. Thyroid size and thyroid function during pregnancy: An analysis. *Eur. J. Endocrinol.* **1998**, *138*, 536–542. [CrossRef]
33. Nizar, A.M.; Battikhi, Z.W.; Battikhi, B.E. Correlation of Serum 25-HydroxyVitamin D and Thyroid Hormones in Pregnant Women in Amman-Jordan. *J. Microbiol. Exp.* **2017**, *4*, 00099. [CrossRef]
34. Prietl, B.; Treiber, G.; Pieber, T.R.; Amrein, K. Vitamin D and immune function. *Nutrients* **2013**, *5*, 2502–2521. [CrossRef] [PubMed]
35. Chen, W.; Lin, H.; Wang, M. Immune intervention effects on the induction of experimental autoimmune thyroiditis. *J. Huazhong Univ. Sci. Technol. Med. Sci.* **2002**, *22*, 343–345, 354. [CrossRef] [PubMed]
36. Fournier, C.; Gepner, P.; Sadouk, M.; Charreire, J. In vivo beneficial effects of cyclosporin A and 1,25-dihydroxyVitamin D3 on the induction of experimental autoimmune thyroiditis. *Clin. Immunol. Immunopathol.* **1990**, *54*, 53–63. [CrossRef]
37. Misharin, A.; Hewison, M.; Chen, C.R.; Lagishetty, V.; Aliesky, H.A.; Mizutori, Y.; Rapoport, B.; McLachlan, S.M. Vitamin D deficiency modulates Graves' hyperthyroidism induced in BALB/c mice by thyrotropin receptor immunization. *Endocrinology* **2009**, *150*, 1051–1060. [CrossRef]
38. Sar, M.; Stumpf, W.E.; DeLuca, H.F. Thyrotropes in the pituitary are target cells for 1,25 dihydroxy Vitamin D3. *Cell Tissue Res.* **1980**, *209*, 161–166. [CrossRef]
39. Kano, K.; Jones, G. Direct in vitro effect of thyroid hormones on 25-hydroxyVitamin D3 metabolism in the perfused rat kidney. *Endocrinology* **1984**, *114*, 330–336. [CrossRef]

Maternal Passive Smoking, Vitamin D Deficiency and Risk of Spontaneous Abortion

Shiqi Lin [1], Jiajia Li [1], Yuan Zhang [2], Xinming Song [1], Gong Chen [1] and Lijun Pei [1,*]

[1] Institute of Population Research and China Center on Population Health and Development, Peking University, Beijing 100871, China
[2] National Research Institute for Health and Family Planning, Beijing 100081, China
* Correspondence: peilj@pku.edu.cn

Abstract: Background: Maternal passive smoking and vitamin D deficiency might elevate risk of spontaneous abortion. The study aimed to investigate the association of co-exposure to passive smoking and vitamin D deficiency with the risk of spontaneous abortion. Methods: A population-based case-control study was performed among non-smoking women in Henan Province, China, with 293 spontaneous abortion cases and 496 liveborn controls with term, normal birthweight. Results: Compared to women without exposure to passive smoking nor vitamin D deficiency, women with deficient vitamin D alone and women with exposure to passive smoking alone had increased risk of spontaneous abortion (OR = 1.76, 95%CI: 1.08~2.89; OR = 1.73, 95%CI: 1.11~2.69, respectively). The risk of spontaneous abortion was even higher for those with co-exposure to passive smoking and vitamin D deficiency (OR = 2.50, 95%CI: 1.63~3.84). A dose-response relationship was found of an incremental risk of spontaneous abortion with rising numbers of exposures to passive smoking and vitamin D deficiency ($p < 0.001$). Conclusion: Co-exposure to passive smoking and vitamin D deficiency was associated with an elevated risk of spontaneous abortion, and the risk of spontaneous abortion rose with rising numbers of exposures. Intervention programs need to specifically target the vulnerable groups of pregnant women with both malnutrition and unfavorable environmental exposure.

Keywords: passive smoking; vitamin D deficiency; spontaneous abortion; co-exposure

1. Introduction

Spontaneous abortion is often accompanied by early and late maternal complications including blood loss, infection and symptomatic complaints, such as pain and bleeding, together with objective difficulties in conceiving [1]. It is also often a sentinel predictor of several adverse outcomes in subsequent pregnancies such as neural defects, recurrent spontaneous abortion or perinatal mortality [2,3]. In China, it is reported that the incidence of spontaneous abortion is around 10~14% [4,5]. Besides genetic and demographic factors, spontaneous abortion can also be attributed to acquired and environmental factors, many of which are modifiable [2].

Cigarettes contain hundreds of toxic substances such as nicotine, cotinine, carbon monoxide, volatile organic compounds or polycyclic aromatic hydrocarbons (PAH), lead and cadmium. With high lipid solubility, a number of these substances could rapidly cross the placenta, accumulate and metabolize in the fetus, causing up to twice the concentration of cotinine on the fetal than on the maternal side [6] and threatening the developing fetus [7]. Currently, evidence from human observational studies of the association between spontaneous abortion and active smoking is more conclusive, yet studies concerning passive smoking are fewer, results are inconsistent, and most were performed in Western countries [8]. In China, the prevalence of passive smoking for non-smoking women was considerable, reaching around 40% in the workplace, 51% in the home and even 76%

in restaurants [9,10]. Women in rural areas or those who are less educated tend to be more easily exposed to passive smoking [11–13]. A large population-based retrospective cohort study in China indicated that women exposed to their husbands' smoking during preconception had an 11% (95% CI: 1.08~1.14) increased risk of spontaneous abortion compared with those without such exposure [14]. Another case-control study also found a rising risk of unexplained recurrent spontaneous abortion among women self-reported to be exposed to passive smoking compared to the non-exposed group [15]. However, more evidence is needed concerning the potential effects and mechanisms of passive smoking on the risk of spontaneous abortion in the Chinese population.

Among pregnant women in China, vitamin D deficiency is prevalent, with an insufficiency prevalence rate of 45% and a deficiency rate of 42% [16]. Circulating vitamin D appears even lower in smokers [17], probably because of tobacco's role in disrupting the vitamin D endocrine system [18] and causing low intake of vitamin D through changing dietary taste. Moreover, maternal vitamin D deficiency might endanger the maintenance of pregnancy and, thus, lead to spontaneous abortion, a conjecture that has been supported by some epidemiological studies [19,20]. Hence, it is likely that co-exposure to passive smoking and vitamin D deficiency corresponds to a higher risk of spontaneous abortion than a single exposure. However, past literature has scarcely probed into this topic. Therefore, based on data from rural Henan Province, China, the present study aimed to explore the relationship among passive smoking, vitamin D deficiency and risk of spontaneous abortion.

2. Materials and Methods

2.1. Study Design and Data Collection

A population-based case-control study was derived from the Birth Defects Monitoring and Comprehensive Intervention Project in Henan Province, China from December 2009 to January 2010. As the fifth most populous province [21], Henan is in central China with latitude/longitude of 31°23′ N–36°22′ N/110°21′ E–116°39′ E. Detailed study design has already been described elsewhere [20,22]. In brief, in order to obtain a representative sample of women of child-bearing age, we conducted a multi-stage cluster sampling of women between 18 and 40 years old with permanent local registered residency. A total of 1151 participants had their serum blood collected, among whom 293 had a spontaneous abortion within one year and 498 had term ($\geq$37 gestational weeks) normal birthweight ($\geq$2500 g and <4000 g) liveborn babies without birth defects during the same period [20]. As our study focused on the effects of passive smoking, we excluded women with active smoking (n = 2). Finally, there were 789 participants included in our study, with 293 spontaneous abortion cases and 496 controls.

After recruitment, participants were interviewed face-to-face by trained healthcare workers about their basic socio-demographic information, as well as their behavioral and dietary habits during pregnancy. During the interview, 8 mL of women's fasting venous blood was also collected, prepared by centrifugation and then stored at -80 °C at Peking University until analysis.

The study protocol was reviewed and approved by the Institutional Review Board of Peking University Health Science Center. All subjects gave written informed consent before completing the questionnaire and collection of blood samples.

2.2. Spontaneous Abortion Cases and Controls

Spontaneous abortion cases in our study were defined as clinically recognized pregnancy loss before 28 gestational weeks. Controls were women delivering liveborn babies with neither birth defects nor preterm birth (<37 gestational weeks), low birthweight (<2500 g) or high birthweight ($\geq$4000 g).

2.3. Maternal Passive Smoking and Vitamin D Deficiency

Maternal passive smoking was defined according to the survey question, "Did you passively inhale cigarette smoke by smokers around you for an average of more than 15 min per day during pregnancy?". Vitamin D was measured quantitatively based on the level of serum 25-hydroxyvitamin D (25(OH)D) concentration in serum samples, which were analyzed using the high-performance liquid chromatography-tandem mass spectrometry (HPLC-MS/MS, Ultimate3000–API 3200 Q TRAP) method. Here we defined vitamin D deficiency as 25(OH)D < 20 ng/mL and sufficiency as $\geq$20 ng/mL as suggested by previous literature [23].

2.4. Covariates

Women's basic characteristics, including age, history of chronic diseases, education, occupation, and diet and behavioral factors, were considered as potential covariates in the analysis. An extreme BMI could have a negative role in reproductive outcomes as well as vitamin D status [2,24] and, thus, was also evaluated as a potential covariate. BMI was calculated as weight divided by the square of height. We used 24 kg/m^2 and 28 kg/m^2 as cut-off points for the "normal weight or underweight", "overweight" and "obesity" groups given the specific body characteristics of Chinese population [25]. Diet referred to vitamin D supplementation (supplementation of vitamin D, cod-liver oil or any multivitamins containing vitamin D), nutritional supplementation (any supplementation of vitamin A, multivitamin B, vitamin B1, vitamin B2, vitamin B6, vitamin B12, vitamin C, vitamin E, cod-liver oil or vitamin D, iron preparations, calcium tablets or zinc), and average frequencies of intake of food that contained relatively high vitamin D, namely, meat, aquatic products, eggs, and milk or dairy products. Behavioral habits were alcohol consumption (drinking alcoholic beverages more than once a month) and physical exercises (referring to any indoor or outdoor health-promoting physical exercises more than once a week for more than 30 min per time). As serum 25(OH)D levels might be influenced by sunlight exposure, the sampling time was also considered.

2.5. Statistical Analysis

Univariate analysis with χ^2 test (or Fisher's exact test when appropriate) was performed to test the differences of socio-demographic characteristics, dietary and behavioral factors as well as sampling time between spontaneous abortion cases and controls and between those with vitamin D deficiency and sufficiency. Significant variables ($p < 0.05$) were then included in later multivariate models.

We conducted a multivariate logistic regression model to investigate the association of passive smoking and vitamin D deficiency with risk of spontaneous abortion. To explore the single and combined effects of maternal passive smoking and vitamin D deficiency, we first divided participants into four groups: (1) women without passive smoking nor vitamin D deficiency; (2) those without passive smoking but with vitamin D deficiency; (3) those without vitamin D deficiency but with passive smoking and (4) those with passive smoking and vitamin D deficiency. The four groups represented a rising degree of the two exposures. Multivariate models were then performed by comparing the latter three groups with the first group to evaluate risk of spontaneous abortion across different combinations of the two risk factors. A trend test was then conducted to determine whether the risk increased with rising degree of exposure combinations. We also conducted an interaction test [26] to determine whether there was an interaction effect between the two factors.

3. Results

The basic characteristics, behavioral and dietary habits and vitamin D status of spontaneous abortion cases and controls were displayed in Table 1. Our study mainly included women $\geq$ 28 years old (62%), achieving junior high school or lower educational attainment (76%) and being a housewife or farmer (81%). Alcoholic consumption was rare among participants, with only 13 (1.7%) reporting drinking over once per month. While passive smoking was prevalent, with over 60% participants demonstrating that they were exposed to smoking air for an average of over 15 min per day. The serum samples were collected after pregnancy outcomes and all in winter (Jan and Dec). Vitamin D deficiency was common, accounting for 49% of all participants. Significant differences were observed between spontaneous abortion cases and controls with regard to BMI, history of chronic diseases, meat intake, milk intake, passive smoking and vitamin D deficiency ($p < 0.05$).

Table 1. Differences in basic characteristics between spontaneous abortion cases and controls.

Variables	Cases (n = 293) n (%)	Controls (n = 496) n (%)	p
Basic characteristics			
Age (years)			0.75
<28	110 (37.5)	192 (38.7)	
≥28	183 (62.5)	304 (61.3)	
Education			0.15
High school or above	61 (20.8)	125 (25.3)	
Junior high or below	232 (79.2)	369 (74.7)	
Occupation			0.74
Unemployed or famers	55 (18.8)	98 (19.8)	
Others	238 (81.2)	398 (80.2)	
Household annual income (RMB [1])			0.34
≥10,000	172 (58.7)	307 (62.2)	
<10,000	121 (41.3)	187 (37.8)	
BMI (kg/m^2)			0.03
<24	170 (58.0)	324 (65.3)	
24–28	79 (27.0)	126 (25.4)	
>28	44 (15.0)	46 (9.3)	
History of chronic diseases			0.002
No	243 (82.9)	449 (90.5)	
Yes	50 (17.1)	47 (9.5)	
Dietary habits			
Nutritional supplement			0.36
No	216 (73.7)	380 (76.6)	
Yes	77 (26.3)	116 (23.4)	
Vitamin D supplement [2]			0.25
No	261 (89.1)	454 (91.5)	
Yes	32 (10.9)	42 (8.5)	
Meat intake			0.02
≥once per week	144 (49.1)	285 (57.6)	
<once per week	149 (50.9)	210 (42.4)	
Aquatic product intake			0.09
≥once per month	51 (17.4)	111 (22.4)	
<once per month	242 (82.6)	384 (77.6)	
Eggs intake			0.15
Everyday	92 (31.4)	157 (31.7)	
4–6 times per week	60 (20.5)	129 (26.1)	
≤3 times per week	141 (48.1)	209 (42.2)	
Milk or dairy products intake			0.006
≥4 times per week	49 (16.7)	100 (20.2)	
<4 times per week but at least once per month	70 (23.9)	159 (32.1)	
Almost never	174 (59.4)	236 (47.7)	
Behavioral factors			

Table 1. *Cont.*

Variables	Cases (n = 293) n (%)	Controls (n = 496) n (%)	p
Alcohol consumption			0.92
No	288 (98.3)	488 (98.4)	
Yes	5 (1.7)	8 (1.6)	
Physical exercise			0.93
No	251 (85.7)	422 (85.4)	
Yes	42 (14.3)	72 (14.6)	
Passive smoking			0.004
No	97 (33.1)	215 (43.4)	
Yes	196 (66.9)	281 (56.6)	
Vitamin D status			0.003
Sufficient	129 (44.0)	273 (55.0)	
Deficient	163 (56.0)	223 (45.0)	
Sampling time			0.34
January 2010	42 (14.3)	84 (16.9)	
December 2009	251 (85.7)	412 (83.1)	

[1] RMB: the Chinese official currency; [2] sufficient: 25(OH)D ≥ 20 ng/mL, deficient: 25(OH)D < 20 ng/mL.

Supplemental Table S1 displays the differences in basic characteristics between different vitamin D statuses. Table 2 describes the results of multivariate analysis for the association of passive smoking and vitamin D deficiency with risk of spontaneous abortion. The multivariate logistic regression analysis showed that women exposed to passive smoking were associated with a 57% (95%CI: 1.15~2.14) higher risk of spontaneous abortion compared to unexposed women; women with vitamin D deficiency were also associated with a higher risk of spontaneous abortion (OR = 1.56, 95%CI: 1.15~2.10).

Table 2. Analysis of association of passive smoking and vitamin D deficiency with risk of spontaneous abortion.

Exposure	cOR(95%CI)	aOR(95%CI) [1]
Passive smoking	1.55(1.14~2.09)	1.57(1.15~2.14)
Vitamin D deficiency [2]	1.56(1.16~2.08)	1.56(1.15~2.10)

[1] Adjusted for BMI, milk or diary product intake, meat intake and history of chronic diseases; [2] vitamin D deficiency: 25(OH)D < 20 ng/mL.

Table 3 showed the different risk of spontaneous abortion across different exposure combinations of passive smoking and vitamin D status. Compared to women without passive smoking nor vitamin D deficiency, a 1.73 (95%CI: 1.11~2.69) times higher risk of spontaneous abortion was observed among those without vitamin D deficiency but with passive smoking, and 1.76 (95%CI: 1.08~2.89) times higher risk for those without passive smoking but with vitamin D deficiency, after adjusting for BMI, history of chronic diseases, meat intake and milk intake. The risk of spontaneous abortion was even higher, accounting for 2.50 (95%CI: 1.63~3.84) times for those with both passive smoking and vitamin D deficiency. There was no statistical interactive effect observed ($p = 0.82$). A significant χ^2_{trend} ($p < 0.001$) indicated a dose-response relationship of an increased risk of spontaneous abortion with rising degree of combined exposure to passive smoking and vitamin D deficiency.

Table 3. Risk of spontaneous abortion across different combination groups of passive smoking and vitamin D status.

Passive smoking	Vitamin D Deficiency [1]	Cases (n = 293)	Controls (n = 497)	aOR (95%CI) [2]	p
No	No	130	46	1.00	
Yes	No	143	83	1.73(1.11~2.69)	<0.05
No	Yes	85	51	1.76(1.08~2.89)	<0.05
Yes	Yes	140	113	2.50(1.63~3.84)	<0.001
χ^2_{trend}					<0.001
Interaction					0.82

[1] Vitamin D deficiency: 25(OH)D < 20 ng/mL; [2] adjusted for BMI, milk or diary product intake, meat intake and history of chronic diseases.

4. Discussion

4.1. Main Findings

With a population-based case-control study performed in rural Henan Province, China, we explored the association between maternal passive smoking, vitamin D status and risk of spontaneous abortion. The findings indicated a dose-response relationship of incremental risk of spontaneous abortion with rising degree of combined exposure to passive smoking and vitamin D deficiency. Our study provided clues of the combined effects of passive smoking and nutritional deficiency on the risk of adverse pregnancy outcomes in a Chinese population of reproductive age.

Our study found that there was an association between maternal exposure to passive smoking and an elevated risk of spontaneous abortion. This result was consistent with another case-control study in China that showed a rising risk of unexplained recurrent spontaneous abortion for passive smokers [15]. A case-control study in Sweden also indicated a higher probability of having a history of spontaneous abortion in women with exposure to passive smoking (defined as plasma cotinine concentrations from 0.1 to 15.0 ng/mL) [27]. Potential mechanisms could be the hazardous substance in tobacco smoke accumulating in women's bodies and crossing the placenta to induce maternal complications and placental pathology [28] affecting the fetal development [7] and, thus, predicting spontaneous abortion [29]. Previous research on the relationship between smoking and spontaneous abortion focuses mainly on active smokers [8]. However, albeit active smoking is relatively rare in pregnant women, passive smoking is still severe in China [9]. Provided that non-smokers with passive smoking generally inhale much smaller amounts of tobacco smoke particles and nicotine than an active smoker [30], our results that passive smoking was associated with a 57% increased risk of spontaneous abortion echoes the warning from the WHO that there is no safe level of tobacco smoke exposure [31]. What is more, nonsmokers with passive smoking are influenced by not only mainstream but also sidestream smoke, which contains different quantities of toxic substances from the former. In other words, passive and active smoking might act differently on maternal and fetal health. As it is well-recognized that the origins of spontaneous abortion are multifactorial and it is hard to observe the whole process and find mechanisms, epidemiological studies are important to provide clues, especially for environmental risk factors. Our study, thus, adds evidence from the Chinese population for avoiding maternal exposure to passive smoking during pregnancy to reduce risk of adverse pregnancy outcomes, including spontaneous abortion.

Furthermore, our findings indicated that the risk of spontaneous abortion increased by 137% for those with co-exposure to passive smoking and vitamin D deficiency (OR = 2.37, 95%CI: 1.54~3.67) compared to those with neither exposure. Furthermore, there was a dose-response relationship of increased risk of spontaneous abortion with the incremental numbers of exposures to passive smoking and vitamin D. Our previous research has already found that women with vitamin D deficiency were more likely to have experienced spontaneous abortion [20]. As stated above, passive smoking might also be associated with a higher risk of spontaneous abortion. What is worse, smoking might further lead to vitamin D deficiency [17], probably because smoking brings about disorders of food intake, synthesis, hydroxylation and catabolism of vitamin D [18]. That could explain our finding that a combined exposure of passive smoking and vitamin D deficiency might be related to an even higher risk of spontaneous abortion than single exposure. This co-exposure to malnutrition and unfavorable environment is constantly observed in some socio-economically disadvantaged groups. Explanations have been offered by past researchers that women with low socio-economic status, low educational level or unprofessional jobs are inclined to be exposed to passive smoking and vitamin D deficiency [11–13,22,32]. Our previous study showed that lower maternal socio-economic status (SES) was associated with higher risk of vitamin D deficiency in women of childbearing age in rural northern China [22], and low maternal SES may strengthen the effect of vitamin D deficiency exposure on spontaneous abortion risk [20]. The two studies, along with the present one, thus, call for policy makers and the whole society to offer special attention to periconceptional women in disadvantaged socio-economic groups with overlying exposure to undernutrition and harmful environments.

4.2. Strengths and Limitations

One of the strengths of the present study was that it is a population-based case-control study adopting a representative and relatively large sample, thus increasing the test power. The selection bias was minimized with a multi-stage cluster sampling method. By restricting our subjects to non-smokers, we excluded the potential confounding effects of active smoking. Furthermore, compared to methods using spousal smoking as a surrogate of exposure to passive smoking, our method, which asked women whether they were surrounded by a smoking environment, was more direct because, with the spread of health knowledge today, many smokers would avoid smoking at home, especially with their pregnant wives or children.

The limitations of our study should also be acknowledged. First, we regarded the measurement of vitamin D level after the pregnancy outcomes as an estimate of vitamin D exposure during pregnancy by assuming a stable serum 25(OH)D level. Admittedly, this was a very strong assumption and serum 25(OH)D does change over time when sunlight, temperature, weight status, nutritional supplementation and other factors change. A longitudinal study that tracked serum 25(OH)D levels found a low degree of agreement in two waves with a 14-year interval [33]. However, we measured the serum 25(OH)D about one year after the pregnancy outcomes, a relatively short period during which serum 25(OH)D level usually had a high consistency according to past research [34,35]. Additionally, vitamin D supplementation was not a prevalent practice among young women in China, as can be indicated in our study and others that only a very small proportion of women took vitamin D supplementation (9% in our study and 9% in another one conducted in 2010–2012 [16]). What is more, the effects of vitamin D deficiency are presumably cumulative instead of temporal. Therefore, our way of estimating cumulative vitamin D exposure during pregnancy was reasonable. Second, the passive smoking was self-reported instead of by some biomarkers that proved to be a more precise way of exposure measurement [36]. However, many past researchers have implied that self-reported questions concerning passive smoking status had a high consistency to nicotine in biomarkers and, thus, could be a reliable way to assess passive smoking in adults [37]. Even if the misclassification was brought about by women's self-report, it is most probably a nondifferential one [38]. Third, our study did not collect more detailed information about the sources and duration of passive smoking exposure, while the degree of exposure might be different with regard to various conditions. Future studies can consider collecting more information on exposure such as whether the exposure comes from home or the workplace and on average how many cigarettes are smoked around the women.

5. Conclusions

In summary, through a population-based case-control study in Henan Province, China, our study investigated the individual and combined effects of maternal passive smoking and vitamin D deficiency during pregnancy on risk of spontaneous abortion. It was found that there was an association of maternal exposure to passive smoking and vitamin D deficiency with an elevated risk of spontaneous abortion. Moreover, compared to women without exposure to passive smoking nor vitamin D deficiency, the risk of spontaneous abortion rose when the exposures increased. Our study speaks to the importance of effective education and public health intervention programs specifically targeting vulnerable groups of pregnant women with both malnutrition and unfavorable environmental exposure.

Supplementary Materials: The following supporting information can be downloaded at: https://www.mdpi.com/article/10.3390/nu14183674/s1, Table S1: Differences of basic characteristics between different vitamin D status.

Author Contributions: Conceptualization, L.P.; methodology, J.L..; software, J.L.; formal analysis, S.L..; investigation, J.L. and Y.Z.; resources, L.P., X.S. and G.C.; data curation, Y.Z.; writing—original draft preparation, S.L..; writing—review and editing, L.P.; supervision, L.P. and X.S.; project administration, L.P. and X.S.; funding acquisition, L.P. All authors have read and agreed to the published version of the manuscript.

Funding: This research was funded by National Key Research and Development Program of China (2018YFC1004303) to Lijun Pei; National Natural Science Foundation of China (41871360) to Lijun Pei; Danone Institute China Diet Nutrition Research & Communication Grant (DIC2015-05) to Lijun Pei.

Institutional Review Board Statement: The study protocol was reviewed and approved by Institutional Review Board of Peking University Health Science Center (IRB00001052-08083).

Informed Consent Statement: Informed consent was obtained from all subjects involved in the study.

Data Availability Statement: The data are available from the corresponding author upon reasonable request.

Conflicts of Interest: The funders had no role in the design of the study; in the collection, analyses, or interpretation of data; in the writing of the manuscript or in the decision to publish the results.

References

1. Tsur, A.; Malvasi, A.; Vergari, U.; Carp, H. Spontaneous Abortion Complications. In *Management and Therapy of Early Pregnancy Complications: First and Second Trimesters*; Malvasi, A., Tinelli, A., Di Renzo, G.C., Eds.; Springer International Publishing: Cham, Switzerland, 2016; pp. 29–50. [CrossRef]
2. Quenby, S.; Gallos, I.D.; Dhillon-Smith, R.K.; Podesek, M.; Stephenson, M.D.; Fisher, J.; Brosens, J.J.; Brewin, J.; Ramhorst, R.; Lucas, E.S.; et al. Miscarriage matters: The epidemiological, physical, psychological, and economic costs of early pregnancy loss. *Lancet* **2021**, *397*, 1658–1667. [CrossRef]
3. Pei, L.; Wu, J.; Li, J.; Mi, X.; Zhang, X.; Li, Z.; Zhang, Y. Effect of periconceptional folic acid supplementation on the risk of neural tube defects associated with a previous spontaneous abortion or maternal first-trimester fever. *Hum. Reprod.* **2019**, *34*, 1587–1594. [CrossRef] [PubMed]
4. Zeng, L.X.; Yan, H.; Chen, Z.J. Study on the current status and risk factors of spontaneous abortion of women at reproductive age in rural areas of Xianyang district, Shaanxi province. *Chin. J. Epidemiol.* **2007**, *28*, 19–23.
5. Liang, R.Y.; Ye, R.W.; Li, H.T.; Ren, A.G.; Liu, J.M. Study on the current status of spontaneous abortion of primigravid women in Jiaxing of Zhejiang province, China. *Chin. J. Epidemiol.* **2010**, *31*, 755–758.
6. Sastry, B.V.; Chance, M.B.; Hemontolor, M.E.; Goddijn-Wessel, T.A. Formation and retention of cotinine during placental transfer of nicotine in human placental cotyledon. *Pharmacology* **1998**, *57*, 104–116. [CrossRef]
7. McDonnell, S.L.; Baggerly, K.A.; Baggerly, C.A.; Aliano, J.L.; French, C.B.; Baggerly, L.L.; Ebeling, M.D.; Rittenberg, C.S.; Goodier, C.G.; Mateus Niño, J.F.; et al. Maternal 25(OH)D concentrations ≥40 ng/mL associated with 60% lower preterm birth risk among general obstetrical patients at an urban medical center. *PLoS ONE* **2017**, *12*, e0180483. [CrossRef]
8. Pineles, B.L.; Park, E.; Samet, J.M. Systematic Review and Meta-Analysis of Miscarriage and Maternal Exposure to Tobacco Smoke During Pregnancy. *Am. J. Epidemiol.* **2014**, *179*, 807–823. [CrossRef]
9. Parascandola, M.; Xiao, L. Tobacco and the lung cancer epidemic in China. *Transl. Lung Cancer Res.* **2019**, *8*, S21–S30. [CrossRef]
10. Xiao, L.; Jiang, Y.; Zhang, J.; Parascandola, M. Secondhand Smoke Exposure among Nonsmokers in China. *Asian Pac. J. Cancer Prev.* **2020**, *21*, 17–22. [CrossRef] [PubMed]

1. Gao, C.S.; Yao, Y.; Niu, H.K.; Li, L.; Li, M.Q.; Qu, Y.M.; Wang, R.; Zhang, P.; Li, M.; Yan, S.M.; et al. Urban-rural differences in related factors of second-hand smoke exposure: A cross-sectional study of adult non-smokers in Northeast China. *J. Public Health* **2019**, *41*, 321–328. [CrossRef] [PubMed]
2. Nan, X.; Lu, H.W.; Wu, J.; Xue, M.M.; Guo, W.D.; Wang, X.M. Prevalence, knowledge and education level associated with secondhand smoke exposure among never-smoking women in Inner Mongolia, Northern China. *Tob. Induc. Dis.* **2020**, *18*, 35. [CrossRef] [PubMed]
3. Wei, X.L.; Zhang, Z.Z.; Song, X.L.; Xu, Y.J.; Wu, W.; Lao, X.Q.; Ma, W.J. Household Smoking Restrictions Related to Secondhand Smoke Exposure in Guangdong, China: A Population Representative Survey. *Nicotine Tob. Res.* **2014**, *16*, 390–396. [CrossRef] [PubMed]
4. Wang, L.; Yang, Y.; Liu, F.; Yang, A.; Xu, Q.; Wang, Q.; Shen, H.; Zhang, Y.; Yan, D.; Peng, Z.; et al. Paternal smoking and spontaneous abortion: A population-based retrospective cohort study among non-smoking women aged 20–49 years in rural China. *J. Epidemiol. Community Health* **2018**, *72*, 783. [CrossRef]
5. Zhang, B.Y.; Wei, Y.S.; Niu, J.M.; Li, Y.; Miao, Z.L.; Wang, Z.N. Risk factors for unexplained recurrent spontaneous abortion in a population from southern China. *Int. J. Gynecol. Obstet.* **2010**, *108*, 135–138. [CrossRef]
6. Hu, Y.; Wang, R.; Mao, D.; Chen, J.; Li, M.; Li, W.; Yang, Y.; Zhao, L.; Zhang, J.; Piao, J.; et al. Vitamin D Nutritional Status of Chinese Pregnant Women, Comparing the Chinese National Nutrition Surveillance (CNHS) 2015–2017 with CNHS 2010–2012. *Nutrients* **2021**, *13*, 2237. [CrossRef]
7. Brot, C.; Jorgensen, N.R.; Sorensen, O.H. The influence of smoking on vitamin D status and calcium metabolism. *Eur. J. Clin. Nutr.* **1999**, *53*, 920–926. [CrossRef]
8. Mousavi, S.E.; Amini, H.; Heydarpour, P.; Chermahini, F.A.; Godderis, L. Air pollution, environmental chemicals, and smoking may trigger vitamin D deficiency: Evidence and potential mechanisms. *Environ. Int.* **2019**, *122*, 67–90. [CrossRef]
9. Andersen, L.B.; Jørgensen, J.S.; Jensen, T.K.; Dalgård, C.; Barington, T.; Nielsen, J.; Beck-Nielsen, S.S.; Husby, S.; Abrahamsen, B.; Lamont, R.F.; et al. Vitamin D insufficiency is associated with increased risk of first-trimester miscarriage in the Odense Child Cohort. *Am. J. Clin. Nutr.* **2015**, *102*, 633–638. [CrossRef] [PubMed]
10. Lin, S.; Zhang, Y.; Jiang, L.; Li, J.; Chai, J.; Pei, L.; Shang, X. Interactive Effects of Maternal Vitamin D Status and Socio-Economic Status on the Risk of Spontaneous Abortion: Evidence from Henan Province, China. *Nutrients* **2022**, *14*, 291. [CrossRef]
11. National Bureau of Statistics of China. National Data: Annual Population by Region. Available online: https://data.stats.gov.cn/english/easyquery.htm?cn=E0103 (accessed on 6 March 2022).
12. Lin, S.; Jiang, L.; Zhang, Y.; Chai, J.; Li, J.; Song, X.; Pei, L. Socioeconomic status and vitamin D deficiency among women of childbearing age: A population-based, case-control study in rural northern China. *BMJ Open* **2021**, *11*, e042227. [CrossRef]
13. Holick, M.F.; Binkley, N.C.; Bischoff-Ferrari, H.A.; Gordon, C.M.; Hanley, D.A.; Heaney, R.P.; Murad, M.H.; Weaver, C.M. Evaluation, treatment, and prevention of vitamin D deficiency: An Endocrine Society clinical practice guideline. *J. Clin. Endocrinol. Metab.* **2011**, *96*, 1911–1930. [CrossRef]
14. Di Filippo, L.; De Lorenzo, R.; Giustina, A.; Rovere-Querini, P.; Conte, C. Vitamin D in Osteosarcopenic Obesity. *Nutrients* **2022**, *14*, 1816. [CrossRef] [PubMed]
15. Qin, Y.; Melse-Boonstra, A.; Pan, X.; Yuan, B.; Dai, Y.; Zhao, J.; Zimmermann, M.B.; Kok, F.J.; Zhou, M.; Shi, Z. Anemia in relation to body mass index and waist circumference among Chinese women. *Nutr. J.* **2013**, *12*, 10. [CrossRef] [PubMed]
16. Greenland, S. Tests for interaction in epidemiologic studies: A review and a study of power. *Stat. Med.* **1983**, *2*, 243–251. [CrossRef] [PubMed]
17. George, L.; Granath, F.; Johansson, A.L.; Annerén, G.; Cnattingius, S. Environmental tobacco smoke and risk of spontaneous abortion. *Epidemiology* **2006**, *17*, 500–505. [CrossRef]
18. Dušková, M.; Hruškovičová, H.; Šimůnková, K.; Stárka, L.; Pařízek, A. The effects of smoking on steroid metabolism and fetal programming. *J. Steroid Biochem. Mol. Biol.* **2014**, *139*, 138–143. [CrossRef]
19. Odendaal, H.J. Strong Association Between Placental Pathology and Second-trimester Miscarriage. *Arch. Obstet. Gynaecol.* **2021**, *2*, 51–56.
20. Remmer, H. Passively inhaled tobacco smoke: A challenge to toxicology and preventive medicine. *Arch. Toxicol.* **1987**, *61*, 89–104. [CrossRef]
21. WHO. Tobacco. Available online: https://www.who.int/news-room/fact-sheets/detail/tobacco (accessed on 6 May 2022).
22. Gan, W.Q.; Mannino, D.M.; Jemal, A. Socioeconomic disparities in secondhand smoke exposure among US never-smoking adults: The National Health and Nutrition Examination Survey 1988–2010. *Tob. Control* **2015**, *24*, 568–573. [CrossRef]
23. Kubiak, J.; Kamycheva, E.; Jorde, R. Tracking of serum 25-hydroxyvitamin D during 21 years. *Eur. J. Clin. Nutr.* **2021**, *75*, 1069–1076. [CrossRef]
24. Saliba, W.; Barnett, O.; Stein, N.; Kershenbaum, A.; Rennert, G. The longitudinal variability of serum 25(OH)D levels. *Eur. J. Intern. Med.* **2012**, *23*, e106–e111. [CrossRef] [PubMed]
25. Jorde, R.; Sneve, M.; Hutchinson, M.; Emaus, N.; Figenschau, Y.; Grimnes, G. Tracking of serum 25-hydroxyvitamin D levels during 14 years in a population-based study and during 12 months in an intervention study. *Am. J. Epidemiol.* **2010**, *171*, 903–908. [CrossRef] [PubMed]
26. Benowitz, N.L. Biomarkers of environmental tobacco smoke exposure. *Environ. Health Perspect.* **1999**, *107*, 349–355. [CrossRef] [PubMed]

37. Avila-Tang, E.; Elf, J.L.; Cummings, K.M.; Fong, G.T.; Hovell, M.F.; Klein, J.D.; McMillen, R.; Winickoff, J.P.; Samet, J.M. Assessing secondhand smoke exposure with reported measures. *Tob. Control* **2013**, *22*, 156. [CrossRef] [PubMed]
38. Ahlborg, G., Jr.; Bodin, L. Tobacco Smoke Exposure and Pregnancy Outcome among Working Women: A Prospective Study at Prenatal Care Centers in Örebro County, Sweden. *Am. J. Epidemiol.* **1991**, *133*, 338–347. [CrossRef] [PubMed]

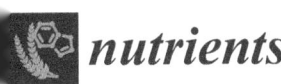

Article

The Associations of Maternal Hemoglobin Concentration in Different Time Points and Its Changes during Pregnancy with Birth Weight Outcomes

Zhicheng Peng [1,2], Shuting Si [1,2], Haoyue Cheng [1,2], Haibo Zhou [1,2], Peihan Chi [1,2], Minjia Mo [1,2], Yan Zhuang [1,2], Hui Liu [3] and Yunxian Yu [1,2,*]

1. Department of Public Health, and Department of Anesthesiology, Second Affiliated Hospital of Zhejiang University School of Medicine, Hangzhou 310058, China; 22018678@zju.edu.cn (Z.P.); 21818499@zju.edu.cn (S.S.); 3150101365@zju.edu.cn (H.C.); 11918158@zju.edu.cn (H.Z.); 22118872@zju.edu.cn (P.C.); minjiamo@zju.edu.cn (M.M.); yanzhuang@zju.edu.cn (Y.Z.)
2. Department of Epidemiology & Health Statistics, School of Public Health, School of Medicine, Zhejiang University, Hangzhou 310058, China
3. Sir Run Run Shaw Hospital, School of Medicine, Zhejiang University, Hangzhou 310058, China; lhui2010@zju.edu.cn
* Correspondence: yunxianyu@zju.edu.cn

Abstract: Maternal hemoglobin (Hb) is related to nutritional status, which affects neonatal birth weight. However, it is very common for maternal Hb to fluctuate during pregnancy. To evaluate the associations of maternal Hb in different time points and its changes during pregnancy with neonatal birth weight, small for gestational age (SGA)/low birth weight (LBW) and large for gestational age (LGA)/macrosomia, we conducted this study by using data from the Electronic Medical Record System (EMRS) database of Zhoushan Maternal and Child Care Hospital in Zhejiang province, China. The pregnancy was divided into five periods: first, early-second, mediate-second, late-second, early-third and late-third trimesters; we further calculated the maternal Hb changes during pregnancy. Overall, the socio-demographic characteristics, health-related information and childbirth-related information of 24,183 mother–infant pairs were obtained. The average Hb concentration during the different periods were 123.95 ± 10.14, 117.95 ± 9.84, 114.31 ± 9.03, 113.26 ± 8.82, 113.29 ± 8.68 and 115.01 ± 8.85 g/L, respectively. Significant dose–response relationships between maternal Hb and birth weight were observed in the first, late-second and later trimesters (p non-linear < 0.05). Maternal Hb < 100 g/L was related to a high risk of LGA/macrosomia in the late-second (OR: 1.47, 95% CI: 1.18, 1.83) and later trimesters; additionally, high maternal Hb (>140 g/L) increased the risk of SGA/LBW in the first (OR: 1.26, 95% CI: 1.01, 1.57) and late-third trimesters (OR: 1.96, 95% CI: 1.20, 3.18). In addition, the increase in maternal Hb from the late-second to late-third trimesters had a positive correlation with SGA/LBW. In conclusion, maternal Hb markedly fluctuated during pregnancy; the negative dose–response association of maternal Hb in the late-second and third trimesters, and Hb change during pregnancy with neonatal birth weight outcomes were observed, respectively. Furthermore, the phenomenon of high Hb in the first trimester and after the late-second trimester and the increase of maternal Hb from the late-second to late-third trimesters more significantly increasing the risk of SGA/LBW should especially be given more attention. Its biological mechanism needs to be further explored.

Keywords: maternal hemoglobin; neonatal; birth weight; SGA/LBW; LGA/macrosomia; pregnancy

Citation: Peng, Z.; Si, S.; Cheng, H.; Zhou, H.; Chi, P.; Mo, M.; Zhuang, Y.; Liu, H.; Yu, Y. The Associations of Maternal Hemoglobin Concentration in Different Time Points and Its Changes during Pregnancy with Birth Weight Outcomes. *Nutrients* 2022, 14, 2542. https://doi.org/10.3390/nu14122542

Academic Editor: Tim Green

Received: 22 April 2022
Accepted: 15 June 2022
Published: 19 June 2022

Publisher's Note: MDPI stays neutral with regard to jurisdictional claims in published maps and institutional affiliations.

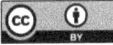

Copyright: © 2022 by the authors. Licensee MDPI, Basel, Switzerland. This article is an open access article distributed under the terms and conditions of the Creative Commons Attribution (CC BY) license (https://creativecommons.org/licenses/by/4.0/).

1. Introduction

Neonatal birth weight has been obtaining wide attention as it is a strong predictor of neonatal and perinatal mortality and disability, as well as birth weight percentiles, are used to predict the risk of growth disorders in newborns [1]. The global prevalence of low birth weight (LBW) was 14.6% in 2015 [2], and it was estimated that approximately 32.4 million infants that were small for gestational age (SGA) were born in low-income and middle-income countries in 2010 [3]. Both LBW and SGA were associated with short-term and long-term adverse outcomes, such as infection, respiratory depression, jaundice, obesity, insulin resistance and type 2 diabetes [1,4,5]. In addition, the prevalence of large for gestational age (LGA) and macrosomia is also increasing, especially in developing countries [6,7]. LGA and macrosomia are also considered factors that can increase the risk of early obesity, metabolic diseases [8], diabetes and early cardiovascular disease [9,10]. Growth restriction and excessive growth were two extremes of fetal development, both of which were associated with neonatal mortality and other adverse outcomes. Therefore, it is essential to identify the early factors that might influence neonatal birth weight and alert the need for an intervention.

Maternal nutritional status during pregnancy is one of the critical influencing factors of neonatal birth weight [11]. Both restricted growth and excessive growth of neonates were derived from altered metabolism in the uterus [12], which was closely related to maternal nutritional status. Hemoglobin (Hb) concentration plays an important role in maternal nutrition, especially the iron condition [13], and it can help to identify the neonatal adverse outcomes and alert the need for intervention measures as early as possible. Generally, hemoglobin testing is contained in routine blood examinations during pregnancy, and it is applied to screen for anemia in clinical practice [14]. However, the relationships of maternal Hb in different time points during pregnancy with fetal growth were controversial.

A retrospective analysis of Chinese pregnant women of Zhuang nationality reported a positive correlation between maternal Hb in the first trimester and birth weight and a negative correlation between Hb in the third trimester and birth weight [15]. Another study measured maternal Hb concentration at least once during pregnancy and found that the lowest maternal Hb during pregnancy might have an inverted U-shaped relationship with neonatal birth weight [16]. Furthermore, the results of meta-analyses suggested that in low-income countries, 25% of low birth weight (LBW) can be attributed to anemia (Hb < 110 g/L) [17]. Some other studies found that maternal Hb < 110 g/L in the first trimester was associated with neonatal adverse outcomes, including LBW, SGA and neonatal mortality [18,19], though no significant associations were observed in the second and third trimesters [19,20]. Nevertheless, another retrospective cohort analysis of 173,031 pregnant women found that anemia in the first and second trimesters was not associated with SGA [21]. In addition, a study found a faint U-shaped relationship between maternal Hb concentration at ≤20 weeks of gestational age and risk of neonatal adverse outcomes (including preterm deliveries, SGA) [22]. However, another study from Northwest China showed a U-shaped relationship between Hb concentration in the third trimester and the risk of SGA/LBW, as well as an inverted U-shaped relationship between maternal Hb and neonatal birth weight [23]. Meanwhile, several studies reported the association between Hb reduction and birth outcomes [24,25]. However, the definition of gestational age for maternal Hb measurements was not precise in all studies, which was considered a confounding factor affecting the association between maternal Hb and birth outcomes [26]. The maternal plasma volume generally expands from 10 weeks of gestational age and then reaches the peak at about 34–36 gestational weeks; after that, it keeps the peak or slowly returns to the level found at 10 weeks of gestational age [27]. Although the volume of red blood cells also increases during pregnancy, the increased plasma volume is larger, and then results in a decline in Hb concentration during pregnancy [25]. In addition, the ability of the placenta to adapt the uterine nutrition, which was thought to maximize fetal growth and viability at birth, also depended on the gestational timing [28,29].

However, whether there was a different effect of Hb measured at the different periods on the birth weight and the association of maternal Hb concentration changes during pregnancy with birth weight outcomes were unclear due to the fluctuation of maternal Hb concentration and change in placental adaptability during pregnancy. The present study defined five time points for maternal Hb measurement and aimed to explore the associations between maternal Hb concentrations in different time points during pregnancy and neonatal birth weight outcomes (including birth weight, SGA/LBW and LGA/macrosomia). Moreover, the effects of maternal Hb concentration changes during pregnancy on birth weight outcomes were also assessed.

2. Materials and Methods

2.1. Data Sources

The data were obtained from a comprehensive Electronic Medical Record System (EMRS) in Zhoushan Maternal and Child Care Hospital, which is a non-private-sector hospital. The EMRS was a municipal system and was established in Zhoushan in 2001 and included a prenatal health dataset and birth registration information dataset. In total, 78,297 pregnant women from January 2001 to May 2018 were recorded in the EMRS. From 2001 to 2009, the EMRS only included the data of the Zhoushan Maternal and Child Care Hospital, and after 2010, it contained the data of all the maternal and children's health care in Zhoushan city. However, the routine blood data, which included maternal Hb levels, was only available in the data from Zhoushan Maternal and Child Care Hospital.

Maternal information about socio-demographic characteristics (e.g., maternal age, educational level, parity, last menstrual period, follow-up date) and health-related characteristics (e.g., maternal weight and height; laboratory parameters, such as Hb and glucose levels; systolic and diastolic blood pressure during pregnancy; liver and kidney disease) were extracted from the prenatal health dataset and birth information (e.g., neonatal gender, birth weight, gestational age at delivery, mode of delivery) of newborns was extracted from the birth registration information dataset. A unique personal identification number was provided to link both datasets. The study protocol was approved by the institutional review board of Zhejiang University School of Medicine.

2.2. Study Population

The pregnant women received their first prenatal check-up before 14 weeks of gestational age. Then, they attended check-ups every four weeks in the first and second trimesters, and then every two weeks before 37 weeks of gestational age according to the guidelines. Pregnant women who met the following criteria were included in the study: (1) maternal age > 18 years old, (2) singleton pregnancy, (3) pregnant women with at least one record of hemoglobin concentration during pregnancy and (4) pregnant women who delivered their baby after 32 weeks of gestational age. The exclusion criteria included (1) women with hypertensive disorders or gestational diabetes mellitus (GDM), (2) maternal BMI in the first trimester of >40 kg/m^2 or <15 kg/m^2 and (3) missing data for maternal Hb during pregnancy or neonatal birth weight.

2.3. Definition of Exposure

The maternal Hb concentration was measured through routine blood tests during pregnancy. Due to fluctuations in the maternal Hb concentration during pregnancy, the gestational period was divided into six time periods to explore the effects of Hb concentration in different time points during pregnancy on the birth outcomes: first (5–13 weeks of gestational age), early-second (14–17 weeks of gestational age), mediate-second (18–22 weeks of gestational age), late-second (23–27 weeks of gestational age), early-third (28–31 weeks of gestational age) and late-third trimesters (from 32 weeks of gestational age to the time of delivery). Meanwhile, the mean Hb concentrations around 100 and 140 g/L were classified into 6 categories using intervals of 10 g/L: <100 g/L, 100~109 g/L, 110~119 g/L, 120~129 g/L, 130~139 g/L and ≥140 g/L. A similar classification was also reported in some other studies [30,31].

The maternal Hb concentration reaches a minimum in the late-second to early-third trimesters and then rises in the late-third trimester [32,33]. When we evaluated the changes in Hb concentration during pregnancy, the Hb concentrations in the late-second trimester and late-third trimester were chosen, which might appropriately reflect the changes in maternal Hb during pregnancy. Therefore, the changes in Hb concentration from the first to late-second trimesters, from the first to late-third trimesters and from the late-second to late-third trimesters were evaluated using Hbfs (Hb in the late-second minus Hb in first), Hbft (Hb in the late-third minus Hb in first) and Hbst (Hb in the late-third minus Hb in late-second). Furthermore, Hbfs, Hbft and Hbst were divided into four categories based on their quartiles.

2.4. Definition of Outcome

The data on birth outcomes were obtained from the birth registration information datasets. SGA and LGA were defined as the top and bottom ten percent of gestational age- and gender-specific birth weights, respectively. LBW and macrosomia were defined as infant birth weight <2500 g and ≥4000 g, respectively [7]. The compound outcomes were defined as the following: the infants with SGA or LBW were grouped as "Lightweight" and those with LGA or macrosomia were grouped as "Heavyweight"; otherwise, they were grouped as "Normalweight". Furthermore, infants with "Lightweight" and "Heavyweight" were grouped as "TotalAdverse".

2.5. Statistical Analysis

Continuous variables are presented as mean ± standard deviation (SD), while categorical parameters are described as number (N) and percentage (%). The characteristics of study participants in the Lightweight, Heavyweight and Normalweight groups were compared using the analysis of variance (ANOVA) for continuous variables and the chi-square test for categorical variables. A restricted cubic spline (RCS) function with 5 knots was applied to analyze the association of maternal Hb concentration in different time points and its changes during pregnancy with neonatal birth weight outcomes [34]. Multinomial logistic regression models were used to analyze the associations of Hb concentration in different time points and Hb changes during pregnancy with neonatal compound outcomes. The maternal Hb concentration at 110~119 g/L was set as the reference group in each time point and the first quartile (Q1) in Hb change was set as the reference group. The odds ratios (Ors) and 95% confidence intervals (Cis) for "Lightweight" and "Heavyweight" were used to evaluate the relative risk. The covariants included maternal age, maternal education, parity, gestational age of Hb measurement, neonatal gender, gestational age at delivery and mode of delivery; they were adjusted in the above analysis model 1. Besides the covariants in model 1, model 2 was additionally adjusted for maternal early pregnancy BMI and weight gain during pregnancy. Sensitivity analysis was conducted among pregnant women with an early pregnancy BMI < 24 kg/m^2 and pregnant women who delivered their babies after 37 weeks of gestational age. All the statistical analyses were performed in R software (version 4.0.3) and $p < 0.05$ was considered statistically significant.

3. Results

3.1. Population Characteristics

A total of 24,183 mother–infant pairs were included in the final analysis (Figure S1) and the comparison of general information between participants and non-participants is shown in Table S1. The maternal socio-demographic, health-related characteristics and neonatal birth characteristics stratified by the compound outcomes are shown in Table 1. The Lightweight and Heavyweight groups accounted for 8.5% and 11.2%, respectively. There were significant differences in maternal age; maternal education level; primipara; BMI at the first trimester; weight gain; and all neonatal characteristics between the Normalweight, Lightweight and Heavyweight groups.

Table 1. Comparison of maternal and neonatal basic characteristics between groups.

Variables	Normalweight N = 19,413	Lightweight N = 2055	Heavyweight N = 2715	p
Maternal Characteristics				
Maternal age, years, mean ± SD	26.62 ± 3.70	26.49 ± 3.59	26.91 ± 3.94	<0.001
Education, N (%)				0.006
Primary school or below	335 (1.7)	51 (2.5)	55 (2.1)	
Junior high school	6603 (34.3)	682 (33.4)	985 (36.7)	
Senior high school	4915 (25.6)	488 (23.9)	671 (25.0)	
College or above	7383 (38.4)	820 (40.2)	971 (36.2)	
Primipara, N (%)				<0.001
Yes	11,622 (59.9)	1221 (59.4)	1638 (60.3)	
No	1855 (9.6)	138 (6.7)	367 (13.5)	
Unknown	5936 (30.6)	696 (33.9)	710 (26.2)	
BMI at 1st trimester, kg/m^2, mean ± SD	20.58 ± 2.53	19.95 ± 2.48	21.83 ± 2.85	<0.001
BMI categories, N (%)				<0.001
Underweight (<18.5)	13,820 (71.2)	1295 (63.0)	1928 (71.0)	
Normalweight (18.5–23.9)	3878 (20.0)	616 (30.0)	242 (8.9)	
Overweight (24.0–27.9)	1458 (7.5)	128 (6.2)	462 (17.0)	
Obesity (≥28.0)	257 (1.3)	16 (0.8)	83 (3.1)	
WG * during pregnancy, kg, mean ± SD	13.88 ± 3.79	12.61 ± 3.95	15.41 ± 4.06	<0.001
Neonatal Characteristics				
Gender of newborn, N (%)				<0.001
Male	10,208 (52.6)	878 (42.7)	1769 (65.2)	
Female	9205 (47.4)	1177 (57.3)	946 (34.8)	
Mode of delivery, N (%)				<0.001
Vaginal	7838 (40.4)	956 (46.5)	599 (22.1)	
Cesarean	10,515 (54.2)	995 (48.4)	1953 (71.9)	
Forceps	205 (1.1)	30 (1.5)	25 (0.9)	
Others	855 (4.4)	74 (3.6)	138 (5.1)	
GA * at delivery, weeks, mean ± SD	39.15 ± 1.17	38.59 ± 2.07	39.34 ± 1.35	<0.001
Birth weight, g, mean ± SD	3.38 ± 0.29	2.64 ± 0.31	4.14 ± 0.31	<0.001
Preterm, N (%)				<0.001
No	19,048 (98.1)	1760 (85.6)	2637 (97.1)	
Yes	365 (1.9)	295 (14.4)	78 (2.9)	

Lightweight, small for gestational age (SGA) or low birth weight (LBW); Heavyweight, large for gestational age (LGA) or macrosomia; * WG, weight gain; GA, gestational age.

3.2. Maternal Hb Status in Different Time Points and Hb Changes during Pregnancy

In the first, early-second, mediate-second, late-second, early-third and late-third trimesters, the averages of the maternal Hb concentrations were 123.95 ± 10.14, 117.95 ± 9.84, 114.31 ± 9.03, 113.26 ± 8.82, 113.29 ± 8.68 and 115.01 ± 8.85 g/L, respectively; the proportions of maternal Hb concentrations <110 g/L were 6.8%, 17.5%, 28.8%, 32.7%, 33.4% and 27.3%, respectively. Before the late-second trimester, there was no significant difference in Hb level between the Normalweight, Lightweight and Heavyweight groups, except in the first trimester. However, in the late-second and third trimesters, there were significant differences in the Hb levels between the Normalweight, Lightweight and Heavyweight groups (Figure 1). In addition, the mean values of Hbfs, Hbft and Hbst were significantly different between the Normalweight, Lightweight and Heavyweight groups. The details are presented in Table S2.

3.3. Association of Maternal Hb Level and Its Changes during Pregnancy with Neonatal Birth Weight Outcomes

Multivariate RCS models were used to assess the non-linear relationships of maternal Hb in different time points of pregnancy and its changes during pregnancy with birth outcomes. The non-linear associations of maternal Hb in the early-second and mediate-second trimester with neonatal birth weight were not observed (Figure S2). Meanwhile, the overall association and non-linear relationships between maternal Hb and birth weight were found in the first, late-second, early-third and late-third trimesters ($P_{\text{non-linear}}$ were 0.011, 0.009, <0.001 and <0.001, respectively). An inverted U-shaped association between maternal Hb and birth weight was observed in the first trimester. In addition, the decrease in neonatal weight was steeper in the 105–120 g/L range of maternal Hb and a roughly negative correlation of maternal with neonatal birth weight was observed in the late-second and later trimesters (Figure 2).

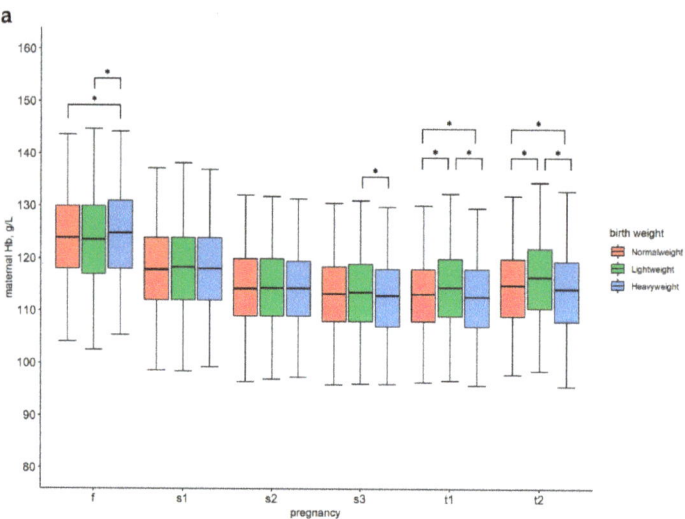

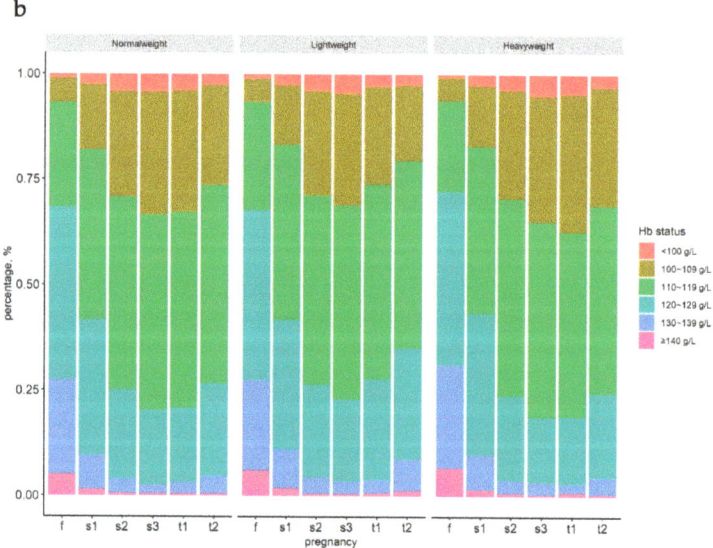

Figure 1. Maternal hemoglobin concentration (**a**) and percentage of maternal hemoglobin status (**b**) stratified by birth weight outcomes at different pregnancy time points. f, first trimester; s1, early-second trimester; s2, mediate-second trimester; s3, late-second trimester; t1, early-third trimester; t2, late-third trimester; * significant difference between the groups.

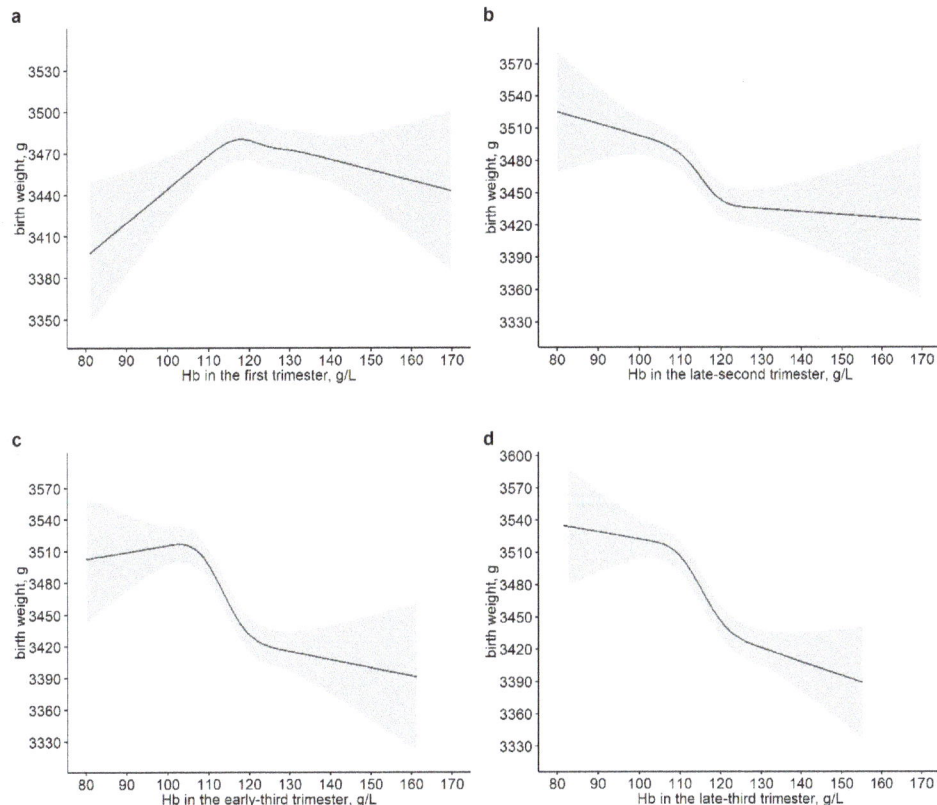

Figure 2. Dose–response associations of maternal hemoglobin in the first trimester (**a**), in the late-second trimester (**b**), in the early-third trimester (**c**) and in the late-third trimester (**d**) with neonatal birth weight. The p-values for overall associations were <0.001. The p-values for non-linear associations were 0.011 (**a**), 0.009 (**b**), <0.001 (**c**) and <0.001 (**d**), respectively. Models were adjusted for maternal age, education, parity, gestational age of hemoglobin measurement, neonatal gender, gestational age at delivery, mode of delivery, maternal BMI in the first trimester and weight gain during pregnancy.

For the compound outcomes, non-linear relationships of maternal Hb in the first, early-second, mediate-second and late-second trimesters with Lightweight, Heavyweight and TotalAdverse were not observed. (Figure S3). In the early-third trimester, significant dose–response associations of maternal Hb with Lightweight and Heavyweight were observed but were not observed in the association of maternal Hb with TotalAdverse. In the late-third trimester, maternal Hb had a significant U-shaped association with Lightweight, and the corresponding maternal Hb where the risk of Lightweight was lowest was about 110 g/L; moreover, when maternal Hb > 120 g/L, the risk of TotalAdverse significantly increased (Figure 3).

In addition, Table 2 displays the associations between maternal Hb concentration in different time points and neonatal compound outcomes. In model 2, compared with women with Hb = 110~119 g/L, those with Hb < 100 g/L had a significantly decreased risk of Lightweight only in the early-third trimester (OR: 0.66, 95% CI: 0.49, 0.88) and those with Hb > 140 g/L had a significantly increased risk of Lightweight only in the first trimester (OR: 1.26, 95% CI: 1.01, 1.57) and late-third trimester (OR: 1.96, 95% CI: 1.20, 3.18); moreover, women with Hb > 120 g/L had a trend of increased risk of Lightweight in the late-third trimester ($P_{trend} < 0.001$). In the mediate-second trimester, compared with women with Hb = 110~119 g/L, pregnant women with Hb = 100~109 g/L had a significantly increased risk of Heavyweight (OR: 1.12, 95% CI: 1.01, 1.25). Compared with women with Hb = 110~119 g/L, women with Hb < 100 had an increased risk of Heavyweight at the late-second and later trimester (late-second trimester: OR: 1.47, 95% CI: 1.18, 1.83; early-third trimester: OR: 1.30, 95% CI: 1.04, 1.63; late-third trimester: OR: 1.38, 95% CI: 1.09, 1.76).

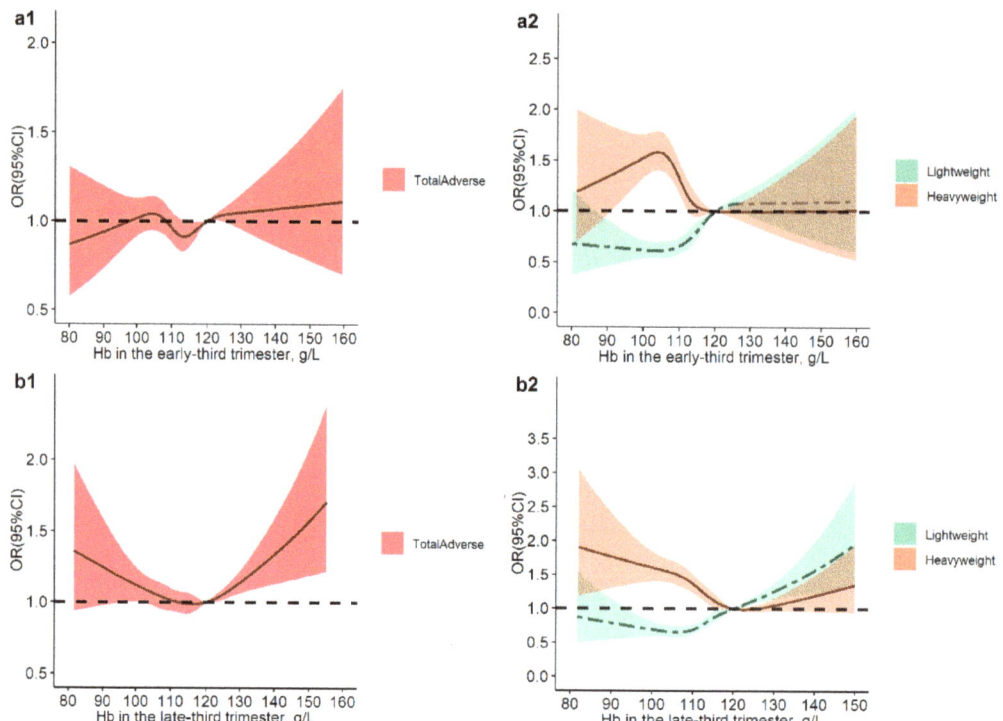

Figure 3. Dose–response associations of maternal hemoglobin in the early-third trimester (**a**) and in the late-third trimester (**b**) with neonatal complex outcomes (including SGA/LBW, LGA/macrosomia and total birth weight adverse outcomes). The *p*-values for overall associations were <0.001. The *p*-values for non-linear associations between Hb and total adverse outcomes were 0.064 (**a1**) and 0.002 (**b1**). The *p*-values for non-linear associations between Hb and SGA/LBW were 0.003 (**a2**) and 0.028 (**b2**), while the *p*-values for non-linear associations between Hb and LGA/macrosomia were <0.001 (**a2**) and <0.001 (**b2**). The models were adjusted for maternal age, education, parity, gestational age of hemoglobin measurement, neonatal gender, gestational age at delivery, mode of delivery, maternal BMI in the first trimester and weight gain during pregnancy. Hemoglobin at 120 g/L was set as the reference level.

On the other hand, there was a positive correlation between maternal Hb reduction during pregnancy and neonatal birth weight, where a non-linear dose–response relationship was found between Hbst and neonatal birth weight ($P_{non\text{-}linear}$ was <0.001) (Figure 4), but not found between Hbfs, Hbft and Hbst and the compound outcomes (Figure S4). A negative association of the decline in maternal Hb with the risk of Lightweight was found in the first to late-second trimesters, first to late-third trimesters and late-second to late-third trimesters; however, a significant association between the decline in Hb and Heavyweight was not observed in the late-second to late-third trimesters. Compared with pregnant women with Hbfs in Q1, those with Hbfs in Q2 had a significantly decreased risk of Heavyweight (OR: 0.83, 95% CI: 0.73, 0.94). In addition, as the maternal Hb decreased more during pregnancy, the risk of Lightweight was lower (all P_{trend} < 0.001) (Table 3). Similar results were observed in pregnant women with early-pregnancy BMI < 24 kg/m^2, pregnant women who delivered their baby after 37 weeks of gestational age and pregnant women who had at least one record of Hb concentration during each defined period (Tables S3–S8).

Table 2. Associations between maternal hemoglobin concentration at different periods and adverse birth outcomes.

Hemoglobin	Normalweight	Lightweight			Heavyweight		
	N (%)	N (%)	Model 1 † OR (95% CI)	Model 2 ‡ OR (95% CI)	N (%)	Model 1 † OR (95% CI)	Model 2 ‡ OR (95% CI)
First trimester							
<100	189 (1.0)	30 (1.5)	1.51 (1.01, 2.25)	1.45 (0.96, 2.18)	17 (0.6)	0.72 (0.44, 1.20)	0.73 (0.43, 1.23)
100~109	1136 (5.9)	136 (6.6)	1.15 (0.93, 1.40)	1.11 (0.91, 1.37)	139 (5.1)	0.97 (0.79, 1.18)	1.03 (0.84, 1.26)
110~119	4830 (24.9)	501 (24.4)	Ref.	Ref.	613 (22.6)	Ref.	Ref.
120~129	7911 (40.8)	821 (40.0)	1.00 (0.89, 1.12)	1.03 (0.91, 1.16)	1115 (41.1)	1.10 (0.99, 1.23)	1.02 (0.92, 1.14)
130~139	4356 (22.4)	447 (21.8)	1.00 (0.87, 1.14)	1.06 (0.92, 1.22)	665 (24.5)	1.17 (1.04, 1.32)	1.05 (0.93, 1.19)
≥140	991 (5.1)	120 (5.8)	1.17 (0.95, 1.46)	1.26 (1.01, 1.57)	166 (6.1)	1.27 (1.05, 1.54)	1.04 (0.86, 1.27)
Early-second trimester							
<100	381 (2.4)	43 (2.6)	1.00 (0.72, 1.40)	0.93 (0.67, 1.31)	60 (2.7)	1.20 (0.90, 1.60)	1.34 (0.99, 1.80)
100~109	2445 (15.3)	230 (13.9)	0.90 (0.76, 1.05)	0.86 (0.73, 1.01)	328 (14.7)	1.01 (0.88, 1.15)	1.12 (0.97, 1.29)
110~119	6407 (40.2)	672 (40.5)	Ref.	Ref.	869 (39.0)	Ref.	Ref.
120~129	5119 (32.1)	533 (32.1)	0.99 (0.88, 1.12)	1.05 (0.93, 1.19)	752 (33.7)	1.06 (0.95, 1.18)	0.96 (0.86, 1.07)
130~139	1323 (8.3)	147 (8.9)	1.08 (0.89, 1.31)	1.20 (0.99, 1.46)	182 (8.2)	0.97 (0.82, 1.16)	0.80 (0.67, 0.96)
≥140	266 (1.7)	33 (2.0)	1.13 (0.77, 1.65)	1.25 (0.85, 1.83)	38 (1.7)	1.07 (0.75, 1.53)	0.87 (0.60, 1.26)
Mediate-second trimester							
<100	694 (4.0)	73 (4.0)	0.98 (0.76, 1.27)	0.87 (0.67, 1.13)	83 (3.4)	0.86 (0.68, 1.10)	1.04 (0.81, 1.33)
100~109	4268 (24.8)	450 (24.5)	1.02 (0.90, 1.15)	0.96 (0.85, 1.09)	608 (25.1)	1.00 (0.90, 1.12)	1.12 (1.00, 1.25)
110~119	7865 (45.6)	815 (44.3)	Ref.	Ref.	1130 (46.7)	Ref.	Ref.
120~129	3720 (21.6)	428 (23.3)	1.10 (0.97, 1.25)	1.17 (1.03, 1.33)	500 (20.7)	0.93 (0.83, 1.04)	0.82 (0.73, 0.93)
130~139	588 (3.4)	61 (3.3)	1.04 (0.79, 1.38)	1.11 (0.83, 1.46)	81 (3.3)	0.92 (0.72, 1.18)	0.79 (0.61, 1.02)
≥140	104 (0.6)	11 (0.6)	0.95 (0.50, 1.80)	1.04 (0.54, 2.00)	16 (0.7)	1.10 (0.64, 1.89)	0.95 (0.55, 1.66)
Late-second trimester							
<100	714 (4.1)	83 (4.6)	1.11 (0.87, 1.42)	0.99 (0.78, 1.27)	111 (4.6)	1.23 (0.99, 1.52)	1.47 (1.18, 1.83)
100~109	4885 (28.4)	497 (27.3)	0.99 (0.88, 1.12)	0.93 (0.82, 1.05)	733 (30.5)	1.15 (1.03, 1.27)	1.29 (1.16, 1.43)
110~119	8036 (46.7)	820 (45.0)	Ref.	Ref.	1068 (44.5)	Ref.	Ref.
120~129	3097 (18.0)	351 (19.3)	1.12 (0.98, 1.28)	1.21 (1.06, 1.39)	412 (17.2)	0.98 (0.86, 1.11)	0.87 (0.76, 0.99)
130~139	395 (2.3)	60 (3.3)	1.49 (1.11, 1.98)	1.59 (1.19, 2.14)	67 (2.8)	1.30 (0.99, 1.71)	1.08 (0.81, 1.43)
≥140	83 (0.5)	10 (0.5)	1.05 (0.53, 2.07)	1.19 (0.59, 2.37)	10 (0.4)	1.01 (0.52, 1.98)	0.89 (0.45, 1.76)
Early-third trimester							
<100	716 (4.2)	58 (3.2)	0.73 (0.55, 0.97)	0.66 (0.49, 0.88)	104 (4.4)	1.12 (0.90, 1.40)	1.30 (1.04, 1.63)
100~109	4929 (29.2)	442 (24.5)	0.84 (0.74, 0.95)	0.80 (0.70, 0.90)	794 (33.3)	1.24 (1.12, 1.37)	1.34 (1.21, 1.49)
110~119	7698 (45.5)	806 (44.6)	Ref.	Ref.	1012 (42.4)	Ref.	Ref.
120~129	3007 (17.8)	429 (23.8)	1.33 (1.17, 1.51)	1.40 (1.23, 1.59)	396 (16.6)	0.99 (0.87, 1.12)	0.87 (0.76, 0.99)
130~139	458 (2.7)	60 (3.3)	1.19 (0.89, 1.58)	1.28 (0.96, 1.70)	61 (2.6)	0.98 (0.74, 1.31)	0.88 (0.66, 1.17)
≥140	94 (0.6)	11 (0.6)	1.02 (0.53, 1.94)	1.04 (0.54, 1.99)	18 (0.8)	1.53 (0.91, 2.56)	1.33 (0.77, 2.30)
Late-third trimester							
<100	529 (2.8)	49 (2.6)	0.98 (0.72, 1.33)	0.92 (0.67, 1.25)	91 (3.5)	1.25 (0.98, 1.58)	1.38 (1.09, 1.76)
100~109	4541 (24.3)	375 (19.8)	0.86 (0.76, 0.98)	0.83 (0.73, 0.94)	741 (28.5)	1.23 (1.11, 1.36)	1.29 (1.16, 1.44)
110~119	8534 (45.8)	819 (43.3)	Ref.	Ref.	1121 (43.2)	Ref.	Ref.
120~129	4080 (21.9)	496 (26.2)	1.26 (1.12, 1.42)	1.31 (1.16, 1.48)	503 (19.4)	0.94 (0.83, 1.05)	0.85 (0.76, 0.96)
130~139	849 (4.6)	131 (6.9)	1.58 (1.30, 1.94)	1.78 (1.45, 2.19)	119 (4.6)	1.06 (0.86, 1.30)	0.90 (0.73, 1.11)
≥140	119 (0.6)	22 (1.2)	1.84 (1.14, 2.96)	1.96 (1.20, 3.18)	21 (0.8)	1.35 (0.84, 2.17)	1.16 (0.71, 1.91)

Lightweight, small for gestational age (SGA) or low birth weight (LBW); Heavyweight, large for gestational age (LGA) or macrosomia. † The model was adjusted for maternal age, education, parity, gestational age of hemoglobin measurement, neonatal gender, gestational age at delivery and mode of delivery. ‡ The model was additionally adjusted for maternal BMI in the first trimester and weight gain during pregnancy.

Table 3. Associations between change of maternal hemoglobin concentrations and adverse birth outcomes.

ΔHb	Normalweight	Lightweight			Heavyweight		
	N (%)	N (%)	Model 1 † OR (95% CI)	Model 2 ‡ OR (95% CI)	N (%)	Model 1 † OR (95% CI)	Model 2 ‡ OR (95% CI)
Hbfs							
Q1 (−50~−17)	4332 (25.2)	444 (24.4)	Ref.	Ref.	724 (30.2)	Ref.	Ref.
Q2 (−17~−11)	4402 (25.6)	429 (23.6)	0.94 (0.82, 1.09)	0.98 (0.85, 1.14)	642 (26.8)	0.90 (0.80, 1.02)	0.83 (0.73, 0.94)
Q3 (−11~−5)	4407 (25.7)	476 (26.2)	1.07 (0.93, 1.25)	1.17 (1.00, 1.36)	537 (22.4)	0.75 (0.66, 0.86)	0.65 (0.57, 0.75)
Q4 (−5~50)	4034 (23.5)	467 (25.7)	1.16 (0.98, 1.38)	1.32 (1.11, 1.57)	495 (20.6)	0.75 (0.65, 0.88)	0.62 (0.53, 0.72)

Table 3. Cont.

ΔHb	Normalweight	Lightweight			Heavyweight		
	N (%)	N (%)	Model 1 † OR (95% CI)	Model 2 ‡ OR (95% CI)	N (%)	Model 1 † OR (95% CI)	Model 2 ‡ OR (95% CI)
Hbft							
Q1 (−50~−16)	4906 (26.3)	391 (20.7)	Ref.	Ref.	831 (32.1)	Ref.	Ref.
Q2 (−16~−9)	4572 (24.6)	438 (23.2)	1.29 (1.11, 1.50)	1.32 (1.14, 1.54)	626 (24.2)	0.82 (0.73, 0.93)	0.78 (0.69, 0.89)
Q3 (−9~−2)	4527 (24.3)	477 (25.2)	1.45 (1.24, 1.69)	1.54 (1.32, 1.80)	579 (22.3)	0.78 (0.69, 0.89)	0.71 (0.63, 0.82)
Q4 (−2~50)	4617 (24.8)	584 (30.9)	1.81 (1.53, 2.14)	1.97 (1.66, 2.33)	555 (21.4)	0.75 (0.65, 0.87)	0.65 (0.56, 0.76)
Hbst *							
Q1 (−50~−3.5)	4362 (26.3)	347 (20.7)	Ref.	Ref.	678 (29.5)	Ref.	Ref.
Q2 (−3.5~2)	4477 (27.0)	431 (25.7)	1.18 (1.01, 1.36)	1.17 (1.01, 1.36)	610 (26.6)	0.91 (0.81, 1.03)	0.93 (0.82, 1.05)
Q3 (2~7)	3727 (22.5)	405 (24.1)	1.34 (1.15, 1.56)	1.33 (1.14, 1.55)	454 (19.8)	0.82 (0.72, 0.93)	0.82 (0.72, 1.01)
Q4 (7~50)	4000 (24.1)	497 (29.6)	1.49 (1.29, 1.73)	1.45 (1.25, 1.68)	555 (24.2)	0.96 (0.85, 1.09)	1.00 (0.88, 1.14)

Lightweight, small for gestational age (SGA) or low birth weight (LBW); Heavyweight, large for gestational age (LGA) or macrosomia; Hbfs, Hb in late-second minus Hb in first; Hbft, Hb in late-third minus Hb in late-third; Hbst, Hb in late-second minus Hb in late-third; Q, quartile. † The model was adjusted for maternal age, education, parity, weeks of gestation at hemoglobin measurement, neonatal gender, gestational age at delivery, mode of delivery and Hb concentration in the first trimester. ‡ The model was additionally adjusted for maternal BMI in the first trimester and weight gain during pregnancy. * Model 1 was adjusted for maternal age, education, parity, weeks of gestation at hemoglobin measurement, neonatal gender, gestational age at delivery, mode of delivery and Hb concentration in the late-second trimester.

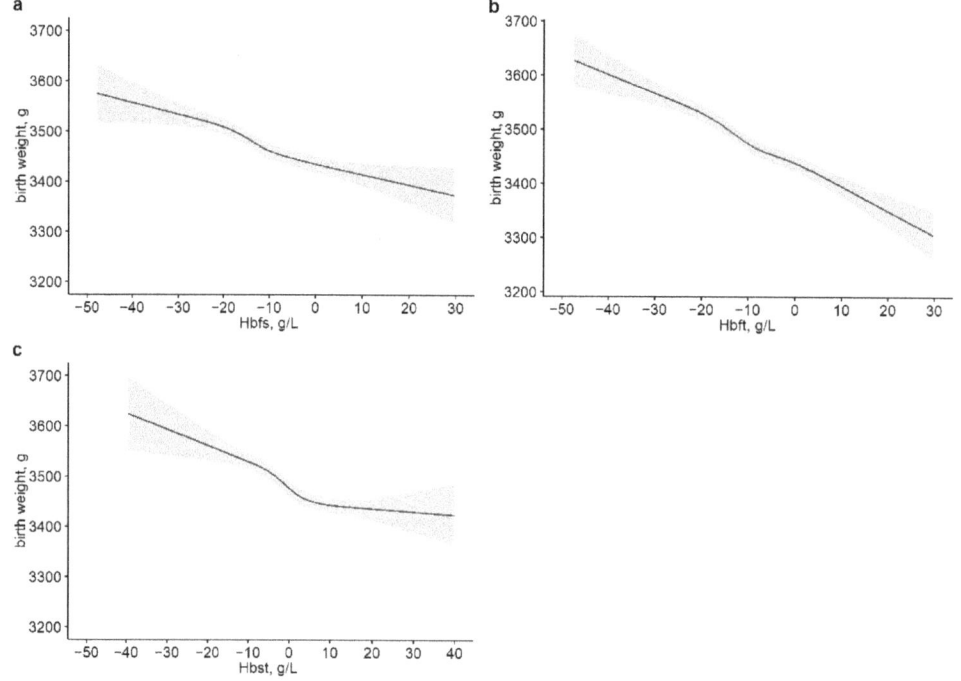

Figure 4. Dose–response associations of maternal hemoglobin change from first to late-second trimesters (**a**), from first to late-third trimesters (**b**) and from late-second to late-third trimesters (**c**) with neonatal birth weight. The p-values for overall associations were <0.001. The p-values for non-linear associations were 0.114 (**a**), 0.390 (**b**) and <0.001 (**c**). Models were adjusted for maternal age, education, parity, neonatal gender, gestational age at delivery, mode of delivery, maternal BMI in the first trimester, weight gain during pregnancy, and Hb concentration in the first trimester or in the late-second trimester. Hbfs, Hb in late-second minus Hb in first; Hbft, Hb in late-third minus Hb in first; Hbst, Hb in late-third minus Hb in late-second.

4. Discussion

This study found a faint inverted U-shaped association between maternal Hb in the first trimester and birth weight, and significant negative associations between maternal Hb and birth weight outcomes (including birth weight, Lightweight and Heavyweight) were mainly observed in the late-second and later trimester. Furthermore, the maternal Hb decline during pregnancy was positively associated with neonatal birth weight and negatively associated with the risk of Lightweight.

In this study, an inverted U-shaped association between maternal Hb in the first trimester and neonatal birth weight was observed. Both extremely low and extremely high maternal Hb in the first trimester might be associated with LBW/SGA. However, many studies found a significant positive correlation between maternal Hb in the first trimester and fetal birth weight, as well as a significant association between low maternal Hb and SGA/LBW [26,35,36]. Other studies did not find a significant association between maternal Hb in the first trimester and birth weight outcomes. A cross-sectional study reported that maternal Hb in the first trimester was interpreted as having little effect on birth weight [37]. Another meta-analysis found that anemia (Hb < 110 g/L) diagnosed before 20 weeks of gestational age did not increase the risk of LBW and SGA [38]; similar results were also shown in a study in Suzhou, China [33]. The associations of maternal Hb in the first trimester with neonatal birth weight outcomes were inconsistent, possibly due to the heterogeneity of a different study population. Another reason for the inconsistency might be unclear iron status and iron supplementation during pregnancy, which is also associated with birth weight outcomes [39].

In addition, the associations of maternal Hb < 100 g/L in the early- and mediate-second trimester with neonatal birth weight and Lightweight were not observed. Similar to our results, some other studies also reported that the associations of maternal Hb in the second trimester with fetal birth weight and LBW were insignificant [26,36]. Some studies reported that severe anemia may cause poor fetal growth in utero because of insufficient oxygen flow to the placental tissue [26], and ultimately, affect fetal birth weight and cause LBW [40]. However, because of the deficient data with few pregnant women Hb < 70 g/L in this study, we were unable to assess the association between severe anemia (Hb < 70 g/L) and birth outcomes. Moreover, in the late-second and later trimester, maternal Hb < 110 g/L was related to the increased birth weight and increased risk of Heavyweight; a review also indicated that low maternal Hb in the late-second trimester was associated with a high risk of LGA [41], which might be due to placental hypertrophy [42]. Additionally, Scanlon et.al reported that a high Hb (>144 g/L) level in the second trimester was associated with SGA [21], which was different from our result showing that maternal Hb > 140 g/L in the second trimester was not related to Lightweight or Heavyweight. This may have been due to the small sample of pregnant women with Hb > 140 g/L in the second trimester in this study.

Maternal Hb concentration in the late-third trimester had a roughly negative association with neonatal birth weight and a faint U-shaped association with Lightweight. When maternal Hb was 100–110 g/L, the risk of Lightweight was the lowest and the risk of Heavyweight was relatively high. Similar to our results, Chen et al. showed that maternal Hb in the third trimester was inversely correlated with neonatal birth weight [15]. Relatively low maternal Hb in the third trimester usually reflects changes in plasma volume rather than poor maternal nutrition or adaptation [43]. However, a recent prospective study from Northwest China showed an inverted U-shaped association between maternal Hb in the third trimester and neonatal birth weight [23], and a significant positive correlation between maternal Hb in the third trimester and birth weight was reported in another study [44]. This may be because, even in the third trimester, maternal Hb in different periods reflects different conditions of the intrauterine environment. As presented in a study, maternal Hb < 110 g/L was related to an increased placental ratio but whether it reflected the placental hypertrophy or restriction of fetal growth was unclear [45]. More studies are needed to explore this mechanism. Maternal high Hb was mainly related to the risk of Lightweight in the late-third trimester. A study from Norway also reported that increased Hb levels were associated with lower placental weight and impaired fetal growth [46]. Abnormally high Hb concentrations during pregnancy usually indicate poor plasma volume expansion, which also leads to an increased risk of LBW [20,21,41,47]. In addition, high Hb might increase blood flow resistance, which reduces maternal blood perfusion and leads to placental dysplasia [48].

On the other hand, we found that the decrease in maternal Hb from first to late-second trimester and from first to late-third trimester was positively correlated with birth weight and negatively correlated with the risk of Lightweight. Similar to our results, preceding studies showed that changes in Hb concentration during pregnancy were associated with adverse birth outcomes. Rasmussen et al. found that a decrease in maternal Hb from the first to second trimester had a strong positive correlation with neonatal birth weight [37]. The same relationship was also observed in the first to third trimesters in other studies [15,24]. Pregnant women with the lowest Hb reduction from early to late pregnancy had an increased risk of LBW and SGA compared with women with an intermediate Hb reduction [15,24]. Changes in Hb during pregnancy were significantly correlated with changes in plasma volume [43,49]. A smaller decrease in maternal Hb from the first trimester may indicate a reduction in plasma volume expansion, which may impair fetoplacental circulation and increase the risk of LBW and SGA [41]. Another possible mechanism was that expansion of the plasma volume may reduce blood viscosity and favor blood flow in the maternal intervillous space [50]. Nevertheless, the positive associations of maternal Hb decline from the first- to late-second trimesters and from the first- to late-third trimesters with Heavyweight were found; we speculated that a larger reduction in Hb levels may indicate more erythropoietin secretion, which was associated with angiogenesis [51]. More studies are necessary to explore this mechanism. The decrease in maternal Hb levels from the late-second to late-third trimesters was related to decreased risk of Lightweight, but not related to Heavyweight. Fetal growth reached a peak in the late-third trimester and the nutrients required by the fetus increased dramatically [52]. Therefore, the reduction in Hb, which implied an increased expansion of plasma volume, may accelerate the transport of nutrients in the body of pregnant women. As far as we know, no study has reported similar results. The above results were shown in pregnant women with early-pregnancy BMI < 24 kg/m^2 or pregnant women who delivered their baby after 37 weeks of gestational age in a sensitivity analysis.

The results of this study showed that the associations of maternal Hb with neonatal birth weight outcomes were different due to the timing of maternal Hb measurements. In addition, maternal Hb change during pregnancy was also strongly associated with birth weight outcomes. Maternal Hb > 120 g/L in the late-third trimester and an increase in maternal Hb from the late-second to late-third trimesters should especially be given more attention. The maternal Hb fluctuated during pregnancy; therefore, the findings in this study were important for clinically identifying the associations of maternal Hb at different time points and its changes during pregnancy with neonatal birth weight outcomes, which could provide recommendations for optimal interventions. Moreover, the research findings might contribute to clinical evidence-based studies to determine the pathological value of maternal Hb in different periods during pregnancy. The association of maternal Hb in different time points with neonatal birth weight outcomes might be partly explained by placental adaptation. Further study should be conducted to explore more biological mechanisms.

5. Strengths and Limitations

There were several strengths to this study. Relatively drastic physiological changes in maternal Hb occurred with the progress of pregnancy; accordingly, even in the second or third trimester, different time points for Hb measurements may lead to heterogeneity in results. We further divided the second and third trimesters into five time periods and explored the relationships between Hb concentrations in different periods and birth weight outcomes. Moreover, we selected the value of Hb concentration in a specific period to calculate the maternal Hb changes during pregnancy, which were more representative. We also collected data on maternal early-pregnancy BMI and weight gain during pregnancy, which were recognized as important factors that had a greater impact on birth weight.

Some limitations to this study should also be taken into consideration. First, the proportion of pregnant women with severe anemia (Hb < 70 g/L) in our data was very low; therefore, we were unable to verify that maternal Hb < 70 g/L was associated with adverse birth weight outcomes [53,54], and the generalizability of the research findings might be limited due to the significant differences between participants and non-participants; therefore, several subgroup analysis and sensitivity analysis were conducted to examine the stability of the results. Second, the information on iron supplementation for pregnant women was mostly missing. The association between iron supplementation and maternal Hb may have had an influence on this study. The relationship between changes in Hb levels and birth weight outcomes was evaluated to diminish the impact. Third, whether maternal low Hb was caused by iron deficiency was unclear. However, iron deficiency is the most common cause of anemia, especially in developing countries [35]; therefore, we can reasonably assume that the majority of pregnant women with low Hb were suffering from iron deficiency. In addition, information on complications such as placental insufficiency was not available, which might affect the association between maternal Hb and neonatal birth weight; further study is needed to eliminate the effect of complications.

6. Conclusions

Maternal Hb markedly fluctuated during pregnancy; a negative dose–response association of maternal Hb in the late-second and third trimesters and a Hb change during pregnancy with neonatal birth weight outcomes were observed. Furthermore, the phenomena of high Hb in the first trimester and after the late-second trimester and the increase in maternal Hb from the late-second to late-third trimesters more significantly increasing the risk of SGA/LBW should especially be given more attention. Its biological mechanism needs to be further explored.

Supplementary Materials: The following are available online at https://www.mdpi.com/article/10.3390/nu14122542/s1. Supplementary Table S1. The comparison of general information between participants and non-participants. Supplementary Table S2. Maternal hemoglobin status in different periods of pregnancy and the change during pregnancy between groups. Supplementary Table S3. Associations between maternal hemoglobin concentration in different periods and adverse birth weight outcomes in women with early-pregnancy BMI < 24 kg/m^2. Supplementary Table S4. Associations between the change in maternal hemoglobin concentration and adverse birth weight outcomes in women with early-pregnancy BMI < 24 kg/m^2. Supplementary Table S5. Associations between maternal hemoglobin concentration in different periods and adverse birth weight outcomes in pregnant women who delivered their baby after 37 weeks of gestational age. Supplementary Table S6. Associations between the change in maternal hemoglobin concentration and adverse birth weight outcomes in pregnant women who delivered their baby after 37 weeks of gestational age. Supplementary Table S7. Associations between maternal hemoglobin concentration at different periods and adverse birth weight outcomes in pregnant women who had at least one record of Hb concentration during each defined period. Supplementary Table S8. Associations between the change in maternal hemoglobin concentration and adverse birth weight outcomes in pregnant women who had at least one record of Hb concentration during each defined period. Supplementary Figure S1. The flow chart of participants. Supplementary Figure S2. Dose–response association of maternal hemoglobin in the early-second trimester (a) and the mediate-second trimester (b) with neonatal birth weight. Supplementary Figure S3. Dose–response association of maternal hemoglobin in the first trimester (a), early-second trimester (b), mediate-second trimester (c) and late-second trimester (d) with neonatal complex outcomes (including SGA/LBW, LGA/macrosomia and total birth weight adverse outcomes). Supplementary Figure S4. Dose–response association of maternal hemoglobin change from the first to late-second trimesters (a), first to late-third trimesters (b) and late-second to late-third trimesters (c) with neonatal complex outcomes (including SGA/LBW, LGA/macrosomia and total birth weight adverse outcomes).

Author Contributions: Conceptualization, Y.Y.; Methodology, S.S.; Validation, Z.P.; Resources, H.C. and H.Z.; Formal Analysis, P.C.; Investigation, M.M.; Writing—Original Draft, Z.P.; Writing—Review and Editing, Z.P. and S.S.; Visualization, S.S., Y.Z. and H.L. All authors read and agreed to the published version of the manuscript.

Funding: This study was funded by the Chinese National Natural Science Foundation (81973055), the National Key Research and Development Programme of China (No. 2021YFC2701901), Major research and development projects of the Zhejiang Science and Technology Department (2018C03010), Key Laboratory of Intelligent Preventive Medicine of Zhejiang Province (2020E10004), and Leading Innovative and Entrepreneur Team Introduction Program of Zhejiang (2019R01007).

Institutional Review Board Statement: The study was conducted according to the guidelines of the Declaration of Helsinki and approved by the institutional review board of Zhejiang University School of Medicine on 2 March 2016 ((2016) Lun Shen Yan (Shen 017)).

Informed Consent Statement: Informed consent was obtained from all subjects involved in the study.

Data Availability Statement: The data presented in this study are available on request from the corresponding author. The data are not publicly available because they contain information that could compromise the privacy of research participants.

Acknowledgments: We thank the staff at the Zhoushan Maternal and Child Health Hospital for their help.

Conflicts of Interest: The authors declare no conflict of interest.

References

1. Goldenberg, R.L.; Culhane, J.F. Low birth weight in the United States. *Am. J. Clin. Nutr.* **2007**, *85*, 584s–590s. [CrossRef] [PubMed]
2. Blencowe, H.; Krasevec, J.; de Onis, M.; Black, R.E.; An, X.; Stevens, G.A.; Borghi, E.; Hayashi, C.; Estevez, D.; Cegolon, L.; et al. National, regional, and worldwide estimates of low birthweight in 2015, with trends from 2000: A systematic analysis. *Lancet Glob. Health* **2019**, *7*, e849–e860. [CrossRef]
3. Lee, A.C.; Katz, J.; Blencowe, H.; Cousens, S.; Kozuki, N.; Vogel, J.P.; Adair, L.; Baqui, A.H.; Bhutta, Z.A.; Caulfield, L.E.; et al. National and regional estimates of term and preterm babies born small for gestational age in 138 low-income and middle-income countries in 2010. *Lancet Glob. Health* **2013**, *1*, e26–e36. [CrossRef]
4. Lee, A.C.; Kozuki, N.; Cousens, S.; Stevens, G.A.; Blencowe, H.; Silveira, M.F.; Sania, A.; Rosen, H.E.; Schmiegelow, C.; Adair, L.S.; et al. Estimates of burden and consequences of infants born small for gestational age in low and middle income countries with INTERGROWTH-21(st) standard: Analysis of CHERG datasets. *BMJ* **2017**, *358*, j3677. [CrossRef]
5. Barker, D.J. The developmental origins of chronic adult disease. *Acta Paediatr.* **2004**, *93*, 26–33. [CrossRef]
6. Surkan, P.J.; Hsieh, C.C.; Johansson, A.L.; Dickman, P.W.; Cnattingius, S. Reasons for increasing trends in large for gestational age births. *Obstet. Gynecol.* **2004**, *104*, 720–726. [CrossRef]
7. Li, G.; Kong, L.; Li, Z.; Zhang, L.; Fan, L.; Zou, L.; Chen, Y.; Ruan, Y.; Wang, X.; Zhang, W. Prevalence of macrosomia and its risk factors in china: A multicentre survey based on birth data involving 101,723 singleton term infants. *Paediatr. Perinat. Epidemiol.* **2014**, *28*, 345–350. [CrossRef]
8. Hong, Y.H.; Lee, J.E. Large for Gestational Age and Obesity-Related Comorbidities. *J. Obes. Metab. Syndr.* **2021**, *30*, 124–131. [CrossRef]
9. Giapros, V.; Evagelidou, E.; Challa, A.; Kiortsis, D.; Drougia, A.; Andronikou, S. Serum adiponectin and leptin levels and insulin resistance in children born large for gestational age are affected by the degree of overweight. *Clin. Endocrinol.* **2007**, *66*, 353–359. [CrossRef]
10. Boney, C.M.; Verma, A.; Tucker, R.; Vohr, B.R. Metabolic syndrome in childhood: Association with birth weight, maternal obesity, and gestational diabetes mellitus. *Pediatrics* **2005**, *115*, e290–e296. [CrossRef]
11. Darnton-Hill, I. Global burden and significance of multiple micronutrient deficiencies in pregnancy. *Nestle Nutr. Inst. Workshop Ser.* **2012**, *70*, 49–60. [CrossRef] [PubMed]
12. Das, U.G.; Sysyn, G.D. Abnormal fetal growth: Intrauterine growth retardation, small for gestational age, large for gestational age. *Pediatric. Clin. N. Am.* **2004**, *51*, 639–654. [CrossRef] [PubMed]
13. Means, R.T. Iron Deficiency and Iron Deficiency Anemia: Implications and Impact in Pregnancy, Fetal Development, and Early Childhood Parameters. *Nutrients* **2020**, *12*, 447. [CrossRef]
14. Crispin, P.J.; Sethna, F.; Andriolo, K. Red Cell and Reticulocyte Parameters for the Detection of Iron Deficiency in Pregnancy. *Clin. Lab.* **2019**, *65*. [CrossRef]

15. Chen, J.H.; Guo, X.F.; Liu, S.; Long, J.H.; Zhang, G.Q.; Huang, M.C.; Qiu, X.Q. Impact and changes of maternal hemoglobin on birth weight in pregnant women of Zhuang Nationality, in Guangxi. *Zhonghua Liu Xing Bing Xue Za Zhi Zhonghua Liuxingbingxue Zazhi* **2017**, *38*, 154–157. [CrossRef] [PubMed]
16. Steer, P.; Alam, M.A.; Wadsworth, J.; Welch, A. Relation between maternal haemoglobin concentration and birth weight in different ethnic groups. *BMJ* **1995**, *310*, 489–491. [CrossRef] [PubMed]
17. Rahman, M.M.; Abe, S.K.; Rahman, M.S.; Kanda, M.; Narita, S.; Bilano, V.; Ota, E.; Gilmour, S.; Shibuya, K. Maternal anemia and risk of adverse birth and health outcomes in low- and middle-income countries: Systematic review and meta-analysis. *Am. J. Clin. Nutr.* **2016**, *103*, 495–504. [CrossRef]
18. King, J.C. A Summary of Pathways or Mechanisms Linking Preconception Maternal Nutrition with Birth Outcomes. *J. Nutr.* **2016**, *146*, 1437s–1444s. [CrossRef]
19. Rahmati, S.; Delpishe, A.; Azami, M.; Hafezi Ahmadi, M.R.; Sayehmiri, K. Maternal Anemia during pregnancy and infant low birth weight: A systematic review and Meta-analysis. *Int. J. Reprod. Biomed.* **2017**, *15*, 125–134. [CrossRef]
20. Dewey, K.G.; Oaks, B.M. U-shaped curve for risk associated with maternal hemoglobin, iron status, or iron supplementation. *Am. J. Clin. Nutr.* **2017**, *106*, 1694s–1702s. [CrossRef]
21. Scanlon, K.S.; Yip, R.; Schieve, L.A.; Cogswell, M.E. High and low hemoglobin levels during pregnancy: Differential risks for preterm birth and small for gestational age. *Obstet. Gynecol.* **2000**, *96*, 741–748. [CrossRef] [PubMed]
22. Gonzales, G.F.; Steenland, K.; Tapia, V. Maternal hemoglobin level and fetal outcome at low and high altitudes. *Am. J. Physiol. Regul. Integr. Comp. Physiol.* **2009**, *297*, R1477–R1485. [CrossRef] [PubMed]
23. Liu, D.; Li, S.; Zhang, B.; Kang, Y.; Cheng, Y.; Zeng, L.; Chen, F.; Mi, B.; Qu, P.; Zhao, D.; et al. Maternal Hemoglobin Concentrations and Birth Weight, Low Birth Weight (LBW), and Small for Gestational Age (SGA): Findings from a Prospective Study in Northwest China. *Nutrients* **2022**, *14*, 858. [CrossRef] [PubMed]
24. Jwa, S.C.; Fujiwara, T.; Yamanobe, Y.; Kozuka, K.; Sago, H. Changes in maternal hemoglobin during pregnancy and birth outcomes. *BMC Pregnancy Childbirth* **2015**, *15*, 80. [CrossRef]
25. Randall, D.A.; Patterson, J.A.; Gallimore, F.; Morris, J.M.; McGee, T.M.; Ford, J.B. The association between haemoglobin levels in the first 20 weeks of pregnancy and pregnancy outcomes. *PLoS ONE* **2019**, *14*, e0225123. [CrossRef]
26. Bakacak, M.; Avci, F.; Ercan, O.; Köstü, B.; Serin, S.; Kiran, G.; Bostanci, M.S.; Bakacak, Z. The effect of maternal hemoglobin concentration on fetal birth weight according to trimesters. *J. Matern.-Fetal Neonatal Med.* **2015**, *28*, 2106–2110. [CrossRef]
27. Hytten, F. Blood volume changes in normal pregnancy. *Clin. Haematol.* **1985**, *14*, 601–612. [CrossRef]
28. Sibley, C.P.; Brownbill, P.; Dilworth, M.; Glazier, J.D. Review: Adaptation in placental nutrient supply to meet fetal growth demand: Implications for programming. *Placenta* **2010**, *31*, S70–S74. [CrossRef]
29. Sandovici, I.; Hoelle, K.; Angiolini, E.; Constância, M. Placental adaptations to the maternal-fetal environment: Implications for fetal growth and developmental programming. *Reprod. Biomed. Online* **2012**, *25*, 68–89. [CrossRef]
30. Ali, S.A.; Tikmani, S.S.; Saleem, S.; Patel, A.B.; Hibberd, P.L.; Goudar, S.S.; Dhaded, S.; Derman, R.J.; Moore, J.L.; McClure, E.M.; et al. Hemoglobin concentrations and adverse birth outcomes in South Asian pregnant women: Findings from a prospective Maternal and Neonatal Health Registry. *Reprod. Health* **2020**, *17*, 154. [CrossRef]
31. Liu, X.; An, H.; Li, N.; Li, Z.; Zhang, Y.; Zhang, L.; Li, H.; Liu, J.; Ye, R. Preconception Hemoglobin Concentration and Risk of Low Birth Weight and Small-for-Gestational-Age: A Large Prospective Cohort Study in China. *Nutrients* **2022**, *14*, 271. [CrossRef] [PubMed]
32. Milman, N.; Graudal, N.; Nielsen, O.J.; Agger, A.O. Serum erythropoietin during normal pregnancy: Relationship to hemoglobin and iron status markers and impact of iron supplementation in a longitudinal, placebo-controlled study on 118 women. *Int. J. Hematol.* **1997**, *66*, 159–168. [CrossRef]
33. Xiong, X.; Buekens, P.; Fraser, W.D.; Guo, Z. Anemia during pregnancy in a Chinese population. *Int. J. Gynaecol. Obstet. Off. Organ Int. Fed. Gynaecol. Obstet.* **2003**, *83*, 159–164. [CrossRef]
34. Perperoglou, A.; Sauerbrei, W.; Abrahamowicz, M.; Schmid, M. A review of spline function procedures in R. *BMC Med. Res. Methodol.* **2019**, *19*, 46. [CrossRef]
35. Ren, A.; Wang, J.; Ye, R.W.; Li, S.; Liu, J.M.; Li, Z. Low first-trimester hemoglobin and low birth weight, preterm birth and small for gestational age newborns. *Int. J. Gynaecol. Obstet. Off. Organ Int. Fed. Gynaecol. Obstet.* **2007**, *98*, 124–128. [CrossRef] [PubMed]
36. Jung, J.; Rahman, M.M.; Rahman, M.S.; Swe, K.T.; Islam, M.R.; Rahman, M.O.; Akter, S. Effects of hemoglobin levels during pregnancy on adverse maternal and infant outcomes: A systematic review and meta-analysis. *Ann. N. Y. Acad. Sci.* **2019**, *1450*, 69–82. [CrossRef]
37. Rasmussen, S.; Oian, P. First- and second-trimester hemoglobin levels. Relation to birth weight and gestational age. *Acta Obstet. Et Gynecol. Scand.* **1993**, *72*, 246–251. [CrossRef]
38. Xiong, X.; Buekens, P.; Alexander, S.; Demianczuk, N.; Wollast, E. Anemia during pregnancy and birth outcome: A meta-analysis. *Am. J. Perinatol.* **2000**, *17*, 137–146. [CrossRef]
39. Chaparro, C.M.; Suchdev, P.S. Anemia epidemiology, pathophysiology, and etiology in low- and middle-income countries. *Ann. N. Y. Acad. Sci.* **2019**, *1450*, 15–31. [CrossRef]
40. Allen, L.H. Biological mechanisms that might underlie iron's effects on fetal growth and preterm birth. *J. Nutr.* **2001**, *131*, 581s–589s. [CrossRef]
41. Steer, P.J. Maternal hemoglobin concentration and birth weight. *Am. J. Clin. Nutr.* **2000**, *71*, 1285s–1287s. [CrossRef] [PubMed]

42. Huang, A.; Zhang, R.; Yang, Z. Quantitative (stereological) study of placental structures in women with pregnancy iron-deficiency anemia. *Eur. J. Obstet. Gynecol. Reprod. Biol.* **2001**, *97*, 59–64. [CrossRef]
43. Whittaker, P.G.; Macphail, S.; Lind, T. Serial hematologic changes and pregnancy outcome. *Obstet. Gynecol.* **1996**, *88*, 33–39. [CrossRef]
44. Yildiz, Y.; Özgü, E.; Unlu, S.B.; Salman, B.; Eyi, E.G. The relationship between third trimester maternal hemoglobin and birth weight/length; results from the tertiary center in Turkey. *J. Matern.-Fetal Neonatal Med.* **2014**, *27*, 729–732. [CrossRef]
45. Lao, T.T.; Tam, K.F. Placental ratio and anemia in third-trimester pregnancy. *J. Reprod. Med.* **2000**, *45*, 923–928.
46. Larsen, S.; Bjelland, E.K.; Haavaldsen, C.; Eskild, A. Placental weight in pregnancies with high or low hemoglobin concentrations. *Eur. J. Obstet. Gynecol. Reprod. Biol.* **2016**, *206*, 48–52. [CrossRef]
47. Carpenter, R.M.; Billah, S.M.; Lyons, G.R.; Siraj, M.S.; Rahman, Q.S.; Thorsten, V.; McClure, E.M.; Haque, R.; Petri, W.A. U-Shaped Association between Maternal Hemoglobin and Low Birth Weight in Rural Bangladesh. *Am. J. Trop. Med. Hyg.* **2021**, *106*, 424–431. [CrossRef]
48. Leach, L. Placental vascular dysfunction in diabetic pregnancies: Intimations of fetal cardiovascular disease? *Microcirculation* **2011**, *18*, 263–269. [CrossRef]
49. Salas, S.P.; Rosso, P.; Espinoza, R.; Robert, J.A.; Valdés, G.; Donoso, E. Maternal plasma volume expansion and hormonal changes in women with idiopathic fetal growth retardation. *Obstet. Gynecol.* **1993**, *81*, 1029–1033.
50. Stephansson, O.; Dickman, P.W.; Johansson, A.; Cnattingius, S. Maternal hemoglobin concentration during pregnancy and risk of stillbirth. *JAMA* **2000**, *284*, 2611–2617. [CrossRef]
51. Knottnerus, J.A.; Delgado, L.R.; Knipschild, P.G.; Essed, G.G.; Smits, F. Haematologic parameters and pregnancy outcome. A prospective cohort study in the third trimester. *J. Clin. Epidemiol.* **1990**, *43*, 461–466. [CrossRef]
52. Grantz, K.L.; Kim, S.; Grobman, W.A.; Newman, R.; Owen, J.; Skupski, D.; Grewal, J.; Chien, E.K.; Wing, D.A.; Wapner, R.J.; et al. Fetal growth velocity: The NICHD fetal growth studies. *Am. J. Obstet. Gynecol.* **2018**, *219*, 285.E1–285.E36. [CrossRef] [PubMed]
53. Kozuki, N.; Lee, A.C.; Katz, J. Moderate to severe, but not mild, maternal anemia is associated with increased risk of small-for-gestational-age outcomes. *J. Nutr.* **2012**, *142*, 358–362. [CrossRef] [PubMed]
54. Sifakis, S.; Pharmakides, G. Anemia in pregnancy. *Ann. N. Y. Acad. Sci.* **2000**, *900*, 125–136. [CrossRef]

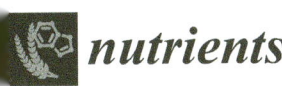

Article

Association of Vitamin D in Different Trimester with Hemoglobin during Pregnancy

Shuting Si [1,2], Zhicheng Peng [1,2], Haoyue Cheng [1,2], Yan Zhuang [1,2], Peihan Chi [1,2], Xialidan Alifu [1,2], Haibo Zhou [1,2], Minjia Mo [1,2] and Yunxian Yu [1,2,*]

[1] Department of Public Health, and Department of Anesthesiology, Second Affiliated Hospital of Zhejiang University School of Medicine, Hangzhou 310058, China; 21818499@zju.edu.cn (S.S.); 22018678@zju.edu.cn (Z.P.); 3150101365@zju.edu.cn (H.C.); yanzhuang@zju.edu.cn (Y.Z.); 22118872@zju.edu.cn (P.C.); 3130100017@zju.edu.cn (X.A.); 11918158@zju.edu.cn (H.Z.); minjiamo@zju.edu.cn (M.M.)

[2] Department of Epidemiology & Health Statistics, School of Public Health, School of Medicine, Zhejiang University, Hangzhou 310058, China

* Correspondence: yunxianyu@zju.edu.cn; Tel.: +86-571-8820-8191

Abstract: The association between vitamin D and hemoglobin has been suggested. Vitamin D can affect erythropoiesis by the induction of erythroid progenitor cell proliferation and enhance iron absorption by regulating the iron-hepcidin-ferroportin axis in monocytes. However, this relationship in pregnant women is scarce. The purpose of this study was to investigate the association between plasma vitamin D levels with hemoglobin concentration in pregnant women considering each trimester and iron supplementation. The data were obtained from Zhoushan Pregnant Women Cohort, collected from 2011 to 2018. Plasma 25(OH)D was measured in each trimester using liquid chromatography–tandem mass spectrometry. Generalized estimating equations and multiple linear regressions were performed. Finally, 2962 pregnant women and 4419 observations in the first trimester were included in this study. Plasma 25(OH)D in first trimester (T1) (β = 0.06, p = 0.0177), second trimester (T2) (β = 0.15, p < 0.0001), and third trimester (T3) (β = 0.12, p = 0.0006) were positively associated with Hb. Association between plasma 25(OH)D levels in T1 and Hb concentration was positively associated with gestational age (β = 0.005, p = 0.0421). Pregnant women with VD deficiency in T1 (OR = 1.42, 95% CI: 1.07–1.88) or T2 (OR = 1.94, 95% CI: 1.30–2.89) presented an increased risk of anemia, compared with women without VD deficiency. Moreover, the significant relationship between VD and Hb was only observed among women with iron supplementation during pregnancy. Plasma 25(OH)D levels in each trimester were positively associated with Hb concentration. Iron supplementation might be an important factor affecting the relationship between VD and Hb.

Keywords: hemoglobin; vitamin D; iron supplementary; pregnancy

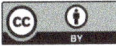

1. Introduction

Anemia is a serious global public health problem particularly affecting young children and pregnant women. In 2019, the global prevalence of anemia among pregnant women aged 15–49 years was 36% (95% CI: 34–9%) and it was 27% (95% CI: 21–35%) in east and southeast Asia [1]. In China, the reported prevalence was relatively low, varying from 10.5% to 23.5% [2–5], but it still cannot be ignored. Because the adverse pregnancy outcomes (such as gestational diabetes, polyhydramnios, preterm birth, low birth weight, neonatal complications, and NICU admission) were significantly higher among pregnant women with anemia [2,6,7]. The most common cause of anemia is poor nutrition, especially iron deficiency. In recent years, it has been suggested that vitamin D (VD) deficiency may also be a key factor. VD insufficiency or deficiency was also prevalent in pregnant women around the world. The prevalence among Asian pregnant women was 45~98% [8], and it was about 96.0% among Chinese pregnant women [9]. As Ellen et al. summarized, epidemiological studies have linked VD deficiency to an increased risk of anemia in various healthy and diseased populations [10–13]. In terms of biological mechanisms, VD affects hemoglobin concentration by regulating erythropoiesis, immune cells, and hepcidin production [14–17]. However, evidence for such an association in pregnant women remains scarce and contradictory. In 2022, one meta-analysis including eight observational studies concluded that VD deficiency might be a risk factor for anemia in pregnancy [18]. However, most studies included in this meta-analysis had moderate or low methodological quality and a limited sample size. Moreover, most studies measured 25(OH)D and hemoglobin (Hb) only once during pregnancy without considering changes in the level of 25(OH)D and Hb throughout pregnancy. Some studies even did not report which trimester or gestational age was to measure 25(OH)D and Hb. In addition, one study was conducted on adolescent pregnant women which might not be able to be extrapolated to adult pregnant women.

Therefore, in this cohort study, we examined plasma 25(OH)D levels across all the three trimesters and extracted each Hb from each prenatal visit to further explore the association of VD in different trimesters as well as the dynamic change of VD with Hb during pregnancy. Meanwhile, whether iron supplementary could influence the association of VD with Hb was explored.

2. Materials and Methods

2.1. Study Design and Participants

This was a prospective cohort study based on the Zhoushan Pregnant Women Cohort (ZPWC) from August 2011 to May 2018. ZPWC is an ongoing prospective cohort conducted in Zhoushan Maternal and Child Health Care Hospital, Zhejiang. Pregnant women were recruited at their first prenatal visit between 8 and 14 gestational weeks. The inclusion and exclusion criteria have been described previously [19]. Briefly, pregnant women aged between 18 and 45 years without serious physical, or mental health disease, threatened abortion or dysontogenesis, and who have conducted plasma 25(OH)D and Hb measurement in T1 and at least two times Hb measurement during pregnancy were included in this study. Before participating in this study, written informed consents were obtained from all pregnant women. The study protocol was approved by the ethics board of Zhejiang University School of Medicine.

2.2. Date and Blood Sample Collection

Pregnant women enrolled in the ZPWC were interviewed with a structured questionnaire face-to-face by a well-trained interviewer to collect information on socio-demographic characteristics, lifestyle, and health behavior in the first trimester (T1: 8th to 13th gestational week). Participants would be followed up in the second trimester (T2: 24th–27th gestational week), third trimester (T3: 32nd–36th gestational week), and 42nd day postpartum with the corresponding questionnaire. At each visit, 5 mL fasting venous blood was drawn and centrifuged at 4 °C. Plasma and white blood cells were separated and stored at −80 °C until use. The Hb concentration was measured during the routine examination, and we extracted it from the electronic medical records system. According to the frequency of blood examination during prenatal visits, Hb may be measured multiple times in T2 and T3. Therefore, we further categorized the Hb concentrations into seven periods (before 14th, 14 to 17th, 18 to 22nd, 23 to 27th, 28 to 31st, 32 to 35th, and 36 to 42nd gestational week).

2.3. Measurement of Plasma 25(OH)

Plasma 25(OH)D2 and 25(OH)D3 concentrations in T1, T2, and T3 were measured by Liquid chromatography–tandem mass spectrometry (API 3200MD (Applied Biosystems/MDS Sciex, Framingham, MA, USA)) and reported in ng/mL, respectively. The lowest sensitivity of the measurement was 2 ng/mL for 25(OH)D2 and 5 ng/mL for 25(OH)D3, respectively. The intra-assay coefficient variances (CVs) were 1.47–7.24% and 2.50–7.59% for 25(OH)D2 and 25(OH)D3, respectively, and the inter-assay CVs were 4.48–6.74% and

4.44–6.76% for 25(OH)D2 and 25(OH)D3, respectively [15]. The 25(OH)D concentrations were the sum of 25(OH)D2 and 25(OH)D3 concentrations.

2.4. Variable Definition

According to the Endocrine Society Clinical Practice Guideline, VD deficiency was defined as 25(OH)D <20 ng/mL [20]. To identify the presence of anemia during pregnancy, we used the anemia criteria from the Centers for Disease Control and Prevention criteria in the United States: <110 g/L in the first trimester, <105 g/L in the second trimester, and <110 g/dL in the third trimester [21]. Gestational age was calculated according to the date of visiting the hospital and conception date (the date of last menstruation and confirmed by B ultrasound). Pre-pregnancy BMI was calculated by dividing the weight in kilograms by the square of height in meters. Considering the duration and intensity of sunshine, we categorized seasons into two groups, summer/autumn (June to November) and winter/spring (December to May). Gravidity was categorized into 1 time, 2 times, 3 times, and ≥ 4 times, and parity was categorized into 0 and ≥ 1 times. Education was categorized into junior high school and below, high school, college, and above. Iron supplementary was categorized into two groups (never, and at least one trimester during pregnancy). The categorical variable was defined as "missing" if there was no response.

2.5. Statistical Analysis

Continuous variables and categorical variables were presented as mean $\pm$ SD and frequency (percentage), respectively. To compare the characteristics between groups, Student's t-test and the Chi-square test were used for continuous variables and categorical variables, respectively. Due to longitudinal repeated measures of Hb during pregnancy, generalized estimating equations (GEE) were used to analyze the association between VD or VD deficiency in each trimester and Hb or anemia during pregnancy after the corresponding 25(OH)D measurement. We also analyzed the interaction between VD and gestational age of Hb measurement on Hb in GEE models. Considering that the iron supplementation could be a key confounder, analyses were further conducted and stratified according to whether iron was supplemented during pregnancy. In addition, the association of VD in each trimester with Hb concentrations in different gestational ages and the association between VD change and Hb change between different trimesters were analyzed using multiple linear regression. Models were adjusted for potential gestational age at Hb measurement, age, gestational age at 25(OH)D measurement, gravidity, parity, season at 25(OH)D measurement, pre-pregnancy BMI, smoking, drinking and tea before pregnancy, sleep quality and physical frequency at trimester of 25(OH)D measurement, weight gain, corresponding baseline Hb, and whether iron was supplementary or not, which were detailed in tables. In GEE models, weight gain was weight at the last Hb test subtracting weight at the corresponding VD measurement, and baseline Hb was defined as the corresponding Hb that detected the nearest VD. In linear models, weight gain was weight at the corresponding Hb test subtracting weight at the corresponding VD measurement, and baseline Hb was defined as the corresponding Hb that detected the nearest VD. The level of $p < 0.05$ was considered statistically significant for all tests in this study. All analyses were performed using R software (version 4.0.2) (http://www.R-project.org accessed on 22 June 2020).

3. Results

Finally, 2962 pregnant women in T1 were included in this study. Of which, 516 pregnant women with data of plasma 25(OH)D and questionnaire in T2 and 293 pregnant women with data of plasma 25(OH)D and questionnaire in T3. In terms of the observation number, there were 4419 observations in T1, 1053 observations in T2, and 337 observations in T3. The prevalence of VD deficiency in T1, T2, and T3 was 65.87%, 48.06%, and 46.42%, respectively. The prevalence of anemia in seven groups (before 14th (n = 2962), 14 to 17th (n = 1156), 18 to 22nd (n = 1058), 23 to 27th (n = 1098), 28 to 31st (n = 696), 32 to 35th (n = 658), and from 36 to 42nd (n = 555) gestational age) was 4.19%, 4.07%, 8.60, 12.39%, 33.33%, 34.65 and 22.70%, respectively. Pregnant women with VD deficiency in T1 had a higher proportion of first pregnancy, nulliparous, drinking before pregnancy, poor sleep quality, 25(OH)D measurement in winter or spring, iron supplementation at T1 and T2 (p < 0.05). Pregnant women with VD deficiency in T1 were younger and had a lower pre-pregnancy BMI, lower Hb, and higher weight gain (p < 0.05) (Table 1).

Table 1. The comparisons of characteristics between pregnant women with and without VD deficiency at T1.

Variables	Vitamin Deficiency at T1		p
	No (n = 1011)	Yes (n = 1951)	
	n (%)		
Gravidity			<0.001
1	406 (40.2)	965 (49.5)	
2	298 (29.5)	496 (25.4)	
3	176 (17.4)	252 (12.9)	
≥4	107 (10.6)	165 (8.5)	
missing	24 (2.4)	73 (3.7)	
Parity			<0.001
0	529 (52.3)	1165 (59.7)	
≥1	301 (29.8)	308 (15.8)	
missing	181 (17.9)	478 (24.5)	
Education			0.5470
Junior high school and below	90 (8.9)	154 (7.9)	
High school	198 (19.6)	364 (18.7)	
College and above	705 (69.7)	1405 (72.0)	
missing	18 (1.8)	28 (1.4)	
Pre-pregnancy smoking			0.0930
No	1006 (99.5)	1927 (98.8)	
Yes	4 (0.4)	23 (1.2)	
missing	1 (0.1)	1 (0.1)	
Pre-pregnancy drinking			0.0190
No	1003 (99.2)	1908 (97.8)	
Yes	5 (0.5)	30 (1.5)	
missing	3 (0.3)	13 (0.7)	
Pre-pregnancy drinking tea			0.3720
No	936 (92.6)	1790 (91.7)	
Yes	71 (7.0)	145 (7.4)	
missing	4 (0.4)	16 (0.8)	
Physical activity frequency at T1			0.2400
Never	859 (85.0)	1654 (84.8)	
<3 times per week	109 (10.8)	236 (12.1)	
≥3 times per week	28 (2.8)	35 (1.8)	
missing	15 (1.5)	26 (1.4)	
Sleep quality at T1			<0.001
Good	214 (21.2)	502 (25.7)	
Normal	774 (76.6)	1352 (69.3)	
Poor	22 (2.2)	94 (4.8)	
missing	1 (0.1)	3 (0.2)	
Season at 25(OH)D measurement			<0.001
summer or autumn	575 (56.9)	726 (37.2)	
winter or spring	436 (43.1)	1225 (62.8)	
Iron supplementary at T1			0.915
No	859 (85.0)	1662 (85.2)	
Yes	152 (15.0)	289 (14.8)	
Iron supplementary at T1 and T2 [†]			0.001
Never	131 (37.2)	382 (47.5)	
At least one trimester	221 (62.8)	422 (52.5)	

Table 1. Cont.

Variables	Vitamin Deficiency at T1		p
	No (n = 1011)	Yes (n = 1951)	
Iron supplementary at T1, T2 an T3 ‡			0.232
Never	58 (29.1)	170 (34.2)	
At least one trimester	141 (70.9)	327 (65.8)	
	Mean ± SD		
Age, year	29.16 ± 3.78	28.39 ± 3.56	<0.001
Pre-pregnancy BMI, kg/m^2	21.33 ± 2.83	21.00 ± 2.80	0.003
Plasma 25(OH)D at T1, ng/L	27.50 ± 7.17	13.38 ± 3.87	<0.001
Gestational age at 25(OH)D measurement, week	11.53 ± 0.89	11.38 ± 0.96	<0.001
Weight gain before HB1, kg	1.30 ± 1.62	1.32 ± 1.84	0.794
Weight gain before HB2, kg	3.35 ± 2.07	3.41 ± 2.12	0.503
Weight gain before HB3, kg	6.08 ± 2.46	6.35 ± 2.65	0.012
Weight gain before HB4, kg	8.27 ± 2.86	8.55 ± 3.13	0.044
Weight gain before HB5, kg	10.43 ± 3.34	10.73 ± 3.49	0.052
Weight gain before HB6, kg	12.17 ± 3.58	12.60 ± 3.64	0.024
HB at T1, g/L	125.96 ± 8.83	125.30 ± 9.06	0.059

HB, hemoglobin; VD, Vitamin D; T1, first trimester; GA, gestational age; HB1, HB of GA from 14 to 17; HB2, HB of GA from 18 to 22; HB3, HB of GA from 23 to 27; HB4, HB of GA from 23 to 27; HB5, HB of GA from 28 to 31; HB6, HB of GA from 36 to 42; † n = 1156; ‡ n = 696; n of HB1 = 1156; n of HB2 = 1058; n of HB3 = 1098; n of HB4 = 696; n of HB5 = 658; n of HB6 = 555.

3.1. Association between Plasma 25(OH)D in Different Trimester and Hemoglobin after Corresponding 25(OH)D Measurement

Due to repeated measurements of Hb during pregnancy, we used GEE models to assess the association of plasma 25(OH)D in each trimester with Hb that was detected during pregnancy but after the corresponding 25(OH)D measurement, respectively. The level of plasma 25(OH)D in T1 (β = 0.06, p = 0.0177), T2 (β = 0.15, p < 0.0001), and T3 (β = 0.12, p = 0.0006) was positively associated with Hb concentrations even if models were adjusted for corresponding confounders, respectively (Table 2). In addition, considering that the association might be different as the gestational age changed, we also created models with the interaction between plasma 25(OH)D in each trimester and the gestational age at the Hb measurement, respectively. Interestingly, we observed that only p for the interaction between plasma 25(OH)D in T1 and gestational age at Hb measurement was statistically significant and revealed that the association of plasma 25(OH)D in T1 with Hb concentrations was positively associated with gestational age (β = 0.005, p = 0.0421). However, no interaction was found between plasma 25(OH)D in T2 (p = 0.2076) or T3 (p = 0.2405) and the gestational age at which Hb was detected after the corresponding 25(OH)D measurement (Table 2).

Iron supplementation may be an important confounding factor. Therefore, we further conducted analyses stratified by whether iron was supplemented or not during pregnancy. As shown in Table 3, we found plasma 25(OH)D in T1 (β = 0.09, p = 0.0016) and T2 (β = 0.17, p < 0.0001) were significantly associated with Hb concentrations that were detected after 25(OH)D measurement among those who received iron supplements during pregnancy. However, the results did not show the interaction between plasma 25(OH)D and iron supplementation. The positive association of plasma 25(OH)D in T3 with Hb concentrations that were detected after the 25(OH)D measurement, and both existed regardless of whether iron supplementation occurred during pregnancy (with iron supplementation, β = 0.08, p = 0.0483; without iron supplementation, β = 0.15, p = 0.0046).

Table 2. The association * between plasma 25(OH)D in different trimesters and hemoglobin during pregnancy after the corresponding 25(OH)D measurement.

Variable	Observation Number	Model 1 β (se)	Model 1 p	Model 2 β (se)	Model 2 p	Model 3 β (se)	Model 3 p
		\multicolumn{6}{c}{Models without interaction}					
25(OH)D in T1 ‡, ng/mL	4419	0.12(0.03)	0.0002	0.08(0.03)	0.0017	0.06(0.03)	0.0177
25(OH)D in T2 ‡, ng/mL	1053	0.17(0.04)	<0.0001	0.16(0.03)	<0.0001	0.15(0.03)	<0.0001
25(OH)D in T3 ‡, ng/mL	337	0.17(0.05)	0.0004	0.12(0.03)	0.0002	0.12(0.03)	0.0006
		\multicolumn{6}{c}{Models with interaction}					
25(OH)D in T1 ‡, ng/mL		−0.01(0.08)	0.9017	−0.05(0.07)	0.4391	−0.07(0.07)	0.2775
GA at Hb measurement, week	4419	−0.23(0.05)	<0.0001	−0.18(0.06)	0.0043	−0.19(0.06)	0.0027
Interaction †		0.005(0.003)	0.0696	0.005(0.003)	0.0464	0.005(0.003)	0.0421
25(OH)D in T2 ‡, ng/mL		−0.05(0.18)	0.7862	−0.07(0.18)	0.7069	−0.07(0.18)	0.6904
GA at Hb measurement, week	1053	0.11(0.15)	0.4503	0.24(0.16)	0.1276	0.25(0.16)	0.1151
Interaction†		0.01(0.01)	0.2314	0.01(0.01)	0.1988	0.01(0.01)	0.2076
25(OH)D in T3 ‡, ng/mL		−0.24(0.31)	0.4366	−0.65(0.50)	0.1914	−1.11(1.05)	0.2929
GA at Hb measurement, week	337	−0.27(0.46)	0.5543	−0.70(0.72)	0.3310	−1.31(1.58)	0.4093
Interaction †		0.01(0.01)	0.1635	0.02(0.01)	0.1122	0.03(0.03)	0.2405

HB, hemoglobin; T1, first trimester; T2, second trimester; T3, third trimester; GA, gestational age. * Analyzed by GEE model; ‡ T1, T2, and T3 were in different models, respectively. † Interaction between VD in each trimester and GA at Hb measurement, respectively. Model 1 was adjusted for GA at HB measurement. Model 2 was adjusted for gestational age at HB measurement, age, gestational age at 25(OH)D measurement, gravidity, parity, season at 25(OH)D measurement, pre-pregnancy BMI, smoking, drinking and tea before pregnancy, sleep quality and physical frequency at trimester of 25(OH)D measurement, weight gain, and corresponding baseline Hb. Model 3 was further adjusted for iron supplementation during pregnancy.

Table 3. The association * between 25(OH)D in different trimester and hemoglobin during pregnancy after corresponding 25(OH)D measurement, stratified by whether iron was supplementary during pregnancy or not.

Variable	Iron Supplementary during Pregnancy — No β (se)	No p	Iron Supplementary during Pregnancy — Yes β (se)	Yes p	p for Interaction
T1 ‡	observation number = 1479		observation number = 2940		
25(OH)D, ng/mL	0.05(0.05)	0.3587	0.09(0.03)	0.0016	0.3140
T2 ‡	observation number = 314		observation number = 759		
25(OH)D, ng/mL	0.09(0.07)	0.2361	0.17(0.03)	<0.0001	0.6991
T3 ‡	observation number = 111		observation number = 226		
25(OH)D, ng/mL	0.15(0.05)	0.0046	0.08(0.04)	0.0486	0.30732

HB, hemoglobin; T1, first trimester; T2, second trimester; T3, third trimester; GA, gestational age. * Analyzed by GEE model; ‡ T1, T2, and T3 were in different models, respectively. Model was adjusted for gestational age at HB measurement, age, gestational age at 25(OH)D measurement, gravidity, parity, season at 25(OH)D measurement, pre-pregnancy BMI, smoking, drinking and tea before pregnancy, sleep quality, and physical frequency at trimester of 25(OH)D measurement, weight gain, and corresponding baseline Hb.

3.2. Association between VD Deficiency in Different Trimester and Anemia after Corresponding 25(OH)D Measurement

Considering the clinical significance, we analyzed the relationship between VD deficiency and anemia. Compared to pregnant women without VD deficiency in T1, pregnant women with VD deficiency in T1 were associated with a higher risk for anemia after the 25(OH)D measurement (OR = 1.42, 95% CI: 1.07–1.88) (Table 4). Similar results of the association between VD deficiency in T2 and anemia were revealed (OR = 1.94, 95% CI: 1.30–2.89) (Table 4). Consistent with the association between plasma 25(OH)D and Hb, we only found that VD deficiency in T1 (OR = 1.68, 95% CI: 1.20–2.34) and T2 (OR = 2.02, 95% CI: 1.27–3.22) was significantly associated with a higher risk for anemia after the 25(OH)D measurement among those who received iron supplements during pregnancy (Table 5).

However, no significant association between VD deficiency in T3 and anemia was observed among the women with or without iron supplementation (Tables 4 and 5).

Table 4. The association * between VD deficiency in different trimesters and anemia during pregnancy after the corresponding 25(OH)D measurement.

VD Deficiency	Anemia after VD Measurement, Observation Number (%)		Model 1		Model 2		Model 3	
	No	Yes	OR (95% CI)	p	OR (95% CI)	p	OR (95% CI)	p
T1 ‡								
No	1097 (84.2)	206 (15.8)	ref.	-	ref.	-	ref.	-
Yes	2452 (78.7)	664 (21.3)	1.54 (1.16–2.04)	0.0025	1.54 (1.16–2.04)	0.0025	1.42 (1.07–1.88)	0.0167
T2 ‡								
No	398 (75.8)	127 (24.2)	ref.	-	ref.	-	ref.	-
Yes	328 (62.1)	200 (37.9)	1.97 (1.38–2.80)	0.0002	1.93 (1.31–2.85)	0.0010	1.94 (1.30–2.89)	0.0011
T3 ‡								
No	157 (82.2)	34 (17.8)	ref.	-	ref.	-	ref.	-
Yes	103 (70.5)	43 (29.5)	1.13 (1.03–1.24)	0.0109	1.05 (0.96–1.14)	0.2650	1.06 (0.97–1.15)	0.2123

HB, hemoglobin; VD, Vitamin D; T1, first trimester; T2, second trimester; T3, third trimester; GA, gestational age. * Analyzed by GEE model; ‡ T1, T2, and T3 were in different models, respectively. Model 1 was adjusted for GA at HB measurement. Model 2 was adjusted for gestational age at HB measurement, age, gestational age at 25(OH)D measurement, gravidity, parity, season at 25(OH)D measurement, pre-pregnancy BMI, smoking, drinking and tea before pregnancy, sleep quality and physical frequency at trimester of 25(OH)D measurement, weight gain, and corresponding baseline Hb. Model 3 was further adjusted for iron supplementation during pregnancy.

Table 5. The association * between VD deficiency in different trimesters and anemia during pregnancy after the corresponding 25(OH)D measurement, stratified by whether iron was supplementary during pregnancy or not.

VD Deficiency	Iron Supplementary during Pregnancy			
	No		Yes	
	OR (95% CI)	p	OR (95% CI)	p
T1 ‡				
No	ref.	-	ref.	-
Yes	1.22 (0.70–2.12)	0.4765	1.68 (1.20–2.34)	0.0024
T2 ‡				
No	ref.	-	ref.	-
Yes	1.14 (0.58–2.25)	0.6981	2.02 (1.27–3.22)	0.0032
T3 ‡				
No	ref.	-	ref.	-
Yes	1.44 (0.38–5.47)	0.5917	0.84 (0.23–3.09)	0.7948

HB, hemoglobin; VD, Vitamin D; T1, first trimester; T2, second trimester; T3, third trimester; GA, gestational age. * Analyzed by GEE model; ‡ T1, T2, and T3 were in different models, respectively. Model was adjusted for gestational age at HB measurement, age, gestational age at 25(OH)D measurement, gravidity, parity, season at 25(OH)D measurement, pre-pregnancy BMI, smoking, drinking and tea before pregnancy, sleep quality, and physical activity frequency at trimester of 25(OH)D measurement, weight gain, and corresponding baseline Hb.

3.3. Association between Plasma 25(OH)D in Different Trimester and Hb in Different Gestational Age after Corresponding 25(OH)D Measurement

In order to further evaluate whether the association of plasma 25(OH)D in different trimesters and Hb concentrations became stronger or not as the gestational age increased, we assessed the association between plasma 25(OH)D in different trimesters and Hb in different gestational ages, respectively. When only adjusted for gestational age at Hb measurement in model 1, the effects of VD per ng/mL in T1 on Hb of gestational age from 14th to 42nd week ranged from 0.02 to 0.17 g/L. After adjustment for corresponding confounders, the relationship that increased with gestational age became less obvious. However, in model 4, when we adjusted for the variables in model 3 but Hb in T1 was instead of baseline Hb, a similar trend to model 1 was observed (Table 6). Consistent with the results of GEE models, we failed to find the changing trend of the association between plasma 25(OH)D in T2 and Hb from 28th to 42nd gestational age or plasma 25(OH)D in T3 and Hb (Supplementary Table S1). When stratified by iron supplementation during pregnancy, the positive associations between plasma 25(OH)D in different trimesters and Hb concentrations in different gestational ages were only observed among those who received iron supplements during pregnancy (Supplementary Table S2).

Table 6. The association between 25(OH)D in the first trimester and hemoglobin in different gestational ages.

Hemoglobin, g/L	n	Model 1 β (se)	p	Model 2 β (se)	p	Model 3 β (se)	p	Model 4 β (se)	p
HB at T1 *	2962	0.17 (0.05)	0.0002	0.06 (0.02)	0.0023	0.06 (0.02)	0.0021	0.06 (0.02)	0.0021
HB of GA from 14 to 17 †	1156	0.02 (0.03)	0.5170	−0.01 (0.02)	0.6885	−0.01 (0.02)	0.5556	−0.01 (0.02)	0.5556
HB of GA from 18 to 22 †	1058	0.06 (0.03)	0.0651	0.04 (0.02)	0.0604	0.04 (0.02)	0.0722	0.02 (0.03)	0.3772
HB of GA from 23 to 27 †	1098	0.10 (0.03)	0.0008	0.04 (0.02)	0.0704	0.04 (0.02)	0.1293	0.04 (0.03)	0.1201
HB of GA from 28 to 31 ‡	696	0.14 (0.04)	0.0005	0.07 (0.03)	0.0158	0.06 (0.03)	0.0622	0.07 (0.04)	0.0627
HB of GA from 32 to 35 ‡	658	0.15 (0.04)	0.0004	0.06 (0.03)	0.0675	0.05 (0.03)	0.1273	0.11 (0.04)	0.0105
HB of GA from 36 to 42 ‡	555	0.17 (0.35)	<0.0001	0.08 (0.03)	0.0245	0.06 (0.03)	0.0916	0.14 (0.05)	0.0036

HB, hemoglobin; T1, first trimester; T2, second trimester; T3, third trimester; GA, gestational age. Model 1 was adjusted for GA at HB measurement. Model 2 was adjusted for age, gestational age at 25(OH)D measurement, gravidity, parity, season at 25(OH)D measurement, pre-pregnancy BMI, smoking, drinking, and tea before pregnancy, sleep quality and physical activity frequency at T1, gestational age and weight gain at the corresponding gestational age of HB measurement and baseline Hb. Model 3 * was further adjusted for iron Supplementary at T1; Model 3 † was further adjusted for iron Supplementary from T1 to T2; Model 3 ‡ was further adjusted for iron Supplementary from T1 to T3. Model 4 was adjusted for the variables in Model 3, but baseline Hb was Hb in T1.

3.4. Association between Plasma 25(OH)D Change and Hemoglobin Change between Different Trimesters

In addition, we also analyzed the association of the plasma 25(OH)D change with hemoglobin change between different trimesters to further confirm the association between plasma 25(OH)D and Hb. The results are shown in Table 7. The change of 25(OH)D from T1 to T2 had no association with the change of Hb from T1 to T2 ($\beta = -0.00$, $p = 0.9225$). However, the change of plasma 25(OH)D from T1 to T3 was positively associated with the change of Hb from T1 to T3 ($\beta = 0.15$, $p = 0.0027$), and the change of plasma 25(OH)D from T2 to T3 was positively associated with the change of Hb from T2 to T3 ($\beta = 0.13$, $p = 0.0312$).

Table 7. The association between plasma 25(OH)D change and hemoglobin change between different trimesters.

25(OH)D Change, ng/mL	n	Crude Model β (se)	p	Model 2 β (se)	p	Model 3 β (se)	p
From T1 to T2				HB change from T1 to T2 †, g/L			
	516	−0.09 (0.03)	0.0013	−0.03 (0.03)	0.3813	−0.00 (0.03)	0.9225
				HB change from T2 to T3 ‡, g/L			
	273	0.15 (0.06)	0.0070	0.15 (0.05)	0.0040	0.11 (0.05)	0.0430
From T2 to T3				HB change from T2 to T3 ‡, g/L			
	216	0.05 (0.06)	0.4253	0.15 (0.06)	0.0153	0.13 (0.06)	0.0312
From T1 to T3				HB change from T1 to T3 ‡, g/L			
	293	0.00 (0.05)	0.9189	0.17 (0.05)	0.0008	0.15 (0.05)	0.0027

HB, hemoglobin; T1, first trimester; T2, second trimester; T3, third trimester; GA, gestational age. Model 2 was adjusted for age, gestational age at later 25(OH)D measurement, gravidity, parity, season at later 25(OH)D measurement, pre-pregnancy BMI, smoking, drinking, and tea before pregnancy, sleep quality and physical activity frequency at later GA, change of gestational age and weight gain at the corresponding gestational age of HB measurement, corresponding baseline HB and 25(OH)D. Model 3 † was further adjusted for iron Supplementary from T1 to T2; Model 3 ‡ was further adjusted for iron supplementation from T1 to T3.

4. Discussion

In the present study, the levels of plasma 25(OH)D in T1, T2, and T3 were positively associated with Hb concentrations after the 25(OH)D measurement and the association of plasma 25(OH)D in T1 and Hb concentration became stronger as the gestational age increased. Meanwhile, pregnant women with VD deficiency in T1 or T2 had an increased risk of anemia, respectively, compared with those without VD deficiency. However, the significant relationship between VD and Hb was only observed among those with iron supplementation during pregnancy.

Some previous studies have reported that pregnant women with VD deficiency had a significantly higher risk of anemia, but in their studies, only one or two measurements of 25(OH)D were conducted [22–26]. However, in our study, we measured 25(OH)D at three trimesters, respectively; meanwhile, we also found that 25(OH)D in T1, T2, and T3 were positively correlated with Hb, respectively. VD deficiency in T1 or T2 was associated with an increased risk of anemia. The finding, that the change of plasma 25(OH)D from T1 to T3 was positively associated with the change of Hb from T1 to T3, further increased the evidence of the relationship between VD and Hb. Thomas et al. [25] found that it could be partly explained by the mediation of erythropoietin, which was recognized in hemodialysis patients clinically [16]. Moreover, VD deficiency might also stimulate immune cells in the bone marrow microenvironment to produce cytokines, resulting in impaired red blood cell production [15]. In addition, hepcidin was also recognized as a key role in the association between VD and Hb. Increased hepcidin could inhibit enterocytes to absorb iron and lead to anemia, but VD could suppress the expression of hepcidin mRNA and enhance iron absorption by regulating the iron-hepcidin-ferroportin axis in monocytes [14,17]. However, one RCT from England reported that VD supplementation (1000 IU/day) from the first trimester had no effect on hepcidin in the third trimester [27]. There were also some studies that found no association between VD deficiency and anemia. One cross-sectional study in Sudan that enrolled 180 pregnant women found no correlation between serum 25(OH)D and Hb level ($r = 0.001$, $p = 0.999$) [28]. Another two cross-sectional studies in Bangladesh and Brazil used VD deficiency as an outcome and also found no association between them [10,29]. We summarized and speculated the reasons for the inconsistent results in the following aspects. First, these three studies were all cross-sectional studies with small sample sizes. Second, the relationship between VD deficiency and anemia was not the main objective of these studies and two of them took VD deficiency as the outcome in statistical models, with the latter results in the low statistical power. Third, the association between VD and anemia could be different in different trimesters. Fourth, they did not consider iron supplementation during pregnancy. In our study, it also could not be ignored that we failed to reveal the statistically significant association between VD deficiency in T3 and anemia after the VD measurement. Perhaps because of the short time interval, the effect of VD on Hb had not been fully shown. As we discovered, the association of plasma 25(OH)D in T1 and Hb became stronger as the gestational age increased. When we adjusted for potential confounders and Hb in T1, a similar trend was observed. To our knowledge, no previous study reported similar results. However, one study found a 6.97-fold increased risk of anemia at delivery in women with vitamin D deficiency [25], which was far stronger than the association between VD deficiency and anemia during pregnancy in previous studies [22,23,26] and the present study. A previous study showed that 25(OH)D3 reached a plateau in the third month in the vitamin D3 supplement group, which indicates that VD supplementation takes more than three months to have the maximal effect [30]. We also found that after adjustment for Hb in T1 (<14 gestational weeks), 25(OH)D in T1 was significantly and positively associated with Hb after 32 gestational weeks rather than that within 32 gestational weeks; furthermore, the dose-response effect of 25(OH)D in T1 and Hb measured in various gestational weeks was observed (Table 6). The time intervals between the VD measurements in T2 or T3 and Hb measurement after corresponding VD measurements were shorter than 3 months. The dose-response effect of 25(OH)D and Hb was not observed. Furthermore, for further demonstrating the dose-response effect between

25(OH)D and Hb, we evaluated the associations between 25(OH)D change and hemoglobin change between different trimesters (Table 7). We also found that the changes in VD level from T1 to T2 had a significant association with the change of Hb from T2 to T3 rather than from T1 to T2. More studies should be conducted to confirm these findings. When we further considered the influence of iron supplementation, we only found a significant correlation between VD and Hb or VD deficiency and anemia in women with iron supplementation during pregnancy. The possible reason partly resulted from the fact that VD might increase Hb by decreasing hepcidin and increasing iron absorption. When iron supplementation was present, it might provide a source for VD to promote iron absorption.

Strengths and Limitations

Our study has some strengths. First, most previous studies focused on plasma 25(OH)D concentration and Hb concentration in a single trimester, but in this study, we evaluated the association between VD in each trimester and Hb at different gestational ages during the whole pregnancy. Meanwhile, we also explored the interaction between plasma 25(OH)D and the gestational age of Hb measurements on Hb levels in GEE models. Second, the association between the change of VD and the change of Hb was also examined to further explore the association. Third, considering the influence of iron supplementation, we also conducted a stratified analysis according to the iron supplementation variable. In addition, we also considered sleep quality, physical activity quality, and several other variables as potential confounders to improve the reliability of results. However, several limitations should be mentioned. First, ferritin, transferrin, etc., were not detected, and we could not distinguish between iron deficiency or anemia. Second, we only adjusted iron supplementation during pregnancy in the model and conducted a stratified analysis, but we did not access the frequency and amount of iron supplementation. Third, the diagnosis criteria of anemia from the Centers for Disease Control and Prevention criteria in the United States were changed across gestational trimesters, such as <110 g/L in the first trimester, <105 g/L in the second trimester, and <110 g/dL in the third trimester, and it may introduce the bias. However, other some studies have used Hb concentration below 110 g/L as the diagnosis criteria for anemia. However, Breymann [31] et al. thought that any Hb below 105 g/L could be regarded as true anemia. Fourth, parathyroid hormone and fibroblast growth factor 23 might have a damaging effect on iron metabolism and confound the association between VD and iron circulation and anemia [32], but they were not measured in our study.

5. Conclusions

In conclusion, the plasma 25(OH)D concentration in each trimester was positively associated with Hb concentration, and the association of plasma 25(OH)D in T1 and Hb became stronger and stronger as the gestational age increased. Iron supplementation might be an important factor affecting the relationship between VD and Hb. Both VD deficiency and anemia are very common among pregnant women. This finding indicates that VD supplementation before conception or early T1 not only improves VD deficiency but is also beneficial for the prevention of anemia, especially in pregnant women with iron supplementation. More studies are warranted to determine the association and mechanisms between VD and Hb.

Supplementary Materials: The following supporting information can be downloaded at: https://www.mdpi.com/article/10.3390/nu14122455/s1, Supplementary Table S1. The association between 25(OH)D in the second and third trimester and hemoglobin in different gestational ages, respectively; Supplementary Table S2. The association between 25(OH)D in different trimesters and hemoglobin in different gestational ages were stratified by whether iron was supplementary during pregnancy or not.

Author Contributions: Conceptualization, Y.Y.; Methodology, Y.Z. and P.C.; Validation, Z.P.; Resources, H.C.; Formal Analysis, S.S.; Investigation, X.A.; Writing—original draft, S.S.; Writing—

Review and Editing, Y.Y.; Visualization, H.Z. and M.M. All authors have read and agreed to the published version of the manuscript.

Funding: This study was funded by the Chinese National Natural Science Foundation (81973055), the National Key Research and Development Program of China (No. 2021YFC2701901), Major research and development projects of Zhejiang Science and Technology Department (2018C03010), Key Laboratory of Intelligent Preventive Medicine of Zhejiang Province (2020E10004) and Leading Innovative and Entrepreneur Team Introduction Program of Zhejiang (2019R01007).

Institutional Review Board Statement: The study was conducted according to the guidelines of the Declaration of Helsinki and approved by the institutional review board of Zhejiang University School of Medicine (No. 2011-1-005).

Informed Consent Statement: Written informed consent was obtained from all participants included in the study.

Data Availability Statement: The data presented in this study are available on request from the corresponding author. The data are not publicly available because they contain information that could compromise the privacy of research participants.

Acknowledgments: We thank all pregnant women who participated in this study. We acknowledge the support from Zhoushan Maternal and Child Care Hospital and fellows there who conducted and managed the cohort.

Conflicts of Interest: The authors declare no conflict of interest.

References

1. Stevens, G.A.; Paciorek, C.J.; Flores-Urrutia, M.C.; Borghi, E.; Namaste, S.; Wirth, J.P.; Suchdev, P.S.; Ezzati, M.; Rohner, F.; Flaxman, S.R.; et al. National, regional, and global estimates of anaemia by severity in women and children for 2000-19: A pooled analysis of population-representative data. *Lancet Glob. Health* **2022**, *10*, e627–e639. [CrossRef]
2. Lin, L.; Wei, Y.; Zhu, W.; Wang, C.; Su, R.; Feng, H.; Yang, H.; on behalf of the Gestational Diabetes Mellitus Prevalence Survey (GPS) Study Group. Prevalence, risk factors and associated adverse pregnancy outcomes of anaemia in Chinese pregnant women: A multicentre retrospective study. *BMC Pregnancy Childbirth* **2018**, *18*, 111. [CrossRef] [PubMed]
3. Wu, Y.; Ye, H.; Liu, J.; Ma, Q.; Yuan, Y.; Pang, Q.; Liu, J.; Kong, C.; Liu, M. Prevalence of anemia and sociodemographic characteristics among pregnant and non-pregnant women in southwest China: A longitudinal observational study. *BMC Pregnancy Childbirth* **2020**, *20*, 535. [CrossRef] [PubMed]
4. Xu, X.; Liu, S.; Rao, Y.; Shi, Z.; Wang, L.; Sharma, M.; Zhao, Y. Prevalence and Sociodemographic and Lifestyle Determinants of Anemia during Pregnancy: A Cross-Sectional Study of Pregnant Women in China. *Int. J. Environ. Res. Public Health* **2016**, *13*, 908. [CrossRef] [PubMed]
5. Zhao, S.Y.; Jing, W.Z.; Liu, J.; Liu, M. Prevalence of anemia during pregnancy in China, 2012–2016: A Meta-analysis. *Zhonghua Yu Fang Yi Xue Za Zhi* **2018**, *52*, 951–957. [CrossRef]
6. Jacobson, D.L.; Neri, D.; Gaskins, A.; Yee, L.; Mendez, A.J.; Hendricks, K.; Siminski, S.; Zash, R.; Hyzy, L.; Jao, J.; et al. Maternal anemia and preterm birth among women living with HIV in the United States. *Am. J. Clin. Nutr.* **2021**, *113*, 1402–1410. [CrossRef]
7. Rahman, M.M.; Abe, S.K.; Rahman, M.S.; Kanda, M.; Narita, S.; Bilano, V.; Ota, E.; Gilmour, S.; Shibuya, K. Maternal anemia and risk of adverse birth and health outcomes in low- and middle-income countries: Systematic review and meta-analysis. *Am. J. Clin. Nutr.* **2016**, *103*, 495–504. [CrossRef]
8. Hossein-nezhad, A.; Holick, M.F. Vitamin D for health: A global perspective. *Mayo Clin. Proc.* **2013**, *88*, 720–755. [CrossRef]
9. Yun, C.; Chen, J.; He, Y.; Mao, D.; Wang, R.; Zhang, Y.; Yang, C.; Piao, J.; Yang, X. Vitamin D deficiency prevalence and risk factors among pregnant Chinese women. *Public Health Nutr.* **2017**, *20*, 1746–1754. [CrossRef]
10. Ahmed, F.; Khosravi-Boroujeni, H.; Khan, M.R.; Roy, A.K.; Raqib, R. Prevalence and Predictors of Vitamin D Deficiency and Insufficiency among Pregnant Rural Women in Bangladesh. *Nutrients* **2021**, *13*, 449. [CrossRef]
11. Liu, T.; Zhong, S.; Liu, L.; Liu, S.; Li, X.; Zhou, T.; Zhang, J. Vitamin D deficiency and the risk of anemia: A meta-analysis of observational studies. *Ren. Fail.* **2015**, *37*, 929–934. [CrossRef] [PubMed]
12. Smith, E.M.; Tangpricha, V. Vitamin D and anemia: Insights into an emerging association. *Curr. Opin. Endocrinol. Diabetes Obes.* **2015**, *22*, 432–438. [CrossRef] [PubMed]
13. Syed, S.; Michalski, E.S.; Tangpricha, V.; Chesdachai, S.; Kumar, A.; Prince, J.; Ziegler, T.R.; Suchdev, P.S.; Kugathasan, S. Vitamin D Status Is Associated with Hepcidin and Hemoglobin Concentrations in Children with Inflammatory Bowel Disease. *Inflamm. Bowel Dis.* **2017**, *23*, 1650–1658. [CrossRef] [PubMed]
14. Bacchetta, J.; Zaritsky, J.J.; Sea, J.L.; Chun, R.F.; Lisse, T.S.; Zavala, K.; Nayak, A.; Wesseling-Perry, K.; Westerman, M.; Hollis, B.W.; et al. Suppression of iron-regulatory hepcidin by vitamin D. *J. Am. Soc. Nephrol.* **2014**, *25*, 564–572. [CrossRef] [PubMed]

15. Icardi, A.; Paoletti, E.; De Nicola, L.; Mazzaferro, S.; Russo, R.; Cozzolino, M. Renal anaemia and EPO hyporesponsiveness associated with vitamin D deficiency: The potential role of inflammation. *Nephrol. Dial. Transplant.* **2013**, *28*, 1672–1679. [CrossRef] [PubMed]
16. Kumar, V.A.; Kujubu, D.A.; Sim, J.J.; Rasgon, S.A.; Yang, P.S. Vitamin D supplementation and recombinant human erythropoietin utilization in vitamin D-deficient hemodialysis patients. *J. Nephrol.* **2011**, *24*, 98–105. [CrossRef]
17. Stallhofer, J.; Veith, L.; Diegelmann, J.; Probst, P.; Brand, S.; Schnitzler, F.; Olszak, T.; Torok, H.; Mayerle, J.; Stallmach, A.; et al. Iron Deficiency in Inflammatory Bowel Disease Is Associated with Low Levels of Vitamin D Modulating Serum Hepcidin and Intestinal Ceruloplasmin Expression. *Clin. Transl. Gastroenterol.* **2022**, *13*, e00450. [CrossRef]
18. Lima, M.S.; Pereira, M.; Castro, C.T.; Santos, D.B. Vitamin D deficiency and anemia in pregnant women: A systematic review and meta-analysis. *Nutr. Rev.* **2022**, *80*, 428–438. [CrossRef]
19. Shen, Y.; Pu, L.; Si, S.; Xin, X.; Mo, M.; Shao, B.; Wu, J.; Huang, M.; Wang, S.; Muyiduli, X.; et al. Vitamin D nutrient status during pregnancy and its influencing factors. *Clin. Nutr.* **2020**, *39*, 1432–1439. [CrossRef]
20. Holick, M.F.; Binkley, N.C.; Bischoff-Ferrari, H.A.; Gordon, C.M.; Hanley, D.A.; Heaney, R.P.; Murad, M.H.; Weaver, C.M.; Endocrine, S. Evaluation, treatment, and prevention of vitamin D deficiency: An Endocrine Society clinical practice guideline. *J. Clin. Endocrinol. Metab.* **2011**, *96*, 1911–1930. [CrossRef]
21. Centers for Disease Control and Prevention. Recommendations to prevent and control iron deficiency in the United States. Centers for Disease Control and Prevention. *MMWR Recomm. Rep.* **1998**, *47*, 1–29.
22. Bener, A.; Al-Hamaq, A.O.; Saleh, N.M. Association between vitamin D insufficiency and adverse pregnancy outcome: Global comparisons. *Int. J. Womens Health* **2013**, *5*, 523–531. [CrossRef] [PubMed]
23. Finkelstein, J.L.; Mehta, S.; Duggan, C.P.; Spiegelman, D.; Aboud, S.; Kupka, R.; Msamanga, G.I.; Fawzi, W.W. Predictors of anaemia and iron deficiency in HIV-infected pregnant women in Tanzania: A potential role for vitamin D and parasitic infections. *Public Health Nutr.* **2012**, *15*, 928–937. [CrossRef]
24. Takaoka, N.; Nishida, K.; Sairenchi, T.; Umesawa, M.; Noguchi, R.; Someya, K.; Kobashi, G. Changes in vitamin D status considering hemodilution factors in Japanese pregnant women according to trimester: A longitudinal survey. *PLoS ONE* **2020**, *15*, e0239954. [CrossRef] [PubMed]
25. Thomas, C.E.; Guillet, R.; Queenan, R.A.; Cooper, E.M.; Kent, T.R.; Pressman, E.K.; Vermeylen, F.M.; Roberson, M.S.; O'Brien, K.O. Vitamin D status is inversely associated with anemia and serum erythropoietin during pregnancy. *Am. J. Clin. Nutr.* **2015**, *102*, 1088–1095. [CrossRef] [PubMed]
26. Yuan, Y.; Cai, Z.; Dai, Y.; Hong, Q.; Wang, X.; Zhu, L.; Xu, P.; You, L.; Wang, X.; Ji, C.; et al. Association of Maternal Serum 25-Hydroxyvitamin D Concentrations with Risk of Gestational Anemia. *Cell. Physiol. Biochem.* **2017**, *43*, 1526–1532. [CrossRef]
27. Braithwaite, V.S.; Crozier, S.R.; D'Angelo, S.; Prentice, A.; Cooper, C.; Harvey, N.C.; Jones, K.S.; Group, M.T. The Effect of Vitamin D Supplementation on Hepcidin, Iron Status, and Inflammation in Pregnant Women in the United Kingdom. *Nutrients* **2019**, *11*, 190. [CrossRef]
28. Gaffer, A.A.; Rayis, D.A.; Elhussein, O.G.; Adam, I. Vitamin D status in Sudanese pregnant women: A cross-sectional study. *Trans. R. Soc. Trop. Med. Hyg.* **2019**, *113*, 569–571. [CrossRef]
29. Pereira-Santos, M.; Queiroz Carvalho, G.; David Couto, R.; Barbosa Dos Santos, D.; Marlucia Oliveira, A. Vitamin D deficiency and associated factors among pregnant women of a sunny city in Northeast of Brazil. *Clin. Nutr. ESPEN* **2018**, *23*, 240–244. [CrossRef]
30. Best, C.M.; Riley, D.V.; Laha, T.J.; Pflaum, H.; Zelnick, L.R.; Hsu, S.; Thummel, K.E.; Foster-Schubert, K.E.; Kuzma, J.N.; Cromer, G.; et al. Vitamin D in human serum and adipose tissue after supplementation. *Am. J. Clin. Nutr.* **2020**, *113*, 83–91. [CrossRef]
31. Breymann, C. Iron Deficiency Anemia in Pregnancy. *Semin. Hematol.* **2015**, *52*, 339–347. [CrossRef] [PubMed]
32. Arabi, S.M.; Ranjbar, G.; Bahrami, L.S.; Vafa, M.; Norouzy, A. The effect of vitamin D supplementation on hemoglobin concentration: A systematic review and meta-analysis. *Nutr. J.* **2020**, *19*, 11. [CrossRef] [PubMed]

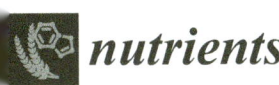

Article

The Association of Vitamin D and Its Pathway Genes' Polymorphisms with Hypertensive Disorders of Pregnancy: A Prospective Cohort Study

Shuting Si [1,2,†], Minjia Mo [1,2,†], Haoyue Cheng [1,2], Zhicheng Peng [1,2], Xialidan Alifu [1,2], Haibo Zhou [1,2], Peihan Chi [1,2], Yan Zhuang [1,2] and Yunxian Yu [1,2,*]

1. Department of Public Health, and Department of Anesthesiology, Second Affiliated Hospital of Zhejiang University School of Medicine, Hangzhou 310058, China; 21818499@zju.edu.cn (S.S.); minjiamo@zju.edu.cn (M.M.); 3150101365@zju.edu.cn (H.C.); 22018678@zju.edu.cn (Z.P.); 3130100017@zju.edu.cn (X.A.); 11918158@zju.edu.cn (H.Z.); 22118872@zju.edu.cn (P.C.); yanzhuang@zju.edu.cn (Y.Z.)
2. Department of Epidemiology & Health Statistics, School of Public Health, School of Medicine, Zhejiang University, Hangzhou 310058, China
* Correspondence: yunxianyu@zju.edu.cn; Tel.: +86-571-8820-8191
† These authors contributed equally to this work.

Abstract: **Objective:** We aimed to explore the effect of single nucleotide polymorphism (SNP) in the genes of the vitamin D (VitD) metabolic pathway and its interaction with VitD level during pregnancy on the development of hypertensive disorders of pregnancy (HDP). **Methods:** The study was conducted in the Zhoushan Maternal and Child Health Care Hospital, China, from August 2011 to May 2018. The SNPs in VitD metabolic pathway-related genes were genotyped. Plasma 25-hydroxyvitamin vitamin D (25(OH)D) levels was measured at first (T1), second (T2), and third (T3) trimesters. The information of systolic blood pressure (SBP) and diastolic blood pressure (DBP), and the diagnosis of HDP were extracted from the electronic medical record system. Multivariable linear and logistic regression models and crossover analysis were applied. **Results:** The prospective cohort study included 3699 pregnant women, of which 105 (2.85%) were diagnosed with HDP. After adjusting for potential confounders, VitD deficiency at T2, as well as the change of 25(OH)D level between T1 and T2, were negatively associated with DBP at T2 and T3, but not HDP. Polymorphisms in *CYP24A1*, *GC*, and *LRP2* genes were associated with blood pressure and HDP. In addition, VitD interacted with *CYP24A1*, *GC*, and *VDR* genes' polymorphisms on blood pressure. Furthermore, participants with polymorphisms in *CYP24A1*-rs2248137, *LRP2*-rs2389557, and *LRP2*-rs4667591 and who had VitD deficiency at T2 showed an increased risk of HDP. **Conclusions:** The individual and interactive association between VitD deficiency during pregnancy and SNPs in the genes of the VitD metabolic pathway on blood pressure and HDP were identified.

Keywords: vitamin D; SNPs; hypertensive disorders of pregnancy; prospective cohort study

1. Introduction

Hypertensive disorders of pregnancy (HDP), including gestational hypertension, preeclampsia, eclampsia, pregnancy complicated with chronic hypertension, and chronic hypertension complicated with preeclampsia [1], accounted for nearly 18% of all maternal deaths worldwide [2]. Its increasing prevalence and related risks for maternal and child health as well as cardiovascular diseases later in life has garnered great attention in the field of public health [3,4]. The risk factors for HDP are advanced age, primipara, multiple pregnancy, family history of hypertension, high pre-pregnancy body mass index (BMI), and high basal blood pressure [5].

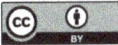

Approximately 5% to 7% of pregnancies are complicated by preeclampsia [6]. While the cause of preeclampsia is not fully discerned, previous studies have suggested that abnormal placentation and angiogenesis were central to the pathogenesis of this syndrome [6]. In recent years, growing evidence of the association between maternal hypovitaminosis D and increased risk of HDP has been suggested [7,8]. Compared to non-pregnant state, there are significant changes in vitamin D (VitD) metabolism during pregnancy, and the serum levels of VitD binding protein (VDBP) [9], as well as the active form, 1,25-dihydroxyvitamin (1,25(OH)$_2$D) [10], increased notably. It is believed that not only the kidneys but also the placenta and decidua produce and secret 1,25(OH)$_2$D during pregnancy [11]. Moreover, VitD receptors and related metabolic enzymes have been discovered in the placenta and decidua [12], indicating a potential role for VitD in implantation and placental function, outside of its well-established role in skeletal health [13].

To date, trial evidence appears insufficient to lean towards a protective effect of VitD supplementation during pregnancy against the risk of preeclampsia owing to small sample size or low study quality [14,15]. In addition, findings from observational studies in regard to the association between maternal VitD status and HDP are discrepant due to the large heterogeneity between study designs, lack of adherence to standardized outcome definitions, and different gestational weeks of VitD detection [8,16]. On the other hand, genetic variants in the VitD metabolic pathway have also been shown to participate in the pathogenesis of blood pressure increase and preeclampsia [8,17], which suggests a possible interaction between VitD and its pathway gene variants for HDP. The concentration or effect of VitD can be highly regulated due to the variation of key protein expression or activity. 25(OH)D is the main circulating metabolism and is considered the biological marker of VitD status. The main metabolic enzymes involved in the synthesis, transport, reabsorption, and inactivation of VitD include 25-hydroxylase (*CYP3A4*), 1-hydroxylase (*CYP27B1*), vitamin D-binding protein (*GC*), 24-hydroxylas and metaling (*LRP2*), and 24-hydroxylase (*CYP24A1*). Moreover, VitD receptor (*VDR*) regulates VitD metabolism through binding 1,25(OH)$_2$D [18].

So far, most studies have only focused on the relationship between VitD status during pregnancy or gene variation in the VitD metabolic pathway and HDP, without considering the possible interaction between them. This study aimed to explore the association of VitD status in three trimesters of pregnancy with the risk of HDP, and to explore the interactive effect between maternal VitD level and genetic variants in the VitD metabolic pathways (*GC*, *CYP24A1*, *CYP3A4*, *CYP27B1*, *LRP2*, *VDR*) on gestational blood pressure and HDP.

2. Materials and Methods

2.1. Study Design and Participants

The Zhoushan Pregnant Women Cohort (ZPWC) is an ongoing prospective cohort, conducted in Zhoushan Maternal and Child Health Care Hospital, Zhejiang. This study was based on the data of ZPWC from August 2011 to May 2018. We recruited pregnant women aged between 18 and 45 years at their first prenatal visit. A more detailed description of the inclusion and exclusion criteria can be seen in a previous study [19]. In addition, pregnant women without extreme/missing information of blood pressure and who measured plasma 25(OH)D levels in the first, second, or third trimester were included in the study. In addition, because gestational hypertension (GH), preeclampsia, and eclampsia are different from pregnancy complicated with chronic hypertension and chronic hypertension complicated with preeclampsia in pathogenesis and clinical treatment, pregnant women with chronic hypertension before pregnancy were also excluded [1]. Informed consent was obtained from all participants before the investigation. The study was conducted according to the guidelines of the Declaration of Helsinki and approved by the Institutional Review Board of Zhoushan Maternal and Child Health Care Hospital on 9 January 2011 (Ethical Approval Code: 2011-05).

2.2. Collection of Data and Blood Sample

The interviewers conducted face-to-face questionnaire surveys. Socio-demographic characteristics, lifestyle, and health behavior in the first (T1: 8th–14th gestational week), second (T2: 24th–28th gestational week), and third (T3: 32nd–36th gestational week) trimester, and 42nd day postpartum were collected. At each visit, professional nurses and inspectors were responsible for drawing and centrifuging fasting venous blood samples under 4 °C and separating the plasma and white blood cells, which were then stored at −80 °C until use.

2.3. Measurement of 25(OH)D Concentrations

Plasma $25(OH)D_2$ and $25(OH)D_3$ concentrations (reported in ng/mL) were measured by Liquid chromatography–tandem mass spectrometry (API 3200MD (Applied Bio-systems/MDS Sciex, Framingham, MA, USA)). The lowest sensitivity of $25(OH)D_2$ and $25(OH)D_3$ was 2 ng/mL and 5 ng/mL, respectively. The intra-assay and inter-assay coefficient variance were 1.47–7.24% and 4.48–6.74% for $25(OH)D_2$ and 2.50–7.59% and 4.44–6.76% for $25(OH)D_3$, respectively [19]. The 25(OH)D concentrations were the sum of $25(OH)D_2$ and $25(OH)D_3$.

2.4. Data Extraction

According to the guidelines of pregnant women prenatal health care, the first check-up and registration was conducted on the 8th–12th gestational week. After registration, 12 check-ups at 16, 20, 24, 28, 30, 32, 34, 36, 37, 38, 39, and 40 weeks of pregnancy were followed, along with a birth check every three days until delivery was performed after the 40th week, and a postpartum visit on the 42th day after delivery. The information including height, gestational age, and follow-up information (e.g., weight, systolic blood pressure (SBP), diastolic blood pressure (DBP), etc.), socio-demographic characteristics (e.g., age, education level, etc.), reproductive history (e.g., gravidity, parity, threatened abortion, and fetal malformation, etc.), history of present diseases (e.g., diabetes, etc.), pregnant complications (such as gestational diabetes mellitus, preeclampsia, and kidney disease, etc.), intrapartum complications (e.g., fetal distress, placenta previa, and placental abruption, etc.), was extracted from an electronic medical recorder system (EMRS).

2.5. Covariates Assessment

According to Endocrine Society Clinical Practice Guidelines, we defined plasma 25(OH)D < 20 ng/mL (50 nmol/L) as VitD deficiency [20], and 25(OH)D concentrations ≥ 20 ng/mL as VitD non-deficiency. The change of 25(OH)D level during pregnancy is defined as a difference of 25(OH)D level between three trimesters. The following parameters were also defined: Pre-pregnancy body mass index (BMI) = weight (kg)/height^2 (m^2), gestational weight gain (continuous) = the weight on the day of VitD test at T1, T2, or T3, the pre-pregnancy weight, educational level (senior high school and below, college and above), gravity (1, ≥2, missing), parity (0, ≥1, missing), basal blood pressure (the level of blood pressure at the first prenatal examination or early pregnancy, continuous), the seasons of blood pressure measurement (divided as followed: spring (March to May), summer (June to August), fall (September to November), and winter (December to February) based on the sunshine intensity and duration in different months [21]).

2.6. HDP Definition

In perinatal care, SBP and DBP would be routinely measured [22]; we extracted the data from EMRS. In a sitting position, blood pressure measurement was performed from the right hand with a standard mercury sphygmomanometer. GH onset was defined as SBP ≥ 140 and/or DBP ≥ 90 mm Hg after the 20th gestational week (according to last menstruation date and B-ultrasound) in at least two consecutive examinations [23]. On the basis of GH, urinary protein ≥ +1 on a dipstick was defined as preeclampsia [1]. Eclampsia was defined as the presence of new-onset grand mal seizures in a woman with preeclampsia [24]. GH, preeclampsia, and eclampsia were combined as the group of HDP in later analysis.

2.7. SNP Selection and Genotyping

VitD-related SNP were selected if they met any one of the following conditions [25,26]: (1) SNPs positively associated with 25(OH)D concentration reported in the literature, and the minimum allele frequency (MAF) $\geq$ 10%; (2) SNPs displayed in the functional region in the NCBI database: exon region, intron splicing point, 5'end and 3'end regulatory regions, and MAF $\geq$ 10%; (3) HapMap Chinese database, including gene regions, SNPs within 1500 bp at the 5'end and 3'end; (4) selected by HaploView, the conditions are: MAF $\geq$ 10%; $R^2 \geq 0.8$. Finally, a total of 34 SNPs in the VitD metabolic pathway were selected (*CYP27B1*: rs10877012, *CYP3A4*: rs2242480, rs4646437, *LRP2*: rs4667591, rs10210408, rs2228171, rs7600336, rs2544381, rs2544390, rs2389557, *GC*: rs16846876, rs12512631, rs17467825, rs2070741, rs2282679, rs3755967, rs2298850, rs4588, rs7041, rs222020, rs1155563, rs2298849, *VDR*: rs2228570, rs7975232, rs11568820, rs2238136, rs2853559, rs4334089, rs10783219, *CYP24A1*: rs6013897, rs2762934, rs2209314, rs6127118, rs2248137).

The conventional phenol–chloroform extraction method was used to extract DNA from the peripheral blood leukocytes, which was then stored in TE-buffer at −80 °C. DNA was diluted to 10 ng/μL using a Nanodrop® ND-1000 Spectrophotometer (Thermo Fisher Scientific Inc., Wilmington, NC, USA) for SNP analysis. A Sequenom MassARRAY iPLEX Gold platform (Sequenom, San Diego, CA, USA) was used for SNP genotyping. The call rate of these SNPs was over 98%, which conformed to the Hardy–Weinberg equilibrium.

2.8. Statistical Analysis

The characteristics between HDP and non-HDP groups were compared by t-test for continuous variables and by chi-squared test for categorical variables. Latent mixture modeling (PROC TRAJ) was used to identify subgroups that shared similar VitD patterns. Model fit was assessed using the Bayesian Information Criterion. We initiated a model with three trajectories, and then compared the BIC to that with two. The model with three trajectories identified fit best [27] (Figure S1). Restricted cubic spline (RCS) analyses were used to characterize the dose-response association and explore the potential linear or nonlinear relationship of 25(OH)D level in three trimesters, the change of 25(OH)D level during pregnancy with blood pressure in three trimesters, and HDP. Multivariable adjusted analyses with three knots were used. Test result for nonlinearity was checked first. If the test for nonlinearity was not significant, test result for overall association and linearity was checked, with a significant result indicating a linear association [28]. Multivariate adjusted RCS analysis showed that there was no nonlinear association of 25(OH)D level in three trimesters, the change of 25(OH)D level during pregnancy with blood pressure, and HDP during pregnancy ($P_{\text{for non-linear}} > 0.05$) (Figures S2–S6). The Hardy–Weinberg equilibrium (HWE) of genotyped SNPs was tested using the χ^2 test.

A multiple linear regression model and a multivariate logistic regression model, combined with a crossover analysis method were utilized to explore the association between VitD and its metabolic pathway-related gene variants as well as their interactions with SBP, DBP, and HDP. The generalized linear model was used to analyze the relationship of the change of 25(OH)D level during pregnancy with SBP and DBP, and the multivariate logistic regression model was used to analyze the association between the changes in 25(OH)D levels and the trajectory of VitD during pregnancy with HDP. Models were adjusted for the following potential confounders: pre-pregnancy BMI, maternal age, gestational weight gain, gestational week, educational level, parity, basal blood pressure, and the seasons of blood pressure measurement.

β (se) for linear regression, ORs, and corresponding 95% CIs for logistic regression were calculated, respectively. All test results were considered statistically significant at a value of $p < 0.05$. RCS analyses were performed using R software (version 3.6.3); the other analyses were performed using SAS (version 9.4, SAS Institute, Cary, NC, USA).

3. Results

3.1. Subject Characteristics

The demographic characteristics of participants with HDP or non-HDP were compared and are shown in Table 1. The prospective cohort study included 3699 pregnant women, of which 105 (2.85%) were diagnosed with HDP. The mean age was 29.30 ± 3.95 years for HDP participants and 28.67 ± 3.64 years for non-HDP participants. Compared with non-HDP participants, HDP women had higher pre-pregnancy BMI (21.16 ± 2.91 kg/m² vs. 23.62 ± 4.05 kg/m², $p < 0.0001$). The SBP and DBP levels in three trimesters were higher in HDP than non-HDP. However, VitD deficiency in three trimesters, educational level, gravity, and parity were not significantly different between the two groups. The characteristics of participants in the SNP analysis are shown in Table 1. Pregnant women with HDP had higher pre-pregnancy BMI than the non-HDP group. There was no significant difference in weight gain and 25(OH)D level in three trimesters, educational level, gravity, and parity between the two groups (Table S1).

Table 1. Baseline characteristics of pregnant women.

Variables	Non-HDP (N = 3594)	HDP (N = 105)	p
Mean ± SD			
Age, years	28.67 ± 3.64	29.30 ± 3.95	0.0811
Pre-pregnancy BMI, kg/m²	21.16 ± 2.91	23.62 ± 4.05	<0.0001
T1 (N = 3302)			
Weight gain, kg	0.01 ± 0.17	0.02 ± 0.14	0.3841
SBP, mmHg	103.53 ± 9.31	112.21 ± 10.58	<0.0001
DBP, mmHg	68.35 ± 6.67	74.48 ± 5.99	<0.0001
25(OH)D, ng/mL	17.85 ± 8.38	17.70 ± 7.10	0.8629
T2 (N = 2479)			
Weight gain, kg	5.61 ± 3.82	6.25 ± 4.50	0.1971
SBP, mmHg	107.17 ± 9.24	116.60 ± 14.44	<0.0001
DBP, mmHg	69.13 ± 7.82	76.61 ± 8.84	<0.0001
25(OH)D, ng/mL	23.28 ± 10.38	22.91 ± 9.60	0.7827
T3 (N = 1549)			
Weight gain, kg	11.91 ± 3.73	11.20 ± 4.69	0.2181
SBP, mmHg	108.86 ± 9.72	123.30 ± 15.68	<0.0001
DBP, mmHg	70.99 ± 7.38	82.43 ± 8.44	<0.0001
25(OH)D, ng/mL	26.53 ± 11.28	26.20 ± 11.01	0.8468
N (%)			
VitD deficiency at T1 [a]	2176 (67.85)	66 (69.47)	0.7386
VitD deficiency at T2 [b]	1067 (44.15)	30 (48.39)	0.5067
VitD deficiency at T3 [c]	476 (31.63)	13 (29.55)	0.7696
Educational level			0.1263
≤High school	957 (26.63)	35 (33.33)	
>High school	2637 (73.37)	70 (66.67)	
Gravity			0.5389
1	1652 (45.97)	43 (40.95)	
≥2	1822 (50.70)	59 (56.19)	
Unknown	120 (3.34)	3 (2.86)	
Parity			0.4887
0	2015 (56.07)	65 (61.90)	
≥1	771 (21.45)	20 (19.05)	
Unknown	808 (22.48)	20 (19.05)	

Abbreviations: HDP, hypertensive disorders in pregnancy; BMI, body mass index; SBP, systolic blood pressure; DBP, diastolic blood pressure; VitD, vitamin D. [a] N = 3302, [b] N = 2479, [c] N = 1549.

3.2. The Association between 25(OH)D in Three Trimesters and HDP

After being adjusted for potential confounders, 25(OH)D level at T1 was negatively associated with SBP (β (se) = −0.05 (0.02), $p = 0.0287$) and DBP (β (se) = −0.05 (0.02), $p = 0.0190$) at T1. In addition, 25(OH)D level at T2 was negatively associated with DBP at

T2 and T3, respectively (β (se) = −0.10 (0.02), $p < 0.0001$, β (se) = −0.07 (0.02), $p = 0.0003$) (Table 2). The association between VitD deficiency in three trimesters with SBP and DBP were consistent with the above results (Table S2). For each 1 ng/mL increase in 25(OH)D changes between T1 and T2, DBP at T2 and T3 decreased by 0.11 (se = 0.02) mmHg and 0.11 (se = 0.02) mmHg, respectively ($p < 0.0001$). (Table 3). Three subgroups of participants with data of 25(OH)D levels in three trimesters were identified by latent mixture modeling. Compared with women whose 25(OH)D levels remained low from T1 to T3, women whose 25(OH)D levels gradually increased at T2 and T3 or whose 25(OH)D levels remained high during pregnancy had lower DBP at T3 (β (se) = −1.13 (0.46), $p = 0.0137$, β (se) = −1.74 (0.74), $p = 0.0195$) (Table 4). However, there was no significant association between 25(OH)D levels, VitD deficiency in three trimesters, the change of 25(OH)D levels, or the VitD trajectory during pregnancy with HDP (Tables S3–S6).

Table 2. Association between 25(OH)D levels in three trimesters with blood pressure.

Trimesters of 25(OH)D	N	SBP, mmHg		DBP, mmHg	
		β (se)	p	β (se)	p
		Blood pressure at T1 (N = 3302)			
T1	3302	−0.02 (0.02)	0.3198	0.02 (0.01)	0.2056
		Blood pressure at T2 (N = 2479)			
T1	2125	−0.05 (0.02)	0.0287	−0.05 (0.02)	0.0190
T2	2479	0.03 (0.02)	0.1675	−0.10 (0.02)	<0.0001
		Blood pressure at T3 (N = 1549)			
T1	1328	0.03 (0.03)	0.2361	−0.02 (0.02)	0.3259
T2	1390	0.04 (0.03)	0.1214	−0.07 (0.02)	0.0003
T3	1549	0.04 (0.02)	0.0541	−0.02 (0.02)	0.2486

Abbreviations: SBP, systolic blood pressure, DBP, diastolic blood pressure. Adjusted for pre-pregnancy BMI, maternal age, gestational weight gain, gestational week, educational level, parity, basal blood pressure, and the seasons of blood pressure measurement.

Table 3. The association between the change of 25(OH)D levels during pregnancy and blood pressure at T2 and T3.

The Change of Trimesters	N	The Change of 25(OH)D Levels, ng/mL *	SBP, mmHg		DBP, mmHg	
			β (se)	p	β (se)	p
			Blood pressure at T2 (N = 2479)			
Between T1 and T2	2125	3.50 (84.59)	0.03 (0.02)	0.1217	−0.11 (0.02)	<0.0001
			Blood pressure at T3 (N = 1549)			
Between T1 and T2	1212	2.40 (81.27)	0.03 (0.03)	0.3142	−0.11 (0.02)	<0.0001
Between T1 and T3	1328	6.59 (98.02)	0.06 (0.03)	0.0294	−0.02 (0.02)	0.3516
Between T2 and T3	1390	3.40 (87.23)	0.02 (0.03)	0.3662	0.04 (0.02)	0.0405

Abbreviations: SBP, systolic blood pressure; DBP, diastolic blood pressure. * Presented as the median (range). Adjusted for pre-pregnancy BMI, maternal age, gestational weight gain, gestational week, educational level, parity, basal blood pressure, the seasons of blood pressure measurement, and 25(OH)D level at T1.

Table 4. The association between the trajectory of VitD during pregnancy and blood pressure at T3.

Trajectory of VitD	N (%)	SBP, mmHg		DBP, mmHg	
		β (se)	p	β (se)	p
Subgroup 1	621 (51.24)	Ref		Ref	
Subgroup 2	469 (38.70)	0.48 (0.60)	0.4216	−1.13 (0.46)	0.0137
Subgroup 3	122 (10.07)	1.58 (0.98)	0.1052	−1.74 (0.74)	0.0195

Abbreviations: SBP, systolic blood pressure; DBP, diastolic blood pressure; VitD, vitamin D. Adjusted for pre-pregnancy BMI, maternal age, gestational weight gain, gestational week, educational level, parity, basal blood pressure, and the seasons of blood pressure measurement.

3.3. The Association between SNP and HDP

The association of each SNP genotype with SBP and DBP at T1, T2, and T3 are shown in Tables S7–S9, respectively. Polymorphisms in *CYP24A1*-rs2248137 was significantly associated with higher SBP at T1 and DBP at T2 and T3. Polymorphisms in *CYP24A1*-rs2762934 were significantly associated with higher DBP at T1 and SBP at T2. Polymorphisms in *LRP2*-rs4667591 were significantly associated with higher SBP at T1 and DBP at T3. Polymorphisms in *GC*-rs2070741, rs222020, and rs2298849 were associated with higher SBP at T2. Polymorphisms in *LRP2*-rs2544390 were associated with higher DBP at T3. Furthermore, polymorphisms in *CYP24A1*-rs2248137, *CYP24A1*-rs2762934, *CYP24A1*-rs6127118, and *GC*-rs2070741 were associated a higher risk of HDP (Table 5). However, there was no significant association between other genes' polymorphisms and HDP.

Table 5. The relationship between single SNP and HDP *.

SNP	Genotypes	N	Case (%)	Crude Model OR (95%CI)	p	Adjusted Model * OR (95%CI)	p
CYP24A1							
rs2209314	TT	941	28 (3.0)	Ref		Ref	
	CT	1309	38 (2.9)	0.97 (0.59–1.60)	0.9198	0.99 (0.60–1.64)	0.9648
	CC	443	4 (0.9)	0.30 (0.10–0.85)	0.024	0.30 (0.10–0.87)	0.026
rs2248137	GG	934	18 (1.9)	Ref		Ref	
	GC	453	20 (4.4)	2.35 (1.23–4.49)	0.0096	2.62 (1.32–5.21)	0.0059
	CC	643	19 (3.0)	1.55 (0.81–2.98)	0.1885	1.80 (0.92–3.53)	0.0869
rs2762934	GG	599	22 (3.7)	Ref		Ref	
	GA	119	5 (4.2)	1.15 (0.43–3.10)	0.7819	1.07 (0.38–3.00)	0.9051
	AA	7	1 (14.3)	4.37 (0.50–37.88)	0.1806	9.98 (1.06–94.04)	0.0444
rs6013897	TT	529	20 (3.8)	Ref		Ref	
	AT	172	8 (4.7)	1.24 (0.54–2.87)	0.6131	1.26 (0.53–3.02)	0.5964
	AA	22	1 (4.5)	1.21 (0.16–9.46)	0.8546	1.53 (0.19–12.57)	0.6905
rs6127118	GG	963	24 (2.5)	Ref		Ref	
	AG	1616	41 (2.5)	1.02 (0.61–1.70)	0.9439	0.96 (0.57–1.61)	0.8736
	AA	119	7 (5.9)	2.45 (1.03–5.80)	0.0426	2.38 (0.98–5.77)	0.0542
CYP27B1							
rs10877012	TT	1125	27 (2.4)	Ref		Ref	
	GT	1204	32 (2.7)	1.11 (0.66–1.87)	0.6925	1.14 (0.67–1.93)	0.6354
	GG	360	12 (3.3)	1.40 (0.70–2.80)	0.3366	1.61 (0.80–3.25)	0.1856
CYP3A4							
rs2242480	CC	1529	41 (2.7)	Ref		Ref	
	CT	1004	26 (2.6)	0.96 (0.59–1.59)	0.8879	0.96 (0.58–1.60)	0.8885
	TT	159	5 (3.1)	1.18 (0.46–3.03)	0.7329	1.37 (0.53–3.56)	0.5164
rs4646437	GG	530	22 (4.2)	Ref		Ref	
	AG	182	7 (3.8)	0.92 (0.39–2.20)	0.8576	0.83 (0.34–2.04)	0.6868
GC							
rs1155563	TT	951	29 (3.0)	Ref		Ref	
	TC	1290	31 (2.4)	0.78 (0.47–1.31)	0.3499	0.76 (0.45–1.29)	0.3091
	CC	450	11 (2.4)	0.80 (0.39–1.61)	0.5262	0.73 (0.36–1.50)	0.3886
rs12512631	TT	463	21 (4.5)	Ref		Ref	
	CT	241	7 (2.9)	0.63 (0.26–1.50)	0.2973	0.77 (0.31–1.89)	0.5683
	CC	18	1 (5.6)	1.24 (0.16–9.75)	0.8393	1.07 (0.13–8.84)	0.9466
rs16846876	AA	1274	38 (3.0)	Ref		Ref	
	AT	1133	25 (2.2)	0.73 (0.44–1.22)	0.2357	0.69 (0.41–1.16)	0.1632
	TT	292	9 (3.1)	1.03 (0.49–2.16)	0.9283	0.89 (0.41–1.93)	0.7745
rs17467825	AA	1254	37 (3.0)	Ref		Ref	
	GA	1150	29 (2.5)	0.85 (0.52–1.39)	0.5208	0.80 (0.48–1.32)	0.3792
	GG	299	6 (2.0)	0.67 (0.28–1.61)	0.375	0.54 (0.22–1.33)	0.181
rs2070741	TT	495	17 (3.4)	Ref		Ref	
	GT	213	8 (3.8)	1.10 (0.47–2.58)	0.8317	1.10 (0.46–2.66)	0.8251
	GG	18	3 (16.7)	5.62 (1.49–21.28)	0.011	4.77 (1.12–20.21)	0.0341

Table 5. Cont.

SNP	Genotypes	N	Case (%)	Crude Model		Adjusted Model *	
				OR (95%CI)	p	OR (95%CI)	p
rs222020	TT	270	10 (3.7)	Ref		Ref	
	CT	344	12 (3.5)	0.94 (0.40–2.21)	0.8867	0.85 (0.35–2.07)	0.7284
	CC	110	6 (5.5)	1.50 (0.53–4.23)	0.4436	1.42 (0.49–4.15)	0.5169
rs2282679	TT	1254	36 (2.9)	Ref		Ref	
	GT	1141	30 (2.6)	0.91 (0.56–1.49)	0.7185	0.87 (0.52–1.43)	0.5726
	GG	306	6 (2.0)	0.68 (0.28–1.62)	0.3808	0.55 (0.22–1.35)	0.1913
rs2298849	AA	1120	27 (2.4)	Ref		Ref	
	GA	1219	38 (3.1)	1.30 (0.79–2.15)	0.3003	1.32 (0.79–2.20)	0.2835
	GG	366	7 (1.9)	0.79 (0.34–1.83)	0.5809	0.82 (0.35–1.90)	0.6376
rs2298850	GG	1229	35 (2.8)	Ref		Ref	
	CG	1151	29 (2.5)	0.88 (0.54–1.45)	0.621	0.84 (0.50–1.39)	0.4891
	CC	305	6 (2.0)	0.68 (0.29–1.64)	0.3967	0.55 (0.22–1.38)	0.2051
rs3755967	CC	1250	36 (2.9)	Ref		Ref	
	CT	1149	30 (2.6)	0.90 (0.55–1.48)	0.6875	0.86 (0.52–1.42)	0.5515
	TT	306	6 (2.0)	0.67 (0.28–1.62)	0.3768	0.54 (0.22–1.35)	0.189
rs4588	GG	1241	36 (2.9)	Ref		Ref	
	GT	1146	29 (2.5)	0.87 (0.53–1.43)	0.5789	0.83 (0.50–1.37)	0.4576
	TT	306	6 (2.0)	0.67 (0.28–1.60)	0.3679	0.54 (0.22–1.34)	0.1819
rs7041	AA	1445	39 (2.7)	Ref		Ref	
	CA	1061	28 (2.6)	0.98 (0.60–1.60)	0.9268	1.03 (0.62–1.70)	0.9026
	CC	195	4 (2.1)	0.76 (0.27–2.14)	0.5968	0.87 (0.30–2.48)	0.7934
LRP2							
rs10210408	CC	895	22 (2.5)	Ref		Ref	
	TC	1325	40 (3.0)	1.24 (0.73–2.09)	0.4322	1.16 (0.68–1.99)	0.5816
	TT	486	10 (2.1)	0.83 (0.39–1.78)	0.6378	0.81 (0.38–1.74)	0.5919
rs2228171	TT	932	24 (2.6)	Ref		Ref	
	CT	394	15 (3.8)	1.50 (0.78–2.89)	0.2279	1.48 (0.75–2.94)	0.2607
	CC	301	8 (2.7)	1.03 (0.46–2.32)	0.9375	1.14 (0.50–2.61)	0.7534
rs2389557	AA	194	8 (4.1)	Ref		Ref	
	GA	363	12 (3.3)	0.79 (0.32–1.98)	0.6218	0.78 (0.31–2.00)	0.6094
	GG	166	9 (5.4)	1.33 (0.50–3.54)	0.5639	1.24 (0.45–3.42)	0.6722
rs2544381	GG	388	20 (5.2)	Ref		Ref	
	CG	284	7 (2.5)	0.46 (0.19–1.12)	0.0862	0.48 (0.19–1.18)	0.108
	CC	52	1 (1.9)	0.36 (0.05–2.75)	0.3249	0.37 (0.05–2.92)	0.349
rs2544390	CC	199	9 (4.5)	Ref		Ref	
	CT	370	14 (3.8)	0.83 (0.35–1.95)	0.6698	0.70 (0.29–1.71)	0.4308
	TT	154	5 (3.2)	0.71 (0.23–2.16)	0.5442	0.68 (0.22–2.15)	0.5131
rs4667591	TT	245	10 (4.1)	Ref		Ref	
	GT	347	11 (3.2)	0.77 (0.32–1.84)	0.5558	0.82 (0.33–2.03)	0.671
	GG	132	8 (6.1)	1.52 (0.58–3.94)	0.3929	1.68 (0.62–4.56)	0.3081
rs7600336	CC	236	8 (3.4)	Ref		Ref	
	TC	342	14 (4.1)	1.22 (0.50–2.95)	0.6643	1.10 (0.44–2.75)	0.8428
	TT	148	6 (4.1)	1.20 (0.41–3.54)	0.7357	1.30 (0.43–3.93)	0.6374
VDR							
rs10783219	AA	998	26 (2.6)	Ref		Ref	
	TA	1275	36 (2.8)	1.09 (0.65–1.81)	0.7512	1.03 (0.61–1.74)	0.8982
	TT	428	9 (2.1)	0.80 (0.37–1.73)	0.5753	0.76 (0.35–1.66)	0.4869
rs11568820	CC	219	6 (2.7)	Ref		Ref	
	TC	350	17 (4.9)	1.81 (0.70–4.67)	0.2182	1.93 (0.72–5.14)	0.19
	TT	153	5 (3.3)	1.20 (0.36–4.00)	0.7675	1.48 (0.43–5.14)	0.5328
rs2228570	GG	212	10 (4.7)	Ref		Ref	
	GA	364	15 (4.1)	0.87 (0.38–1.97)	0.7351	0.86 (0.37–2.00)	0.7204
	AA	148	3 (2.0)	0.42 (0.11–1.55)	0.191	0.41 (0.11–1.56)	0.1905
rs2238136	CC	483	19 (3.9)	Ref		Ref	
	TC	218	10 (4.6)	1.17 (0.54–2.57)	0.6879	1.16 (0.51–2.60)	0.7259

Table 5. Cont.

SNP	Genotypes	N	Case (%)	Crude Model		Adjusted Model *	
				OR (95%CI)	p	OR (95%CI)	p
rs2853559	GG	319	16 (5.0)	Ref		Ref	
	GA	313	10 (3.2)	0.62 (0.28–1.40)	0.2531	0.68 (0.29–1.56)	0.3599
	AA	87	2 (2.3)	0.45 (0.10–1.98)	0.2875	0.40 (0.09–1.84)	0.2418
rs4334089	GG	227	7 (3.1)	Ref		Ref	
	AG	350	15 (4.3)	1.41 (0.56–3.51)	0.4637	1.45 (0.56–3.75)	0.4397
	AA	148	6 (4.1)	1.33 (0.44–4.03)	0.617	1.54 (0.49–4.85)	0.4563
rs7975232	CC	382	11 (2.9)	Ref		Ref	
	CA	285	15 (5.3)	1.87 (0.85–4.14)	0.121	1.84 (0.81–4.20)	0.1458
	AA	60	3 (5.0)	1.78 (0.48–6.56)	0.3894	1.77 (0.46–6.78)	0.4031

Abbreviations: VitD, vitamin D; HDP, hypertensive disorders in pregnancy. * Adjusted for pre-pregnancy BMI, maternal age, gestational weight gain, educational level, parity, and basal blood pressure.

3.4. The Interaction between Single SNP and VitD Deficiency in Three Trimesters on the Risk of HDP

Results of the crossover analysis are shown in Tables S10–S13. Polymorphisms of seven SNPs (rs16846876, rs2282679, rs17467825, rs2298849, rs2298850, rs3755967, and rs4588) in GC gene and VitD deficiency at T2 might exert interactions on DBP at T2. In addition, VDR-rs2228570 and VitD deficiency at T2 might exert interaction on SBP at T2. Furthermore, women with mutations in CYP24A1-rs2248137, LRP2-rs2389557, and LRP2-rs4667591 and had VitD deficiency at T2 showed increased risk of HDP (Table 6).

Table 6. The interaction between SNPs and VitD in three trimesters on the risk of HDP.

SNP	Genotypes	VitD	T1 N	OR (95%CI)	T2 N	OR (95%CI)	T3 N	OR (95%CI)
CYP24A1								
rs2209314	CC/CT	≥20	545	Ref	724	Ref	557	Ref
	TT	≥20	316	1.60 (0.66–3.87)	383	1.41 (0.65–3.08)	294	1.86 (0.80–4.28)
	CC/CT	<20	1026	1.18 (0.57–2.45)	541	1.13 (0.53–2.40)	260	1.20 (0.43–3.29)
	TT	<20	560	1.52 (0.70–3.32)	309	1.41 (0.62–3.18)	145	1.04 (0.28–3.79)
	$P_{interaction}$			0.8774		0.7996		0.5739
rs2248137	GG	≥20	357	Ref	451	Ref	339	Ref
	GC	≥20	117	2.50 (0.81–7.73)	111	4.45 (1.25–15.79) *	106	3.81 (1.11–13.07) *
	CC	≥20	220	1.04 (0.32–3.31)	269	3.90 (1.33–11.41) *	195	2.22 (0.66–7.47)
	GG	<20	480	0.77 (0.28–2.09)	283	2.11 (0.67–6.63)	131	1.17 (0.22–6.23)
	GC	<20	317	1.80 (0.70–4.67)	133	5.42 (1.71–17.23) *	63	1.05 (0.12–9.51)
	CC	<20	377	1.65 (0.64–4.26)	171	1.17 (0.22–6.04)	90	2.47 (0.56–10.81)
	$P_{interaction}$			0.5195		0.1442		0.8045
rs6127118	GG	≥20	288	Ref	405	Ref	316	Ref
	AG/AA	≥20	572	2.01 (0.66–6.10)	702	0.83 (0.38–1.81)	537	2.97 (0.99–8.88)
	GG	<20	582	2.29 (0.77–6.87)	291	0.77 (0.28–2.12)	133	1.86 (0.40–8.58)
	AG/AA	<20	1010	1.63 (0.56–4.77)	558	1.12 (0.52–2.42)	271	2.18 (0.62–7.65)
	$P_{interaction}$			0.855		0.2332		0.5262
CYP27B1								
rs10877012	TT	≥20	363	Ref	445	Ref	331	Ref
	GT	≥20	372	1.14 (0.40–3.23)	510	1.24 (0.53–2.93)	405	1.12 (0.42–2.94)
	GG	≥20	121	2.67 (0.86–8.29)	151	1.84 (0.60–5.61)	115	2.56 (0.83–7.85)
	TT	<20	661	1.28 (0.52–3.15)	361	1.08 (0.41–2.84)	168	0.84 (0.21–3.27)
	GT	<20	725	1.41 (0.59–3.41)	370	1.26 (0.51–3.12)	180	1.32 (0.41–4.21)

Table 6. Cont.

SNP	Genotypes	VitD	T1 N	OR (95%CI)	T2 N	OR (95%CI)	T3 N	OR (95%CI)
	GG	<20	201	1.79 (0.58–5.49)	114	2.80 (0.97–8.10)	54	2.26 (0.45–11.45)
	$P_{interaction}$			0.6139		0.4639		0.9865
CYP3A4								
rs2242480	CC	≥20	490	Ref	644	Ref	504	Ref
	CT	≥20	314	0.89 (0.34–2.31)	404	1.16 (0.51–2.64)	293	1.08 (0.44–2.68)
	TT	≥20	54	1.74 (0.37–8.17)	59	1.57 (0.35–7.15)	52	2.47 (0.66–9.19)
	CC	<20	899	1.04 (0.51–2.13)	480	1.53 (0.75–3.13)	247	1.25 (0.48–3.22)
	CT	<20	604	1.16 (0.54–2.47)	318	0.53 (0.17–1.61)	142	0.51 (0.11–2.33)
	TT	<20	87	1.52 (0.41–5.62)	51	3.13 (0.85–11.47)	17	3.30 (0.39–28.05)
	$P_{interaction}$			0.7911		0.696		0.5117
GC								
rs1155563	TT	≥20	331	Ref	440	Ref	326	Ref
	TC	≥20	401	0.81 (0.31–2.11)	498	1.04 (0.44–2.44)	392	0.45 (0.17–1.15)
	CC	≥20	127	0.81 (0.21–3.09)	167	1.31 (0.44–3.95)	133	0.87 (0.27–2.80)
	TT	<20	531	1.26 (0.55–2.88)	272	1.70 (0.70–4.15)	123	0.21 (0.03–1.65)
	TC	<20	766	0.78 (0.34–1.80)	403	1.02 (0.40–2.55)	199	0.92 (0.33–2.52)
	CC	<20	290	0.89 (0.33–2.42)	172	0.87 (0.26–2.89)	83	0.94 (0.25–3.54)
	$P_{interaction}$			0.9456		0.5655		0.2934
rs16846876	AA	≥20	437	Ref	557	Ref	419	Ref
	AT	≥20	366	1.22 (0.48–3.07)	450	1.18 (0.52–2.70)	353	0.34 (0.12–0.99)
	TT	≥20	58	1.31 (0.27–6.38)	102	1.46 (0.43–4.97)	81	1.83 (0.62–5.37)
	AA	<20	714	1.65 (0.75–3.60)	379	1.71 (0.77–3.79)	168	0.51 (0.14–1.84)
	AT	<20	672	0.87 (0.37–2.07)	362	1.00 (0.40–2.51)	182	1.00 (0.38–2.69)
	TT	<20	206	1.12 (0.37–3.36)	108	0.72 (0.15–3.38)	55	0.48 (0.06–3.85)
	$P_{interaction}$			0.4024		0.3482		0.8437
rs17467825	AA	≥20	447	Ref	578	Ref	430	Ref
	GA	≥20	352	0.79 (0.31–1.99)	437	1.06 (0.48–2.34)	337	0.41 (0.15–1.07)
	GG	≥20	62	0.49 (0.06–3.95)	94	0.59 (0.12–3.00)	88	0.56 (0.13–2.33)
	AA	<20	692	1.15 (0.55–2.38)	347	1.55 (0.71–3.40)	152	0.36 (0.08–1.61)
	GA	<20	691	0.91 (0.43–1.93)	383	0.84 (0.35–2.04)	191	0.85 (0.32–2.25)
	GG	<20	213	0.65 (0.21–1.98)	121	0.81 (0.22–2.96)	62	0.76 (0.17–3.48)
	$P_{interaction}$			0.8118		0.8253		0.2029
rs2282679	TT	≥20	449	Ref	578	Ref	429	Ref
	GT	≥20	349	0.81 (0.32–2.04)	434	1.27 (0.57–2.80)	336	0.42 (0.16–1.10)
	GG	≥20	63	0.47 (0.06–3.80)	98	0.62 (0.12–3.11)	89	0.56 (0.13–2.34)
	TT	<20	688	1.10 (0.53–2.29)	345	1.67 (0.75–3.71)	153	0.36 (0.08–1.60)
	GT	<20	689	0.97 (0.46–2.04)	381	0.92 (0.37–2.25)	188	0.87 (0.33–2.30)
	GG	<20	217	0.65 (0.21–1.97)	123	0.88 (0.24–3.22)	63	0.76 (0.17–3.48)
	$P_{interaction}$			0.7444		0.6979		0.2075
rs2298849	AA	≥20	332	Ref	430	Ref	346	Ref
	GA	≥20	411	3.12 (1.02–9.59) *	511	0.92 (0.41–2.05)	386	0.93 (0.38–2.27)
	GG	≥20	120	1.36 (0.24–7.60)	170	0.43 (0.09–1.95)	124	1.23 (0.37–4.10)
	AA	<20	692	2.29 (0.77–6.85)	378	0.72 (0.29–1.82)	173	1.01 (0.33–3.11)
	GA	<20	700	2.33 (0.78–6.95)	362	1.28 (0.57–2.87)	178	1.25 (0.41–3.82)
	GG	<20	204	1.94 (0.51–7.40)	111	1.01 (0.28–3.70)	54	—
	$P_{interaction}$			0.5918		0.1481		0.4554
rs2298850	GG	≥20	441	Ref	564	Ref	416	Ref
	CG	≥20	354	0.77 (0.31–1.95)	437	1.34 (0.60–3.01)	341	0.41 (0.15–1.10)
	CC	≥20	63	0.46 (0.06–3.71)	99	0.66 (0.13–3.33)	89	0.56 (0.13–2.37)
	GG	<20	672	1.04 (0.50–2.20)	339	1.83 (0.81–4.12)	150	0.38 (0.09–1.70)
	CG	<20	694	0.90 (0.42–1.91)	385	0.85 (0.33–2.20)	191	0.75 (0.26–2.12)
	CC	<20	215	0.64 (0.21–1.96)	122	0.94 (0.25–3.50)	63	0.79 (0.17–3.65)
	$P_{interaction}$			0.759		0.5603		0.2452

Table 6. Cont.

SNP	Genotypes	VitD	T1 N	OR (95%CI)	T2 N	OR (95%CI)	T3 N	OR (95%CI)
rs3755967	CC	≥20	448	Ref	575	Ref	427	Ref
	CT	≥20	351	0.80 (0.32–2.01)	438	1.25 (0.57–2.76)	340	0.41 (0.16–1.08)
	TT	≥20	63	0.47 (0.06–3.78)	98	0.61 (0.12–3.10)	89	0.56 (0.13–2.32)
	CC	<20	685	1.09 (0.52–2.29)	345	1.66 (0.75–3.69)	153	0.36 (0.08–1.58)
	CT	<20	695	0.96 (0.46–2.02)	383	0.91 (0.37–2.24)	189	0.86 (0.33–2.27)
	TT	<20	217	0.64 (0.21–1.96)	123	0.87 (0.24–3.20)	63	0.75 (0.16–3.45)
	$P_{interaction}$			0.7354		0.7072		0.2031
rs4588	GG	≥20	448	Ref	571	Ref	422	Ref
	GT	≥20	348	0.81 (0.32–2.05)	439	1.23 (0.56–2.72)	339	0.40 (0.15–1.07)
	TT	≥20	64	0.45 (0.06–3.57)	98	0.60 (0.12–3.05)	90	0.54 (0.13–2.24)
	GG	<20	676	1.11 (0.53–2.32)	341	1.66 (0.75–3.70)	149	0.37 (0.08–1.65)
	GT	<20	696	0.91 (0.43–1.93)	382	0.80 (0.31–2.05)	192	0.70 (0.25–1.98)
	TT	<20	215	0.65 (0.21–1.99)	124	0.84 (0.23–3.11)	63	0.75 (0.16–3.46)
	$P_{interaction}$			0.8164		0.6081		0.2578
rs7041	AA	≥20	423	Ref	573	Ref	454	Ref
	CA	≥20	358	2.46 (0.96–6.32)	453	0.92 (0.42–2.04)	337	0.65 (0.27–1.58)
	CC	≥20	82	0.97 (0.12–8.11)	84	0.55 (0.07–4.25)	63	0.50 (0.06–3.91)
	AA	<20	892	2.03 (0.87–4.75)	478	1.15 (0.55–2.40)	226	0.80 (0.30–2.13)
	CA	<20	612	1.21 (0.46–3.14)	316	1.04 (0.43–2.50)	158	0.61 (0.17–2.18)
	CC	<20	88	2.18 (0.54–8.77)	56	—	21	—
	$P_{interaction}$			0.2275		0.8097		0.8926
LRP2								
rs10210408	CC	≥20	289	Ref	354	Ref	287	Ref
	TC	≥20	418	1.75 (0.60–5.10)	558	1.45 (0.58–3.62)	415	0.69 (0.29–1.62)
	TT	≥20	155	1.56 (0.40–6.00)	199	1.25 (0.39–4.03)	154	0.30 (0.07–1.42)
	CC	<20	526	1.83 (0.66–5.12)	294	1.10 (0.36–3.33)	127	0.41 (0.09–1.94)
	TC	<20	782	1.64 (0.61–4.40)	399	1.96 (0.79–4.89)	214	0.86 (0.32–2.31)
	TT	<20	290	1.16 (0.34–3.91)	158	0.64 (0.13–3.15)	64	0.44 (0.06–3.55)
	$P_{interaction}$			0.497		0.9331		0.3864
rs2228171	TT	≥20	291	Ref	374	Ref	292	Ref
	CT	≥20	92	0.97 (0.19–4.86)	89	2.33 (0.65–8.38)	63	0.98 (0.21–4.70)
	CC	≥20	84	1.61 (0.39–6.59)	104	0.91 (0.19–4.49)	74	0.37 (0.05–3.00)
	TT	<20	548	1.21 (0.48–3.07)	294	1.06 (0.36–3.16)	140	0.60 (0.16–2.29)
	CT	<20	286	1.68 (0.62–4.56)	96	2.12 (0.59–7.56)	60	—
	CC	<20	194	1.26 (0.38–4.14)	111	2.37 (0.67–8.41)	59	1.22 (0.25–5.97)
	$P_{interaction}$			0.9483		0.4054		0.5358
rs2389557	AA/GA	≥20	113	Ref	102	Ref	87	Ref
	GG	≥20	37	2.15 (0.18–25.61)	35	1.66 (0.22–12.36)	26	2.11 (0.21–20.73)
	AA/GA	<20	433	2.50 (0.55–11.48)	156	1.04 (0.20–5.46)	100	0.55 (0.07–4.57)
	GG	<20	125	3.57 (0.70–18.10)	33	7.09 (1.21–41.47)	18	—
	$P_{interaction}$			0.7002		0.8493		0.2569
rs4667591	TT/GT	≥20	120	Ref	116	Ref	94	Ref
	GG	≥20	31	7.98 (0.64–98.90)	21	6.84 (0.76–61.89)	19	0.90 (0.04–21.95)
	TT/GT	<20	458	4.84 (0.63–37.13)	146	1.74 (0.35–8.58)	93	0.15 (0.01–2.10)
	GG	<20	100	7.64 (0.88–66.52)	44	7.44 (1.11–49.79) *	26	1.60 (0.13–19.78)
	$P_{interaction}$			0.8345		0.7612		0.3993
VDR								
rs10783219	AA	≥20	309	Ref	431	Ref	336	Ref
	TA	≥20	412	1.15 (0.44–3.05)	523	0.80 (0.36–1.77)	397	1.66 (0.67–4.12)
	TT	≥20	140	0.96 (0.24–3.87)	156	0.41 (0.09–1.90)	120	0.77 (0.16–3.86)
	AA	<20	602	1.28 (0.52–3.15)	297	0.78 (0.30–2.02)	145	1.44 (0.41–5.02)
	TA	<20	739	1.15 (0.47–2.78)	419	1.00 (0.45–2.21)	194	0.71 (0.18–2.78)

Table 6. Cont.

SNP	Genotypes	VitD	T1 N	OR (95%CI)	T2 N	OR (95%CI)	T3 N	OR (95%CI)
rs2238136	TT	<20	253	0.90 (0.29–2.80)	135	1.04 (0.33–3.31)	65	2.65 (0.66–10.67)
	$P_{interaction}$			0.8452		0.1733		0.945
	CC	≥20	111	Ref	99	Ref	83	Ref
	TC/TT	≥20	40	4.94 (0.42–58.60)	38	6.78 (0.84–54.44)	30	0.77 (0.06–9.56)
	CC	<20	363	5.26 (0.68–40.67)	126	4.10 (0.66–25.32)	77	0.44 (0.06–3.28)
	TC/TT	<20	196	3.82 (0.45–32.40)	65	2.57 (0.29–22.94)	42	—
	$P_{interaction}$			0.4588		0.0586		0.9648

Abbreviations: VitD, vitamin D; HDP, hypertensive disorders in pregnancy. Adjusted for pre-pregnancy BMI, maternal age, educational level, parity, basal blood pressure. * p < 0.05.

4. Discussion

In the present study, 25(OH)D level at T2, as well as 25(OH)D change between T1 and T2, were significantly inversely associated with DBP at T2 and T3. However, significant associations between maternal VitD deficiency in any trimesters and HDP were not observed. Polymorphism in *CYP24A1*, *GC*, and *LRP2* was associated with blood pressure, and polymorphism in *CYP24A1* and *GC* was associated with increased risk of HDP. Furthermore, interactive effects between VitD deficiency and polymorphisms in *CYP24A1*, *GC*, and *VDR* genes on blood pressure were identified. Women with polymorphisms in *CYP24A1* and *LRP2* genes and had VitD deficiency at T2 showed a higher risk of HDP.

Previous findings on the association between VitD level during pregnancy and HDP were not consistent. A prospective observational study conducted in southern China found that there were no significant differences in the risk of HDP among women with different levels of VitD at 16–20-week gestation [29]. A case-control study conducted in Iran found that pregnant women with VitD deficiency (25(OH)D < 20 ng/mL) had higher blood pressure and increased risk of preeclampsia than those with VitD insufficiency (25(OH)D: 20~30 ng/mL) [8]. The prospective Swedish GraviD cohort study, including 1413 pregnant women, found that 25(OH)D was positively associated with T1 blood pressure [16]; however, both 25(OH)D level at T3 and change in 25(OH)D level from T1 to T3 were significantly and negatively associated with preeclampsia, but not with the risk of GH [30]. Another nested case-control study carried out among Australian pregnant women found that higher levels of VitD (25(OH)D > 75 nmol/L) in early pregnancy (10–14 weeks) could prevent the occurrence of early-onset preeclampsia (p = 0.09); however, women with low levels of 25(OH)D (<37.5 ng/mL) in the first trimester of pregnancy had a tendency toward reduced risk of preeclampsia (p = 0.07) [31]. Conflicting data for an association of VitD during pregnancy with HDP results from a number of sources, including large heterogeneity between study designs, different ethnicities, different subtypes of HDP included in the analysis, variable quality of measurement for 25(OH)D, and inconsistent definition of VitD status [32]. On the other hand, studies have shown that the gene variation of key enzymes in VitD synthesis, transport and metabolism pathway would also affect the levels and effects of 25(OH)D and 1,25(OH)$_2$D [25,33]. Furthermore, genetic mutations in the VitD metabolic pathway were also associated with increased risk of HDP [8].

The active form of VitD (1,25(OH)$_2$D) needs to bind to VDR to exert its biological function. Relevant studies related to genetic variants in the VitD metabolic pathway with HDP were mainly focus on three SNPs (rs2228570, rs731236, and rs1544410) of *VDR* gene. Rezavand et al. [8] found that, compared with *VDR*-rs2228570 TC and TT + TC genotypes, the SBP and DBP of CC genotype were higher, and the risk of preeclampsia increased by 1.72 times. However, no association was found between *VDR*-rs731236, *VDR*-rs1544410, and preeclampsia. Knabl et al. [34] also reported that there was a strong association between the polymorphisms in rs10735810 and rs1544410 of *VDR* and the risk of GH. The polymorphisms in rs10735810 affect plasma renin activity and may be associated with a reduced risk of GH [34]. In this study, VitD deficiency at T2 interacted with the variants of *VDR*-rs2238136 on DBP and *VDR*-rs2228570 on SBP at T2.

The *CYP24A1* gene is located in 20q13-2, which is mainly expressed in the kidney and encodes the catabolic enzymes of 1,25(OH)$_2$D and 25(OH)D [35]. Evidence relating to the association between *CYP24A1* gene polymorphism and susceptibility to hypertension, especially among pregnant women, is scare. A case-control study among the Chinese Han population found that *CYP24A1*-rs56229249 significantly decreased the hypertension risk in homozygote and recessive models [36]. In addition, rs2762940 was related to hypertension risk in men, and rs56229249 was a protective factor against hypertension in women [36]. The comprehensive genetic association study in the Women's Genome Health Study (WGHS) found that *CYP24A1*-rs2296241 showed significant associations with SBP, DBP, mean arterial pressure, and pulse pressure [37]. In this study, we found that gene variants in *CYP24A1*-rs2248137, *CYP24A1*-rs2762934, and *CYP24A1*-rs6127118 were associated with increased risk of HDP. Furthermore, *CYP24A1*-rs6013897 interacted with VitD deficiency at T2 on HDP. On the other hand, *LRP2* is located on 2q24-q31, which is a member of the low-density lipoprotein receptor family and encodes megalin protein. In the kidney, megalin and cubilin combine together with hydroxylate 25(OH)D$_3$ into 1,25(OH)$_2$D$_3$ [38]. Studies regarding the association between *LRP2* genes and VitD with the risk for HDP are still lacking. This study found that the mutations of *LRP2*-rs2389557 and *LRP2*-rs4667591 and VitD deficiency at T2 had a combined effect on the risk of HDP.

The *GC* gene encodes VitD binding protein (VDBP) [39], which is the major transporter of VitD. About 85% to 90% of 25(OH)D is bound to VDBP in circulation [40]. VDBP can aggravate or enhance various biological processes during pregnancy, such as immune regulation, glucose metabolism, and blood pressure regulation [39]. The GC-1 subtype was more common in pregnant women with preeclampsia than in those without preeclampsia, which was considered as a potential early detection genetic marker for women at risk of preeclampsia [41]. In HIV endemic areas of South Africa, compared with women with normal blood pressure, two SNPs of *GC* gene (rs4588 and rs7041) were more common in pregnant women with preeclampsia, and were not related to HIV status [42]. Furthermore, *GC*-rs4588 polymorphism was associated with early-onset (<34 weeks) and late-onset (≥34 weeks of pregnancy) preeclampsia, while *GC*-rs7041 was associated with early-onset eclampsia [42]. A nested case-control study of 170 American women from Massachusetts tracked the levels of VDBP and 25(OH)D throughout pregnancy to examine whether these biomarkers were associated with blood pressure or the risk of preeclampsia, but found no significant correlation of VDBP or 25(OH)D levels with preeclampsia [43]. At present, the combined effect of *GC* gene polymorphism and VitD during pregnancy on HDP is not clear. A study focused on preterm birth found that rs7041 variants interacted with VitD at T2 on the gestational week of delivery and preterm birth [44]. Our study found that the variant of *GC*-rs2070741 was associated with higher SBP at T2 and increased risk of HDP. Mutations at *GC* rs16846876, rs2282679, rs17467825, rs2298849, rs2298850, rs3755967, and rs4588 interacted with VitD deficiency at T2 on higher DBP at T2.

To our knowledge, this is the first prospective cohort study exploring the association between VitD in three trimesters and VitD pathway gene variants as well as their interactions on SBP, DBP, and the risk of HDP. However, limitations could not be neglected. First of all, some subjects had a lack of 25(OH)D data at T2 and T3, and therefore selection bias might exist. However, subgroup analysis of pregnant women with VitD detected at T1 and T2 showed that the results were almost consistent with the results in the whole study population. Secondly, as the prevalence of HDP in this study was relatively low (2.84%), the association between VitD and different HDP subtypes (GH, preeclampsia, eclampsia) could not be explored. However, studies have shown that, although these subtypes can appear alone, they are progressive manifestations of a single process and share common etiology [45,46]. Lastly, the relatively single ethnic population of this study may also limit the extrapolation of findings.

5. Conclusions

This study found that the level of 25(OH)D at T1 and T2 was negatively correlated with DBP at T2. In addition, polymorphisms in VitD metabolic pathway genes, including CYP24A1 and GC, increased the risk of HDP. Furthermore, gene variants in CYP24A1 and LRP2 and VitD deficiency at T2 showed combined effect on the risk of HDP, but the specific mechanism remains to be further investigated. The results of this study provide a scientific basis for the clinical detection of VitD during pregnancy and the supplementation of VitD during pregnancy.

Supplementary Materials: The following supporting information can be downloaded at: https://www.mdpi.com/article/10.3390/nu14112355/s1, Figure S1. Trajectory of 25(OH)D level during pregnancy. Figure S2. Dose-response relationships of 25(OH)D levels at T1 and T2 with blood pressure at T1 and T2. Figure S3. Dose-response relationships of 25(OH)D levels at T1, T2, and T3 with blood pressure at T3. Figure S4. Dose-response relationships of 25(OH)D levels at T1, T2, and T3 with HDP. Figure S5. Dose-response relationships of the change of 25(OH)D levels during pregnancy with blood pressure at T2 and T3. Figure S6. Dose-response relationships between the change of 25(OH)D levels during pregnancy and HDP. Table S1. Baseline characteristics of pregnant women in SNP analysis. Table S2. The relationship of VitD deficiency in three trimesters with blood pressure. Table S3. The association between 25(OH)D levels in three trimesters and HDP. Table S4. The relationship between VitD deficiency in three trimesters with HDP. Table S5. The association between the change of 25(OH)D levels during pregnancy and HDP. Table S6. The association between the trajectory of VitD during pregnancy and HDP. Table S7. The association of single SNP with SBP and DBP at T1. Table S8. The association of single SNP with SBP and DBP at T2. Table S9. The association of single SNP with SBP and DBP at T3. Table S10. The association of single SNP and VitD at T1 with blood pressure at T1. Table S11. The association between single SNP and VitD at T2 with blood pressure at T2. Table S12. The association between single SNP and VitD at T3 with blood pressure at T3. Table S13. The association between single SNP and VitD at T2 with blood pressure at T3.

Author Contributions: Conceptualization, Y.Y.; methodology, M.M.; validation, S.S.; resources, H.C.; formal analysis, Z.P.; investigation, X.A.; writing—review and editing, M.M.; visualization, H.Z., P.C. and Y.Z. All authors have read and agreed to the published version of the manuscript.

Funding: This study was funded by the Chinese National Natural Science Foundation (81973055), the National Key Research and Development Programme of China (No. 2021YFC2701901), and Major research and development projects of the Zhejiang Science and Technology Department (2018C03010), the Key Laboratory of Intelligent Preventive Medicine of Zhejiang Province (2020E10004) and the Leading Innovative and Entrepreneur Team Introduction Program of Zhejiang (2019R01007).

Institutional Review Board Statement: The study was conducted according to the guidelines of the Declaration of Helsinki and approved by the Institutional Review Board of Zhoushan Maternal and Child Health Care Hospital on 9 January 2011 (Ethical Approval Code: 2011-05).

Informed Consent Statement: Informed consent was obtained from all subjects involved in the study.

Data Availability Statement: The data presented in this study are available on request from the corresponding author. The data are not publicly available because they contain information that could compromise the privacy of research participants.

Acknowledgments: We thank all the participants who took part in this study. We acknowledge the support of staff in Zhoushan Maternal and Child Care Hospital, who conducted and managed the cohort.

Conflicts of Interest: The authors declare that they have no conflict of interest.

References

1. American College of Obstetricians and Gynecologists' Task Force on Hypertension in Pregnancy. Hypertension in Pregnancy. *Obstet. Gynecol.* **2013**, *122*, 1122–1131. [CrossRef]
2. Khan, K.S.; Wojdyla, D.; Say, L.; Gülmezoglu, A.M.; Van Look, P.F. WHO analysis of causes of maternal death: A systematic review. *Lancet* **2006**, *367*, 1066–1074. [CrossRef]
3. Say, L.; Chou, D.; Gemmill, A.; Tunçalp, Ö.; Moller, A.-B.; Daniels, J.; Gülmezoglu, A.M.; Temmerman, M.; Alkema, L. Global causes of maternal death: A WHO systematic analysis. *Lancet Glob. Health* **2014**, *2*, E323–E333. [CrossRef]
4. Theilen, L.H.; Meeks, H.; Fraser, A.; Esplin, M.S.; Smith, K.R.; Varner, M.W. Long-term mortality risk and life expectancy following recurrent hypertensive disease of pregnancy. *Am. J. Obstet. Gynecol.* **2018**, *219*, 107.e1–107.e6. [CrossRef]
5. Visintin, C.; Mugglestone, M.A.; Almerie, M.Q.; Nherera, L.M.; James, D.; Walkinshaw, S. On behalf of the Guideline Development Group Management of hypertensive disorders during pregnancy: Summary of NICE guidance. *BMJ* **2010**, *341*, c2207. [CrossRef] [PubMed]
6. Rana, S.; Lemoine, E.; Granger, J.P.; Karumanchi, S.A. Preeclampsia: Pathophysiology, Challenges, and Perspectives. *Circ. Res.* **2019**, *124*, 1094–1112. [CrossRef] [PubMed]
7. Adela, R.; Borkar, R.M.; Mishra, N.; Bhandi, M.M.; Vishwakarma, G.; Varma, B.A.; Ragampeta, S.; Banerjee, S.K. Lower Serum Vitamin D Metabolite Levels in Relation to Circulating Cytokines/Chemokines and Metabolic Hormones in Pregnant Women with Hypertensive Disorders. *Front. Immunol.* **2017**, *8*, 273. [CrossRef]
8. Rezavand, N.; Tabarok, S.; Rahimi, Z.; Vaisi-Raygani, A.; Mohammadi, E.; Rahimi, Z. The effect of VDR gene polymorphisms and vitamin D level on blood pressure, risk of preeclampsia, gestational age, and body mass index. *J. Cell. Biochem.* **2018**, *120*, 6441–6448. [CrossRef]
9. Zhang, J.Y.; Lucey, A.J.; Horgan, R.; Kenny, L.C.; Kiely, M. Impact of pregnancy on vitamin D status: A longitudinal study. *Br. J. Nutr.* **2014**, *112*, 1081–1087. [CrossRef] [PubMed]
10. Ganguly, A.; Tamblyn, J.A.; Finn-Sell, S.; Chan, S.; Westwood, M.; Gupta, J.; Kilby, M.D.; Gross, S.; Hewison, M. Vitamin D, the placenta and early pregnancy: Effects on trophoblast function. *J. Endocrinol.* **2018**, *236*, R93–R103. [CrossRef]
11. Weisman, Y.; Harell, A.; Edelstein, S.; David, M.; Spirer, Z.; Golander, A. 1α,25-Dihydroxyvitamin D3, and 24,25-dihydroxyvitamin D3 in vitro synthesis by human decidua and placenta. *Nature* **1979**, *281*, 317–319. [CrossRef]
12. Zehnder, D.; Evans, K.N.; Kilby, M.D.; Bulmer, J.N.; Innes, B.A.; Stewart, P.M.; Hewison, M. The Ontogeny of 25-Hydroxyvitamin D3 1α-Hydroxylase Expression in Human Placenta and Decidua. *Am. J. Pathol.* **2002**, *161*, 105–114. [CrossRef]
13. Karras, S.N.; Wagner, C.L.; Castracane, V.D. Understanding vitamin D metabolism in pregnancy: From physiology to pathophysiology and clinical outcomes. *Metabolism* **2018**, *86*, 112–123. [CrossRef] [PubMed]
14. De-Regil, L.M.; Palacios, C.; Lombardo, L.K.; Pena-Rosas, J.P. Vitamin D supplementation for women during pregnancy. *Cochrane Database Syst. Rev.* **2016**, *1*, CD008873.
15. Palacios, C.; Kostiuk, L.K.; Pena-Rosas, J.P. Vitamin D supplementation for women during pregnancy. *Cochrane Database Syst. Rev.* **2019**, *7*, CD008873. [CrossRef]
16. Barebring, L.; O'Connell, M.; Winkvist, A.; Johannsson, G.; Augustin, H. Serum cortisol and vitamin D status are independently associated with blood pressure in pregnancy. *J. Steroid Biochem. Mol. Biol.* **2019**, *189*, 259–264. [CrossRef]
17. Magnus, M.C.; Miliku, K.; Bauer, A.; Engel, S.M.; Felix, J.F.; Jaddoe, V.W.V.; ALawlor, D.; London, S.J.; Magnus, P.; McGinnis, R.; et al. Vitamin D and risk of pregnancy related hypertensive disorders: Mendelian randomisation study. *BMJ* **2018**, *361*, k2167. [CrossRef]
18. Barry, E.L.; Rees, J.R.; Peacock, J.L.; Mott, L.A.; Amos, C.I.; Bostick, R.M.; Figueiredo, J.C.; Ahnen, D.J.; Bresalier, R.S.; Burke, C.A.; et al. Genetic variants in CYP2R1, CYP24A1, and VDR modify the efficacy of vitamin D3 supplementation for increasing serum 25-hydroxyvitamin D levels in a randomized controlled trial. *J. Clin. Endocrinol. Metab.* **2014**, *99*, E2133–E2137. [CrossRef] [PubMed]
19. Shao, B.; Mo, M.; Xin, X.; Jiang, W.; Wu, J.; Huang, M.; Wang, S.; Muyiduli, X.; Si, S.; Shen, Y.; et al. The interaction between prepregnancy BMI and gestational vitamin D deficiency on the risk of gestational diabetes mellitus subtypes with elevated fasting blood glucose. *Clin. Nutr.* **2020**, *39*, 2265–2273. [CrossRef]
20. Holick, M.F.; Binkley, N.C.; Bischoff-Ferrari, H.A.; Gordon, C.M.; Hanley, D.A.; Heaney, R.P.; Murad, M.H.; Weaver, C.M. Endocrine Society. Evaluation, Treatment, and Prevention of Vitamin D Deficiency: An Endocrine Society Clinical Practice Guideline. *J. Clin. Endocrinol. Metab.* **2011**, *96*, 1911–1930. [CrossRef]
21. Thorne, H.C.; Jones, K.H.; Peters, S.P.; Archer, S.N.; Dijk, D.-J. Daily and Seasonal Variation in the Spectral Composition of Light Exposure in Humans. *Chrono Int.* **2009**, *26*, 854–866. [CrossRef] [PubMed]
22. Zhao, P.; Diao, Y.; You, L.; Wu, S.; Yang, L.; Liu, Y. The influence of basic public health service project on maternal health services: An interrupted time series study. *BMC Public Health* **2019**, *19*, 824–831. [CrossRef] [PubMed]
23. Brown, M.A.; Magee, L.A.; Kenny, L.C.; Karumanchi, S.A.; McCarthy, F.P.; Saito, S.; Hall, D.R.; Warren, C.E.; Adoyi, G.; Ishaku, S.; et al. Hypertensive Disorders of Pregnancy: ISSHP Classification, Diagnosis, and Management Recommendations for International Practice. *Hypertension* **2018**, *72*, 24–43. [CrossRef]
24. American College of Obstetricians and Gynecologists. Practice ACoO. ACOG practice bulletin. Diagnosis and management of preeclampsia and eclampsia. International journal of gynaecology and obstetrics: The official organ of the International Federation of Gynaecology and Obstetrics. *Obstet. Gynecol.* **2002**, *77*, 67–75.

25. Shao, B.; Jiang, S.; Muyiduli, X.; Wang, S.; Mo, M.; Li, M.; Wang, Z.; Yu, Y. Vitamin D pathway gene polymorphisms influenced vitamin D level among pregnant women. *Clin. Nutr.* **2018**, *37*, 2230–2237. [CrossRef]
26. Wu, J.; Shao, B.; Xin, X.; Luo, W.; Mo, M.; Jiang, W.; Si, S.; Wang, S.; Shen, Y.; Yu, Y. Association of vitamin D pathway gene polymorphisms with vitamin D level during pregnancy was modified by season and vitamin D supplement. *Clin. Nutr.* **2020**, *40*, 3650–3660. [CrossRef]
27. Li, W.; Jin, C.; Vaidya, A.; Wu, Y.; Rexrode, K.; Zheng, X.; Gurol, M.E.; Ma, C.; Wu, S.; Gao, X. Blood Pressure Trajectories and the Risk of Intracerebral Hemorrhage and Cerebral Infarction: A Prospective Study. *Hypertension* **2017**, *70*, 508–514. [CrossRef] [PubMed]
28. Desquilbet, L.; Mariotti, F. Dose-response analyses using restricted cubic spline functions in public health research. *Stat. Med.* **2010**, *29*, 1037–1057. [CrossRef] [PubMed]
29. Zhou, J.; Su, L.; Liu, M.; Liu, Y.; Cao, X.; Wang, Z.; Xiao, H. Associations between 25-hydroxyvitamin D levels and pregnancy outcomes: A prospective observational study in southern China. *Eur. J. Clin. Nutr.* **2014**, *68*, 925–930. [CrossRef]
30. Bärebring, L.; Bullarbo, M.; Glantz, A.; Agelii, M.L.; Jagner; Ellis, J.; Hulthen, L.; Schoenmakers, I.; Augustin, H. Preeclampsia and Blood Pressure Trajectory during Pregnancy in Relation to Vitamin D Status. *PLoS ONE* **2016**, *11*, e0152198. [CrossRef] [PubMed]
31. Schneuer, F.J.; Roberts, C.L.; Guilbert, C.; Simpson, J.M.; Algert, C.S.; Khambalia, A.Z.; Tasevski, V.; Ashton, A.W.; Morris, J.M.; Nassar, N. Effects of maternal serum 25-hydroxyvitamin D concentrations in the first trimester on subsequent pregnancy outcomes in an Australian population. *Am. J. Clin. Nutr.* **2014**, *99*, 287–295. [CrossRef] [PubMed]
32. O'Callaghan, K.M.; Kiely, M. Systematic Review of Vitamin D and Hypertensive Disorders of Pregnancy. *Nutrients* **2018**, *10*, 294. [CrossRef]
33. Wang, T.J.; Zhang, F.; Richards, J.B.; Kestenbaum, B.; van Meurs, J.B.; Berry, D.; Kiel, D.P.; Streeten, E.A.; Ohlsson, C.; Koller, D.L.; et al. Common genetic determinants of vitamin D insufficiency: A genome-wide association study. *Lancet* **2010**, *376*, 180–188. [CrossRef]
34. Knabl, J.; Vattai, A.; Ye, Y.; Jueckstock, J.; Hutter, S.; Kainer, F.; Mahner, S.; Jeschke, U. Role of Placental VDR Expression and Function in Common Late Pregnancy Disorders. *Int. J. Mol. Sci.* **2017**, *18*, 2340. [CrossRef] [PubMed]
35. Sakaki, T.; Kagawa, N.; Yamamoto, K.; Inouye, K. Metabolism of vitamin D3 by cytochromes P450. *Front. Biosci.* **2005**, *10*, 119–134.
36. Bao, Q.; Wang, D.; Zhang, Y.; Bao, L.; Jia, H. The Impact of CYP24A1 Polymorphisms on Hypertension Susceptibility. *Kidney Blood Press. Res.* **2020**, *45*, 28–37. [CrossRef]
37. Wang, L.; Chu, A.; Buring, J.E.; Ridker, P.M.; Chasman, D.I.; Sesso, H.D. Common Genetic Variations in the Vitamin D Pathway in Relation to Blood Pressure. *Am. J. Hypertens.* **2014**, *27*, 1387–1395. [CrossRef]
38. Marzolo, M.-P.; Farfán, P. New Insights into the Roles of Megalin/LRP2 and the Regulation of its Functional Expression. *Biol. Res.* **2011**, *44*, 89–105. [CrossRef]
39. Norman, A.W. *1α,25(OH)2 Vitamin D3Vitamin D Nuclear Receptor (VDR) and Plasma Vitamin D-Binding Protein (DBP) Structures and Ligand Shape Preferences for Genomic and Rapid Biological Responses*; Elsevier Inc.: Amsterdam, The Netherlands, 2008.
40. Bikle, D.D.; Malmstroem, S.; Schwartz, J. Current Controversies: Are Free Vitamin Metabolite Levels a More Accurate Assessment of Vitamin D Status than Total Levels? *Endocrinol. Metab. Clin. N. Am.* **2017**, *46*, 901–918. [CrossRef]
41. Mekbeb, T. The association of serum proteins with preeclampsia. *Ethiop. Med. J.* **1990**, *28*, 1–30.
42. Naidoo, Y.; Moodley, J.; Ramsuran, V.; Naicker, T. Polymorphisms within vitamin D binding protein gene within a Preeclamptic South African population. *Hypertens. Pregnancy* **2019**, *38*, 260–267. [CrossRef]
43. Powe, C.E.; Seely, E.W.; Rana, S.; Bhan, I.; Ecker, J.; Karumanchi, S.A.; Thadhani, R. First trimester vitamin D, vitamin D binding protein, and subsequent preeclampsia. *Hypertension* **2010**, *56*, 758–763. [CrossRef]
44. Wang, S.; Xin, X.; Luo, W.; Mo, M.; Si, S.; Shao, B.; Shen, Y.; Cheng, H.; Yu, Y. Association of vitamin D and gene variants in the vitamin D metabolic pathway with preterm birth. *Nutrition* **2021**, *89*, 111349. [CrossRef] [PubMed]
45. Phoswa, W.N. Dopamine in the Pathophysiology of Preeclampsia and Gestational Hypertension: Monoamine Oxidase (MAO) and Catechol-O-methyl Transferase (COMT) as Possible Mechanisms. *Oxidative Med. Cell. Longev.* **2019**, *2019*, 1–8. [CrossRef] [PubMed]
46. Mammaro, A.; Carrara, S.; Cavaliere, A.; Ermito, S.; Dinatale, A.; Pappalardo, E.M.; Militello, M.; Pedata, R. Hypertensive disorders of pregnancy. *J. Prenat. Med.* **2009**, *3*, 1–5. [PubMed]

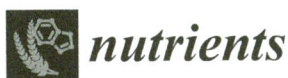

Article

Associations between Maternal Selenium Status and Cord Serum Vitamin D Levels: A Birth Cohort Study in Wuhan, China

Huiqing Gang [1], Hongling Zhang [2], Tongzhang Zheng [3], Wei Xia [1], Shunqing Xu [1] and Yuanyuan Li [1,*]

1. Key Laboratory of Environment and Health, Ministry of Education & Ministry of Environmental Protection, and State Key Laboratory of Environmental Health, School of Public Health, Tongji Medical College, Huazhong University of Science and Technology, Wuhan 430030, China; ganghq342@163.com (H.G.); xiawei@hust.edu.cn (W.X.); xust@hust.edu.cn (S.X.)
2. School of Health and Nursing, Wuchang University of Technology, Wuhan 430000, China; zhanghongling@wut.edu.cn
3. Department of Epidemiology, Brown University, Providence, RI 02912, USA; tongzhang_zheng@brown.edu
* Correspondence: liyuanyuan@hust.edu.cn

Abstract: Serum selenium (Se) has been reported to be associated with serum 25-hydroxyvitamin D [25(OH)D], but epidemiological findings are limited in pregnant women. We aimed to assess the associations between maternal urinary Se concentrations and cord serum 25(OH)D levels. We measured urinary concentrations of Se in the first, second, and third trimesters and cord serum 25(OH)D of 1695 mother-infant pairs from a prospective cohort study in Wuhan, China. The results showed that each doubling of urinary Se concentrations in the first, second, third trimester, and whole pregnancy (average SG-adjusted concentrations across three trimesters) were associated with 8.76% (95% confidence interval (CI): 4.30%, 13.41%), 15.44% (95% CI: 9.18%, 22.06%), 11.84% (95% CI: 6.09%, 17.89%), and 21.14% (95% CI: 8.69%, 35.02%) increases in 25(OH)D levels. Newborns whose mothers with low (<10 μg/L) or medium (10.92–14.34 μg/L) tertiles of urinary Se concentrations in whole pregnancy were more likely to be vitamin D deficient (<20 ng/mL) compared with those with the highest tertile (>14.34 μg/L). Our study provides evidence that maternal Se levels were positively associated with cord serum vitamin D status.

Keywords: cord serum 25(OH)D level; vitamin D deficiency; urinary selenium; repeated measurements

Citation: Gang, H.; Zhang, H.; Zheng, T.; Xia, W.; Xu, S.; Li, Y. Associations between Maternal Selenium Status and Cord Serum Vitamin D Levels: A Birth Cohort Study in Wuhan, China. *Nutrients* **2022**, *14*, 1715. https:// doi.org/10.3390/nu14091715

Academic Editors: Yunxian Yu and Lutz Schomburg

Received: 17 March 2022
Accepted: 14 April 2022
Published: 20 April 2022

Publisher's Note: MDPI stays neutral with regard to jurisdictional claims in published maps and institutional affiliations.

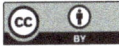

Copyright: © 2022 by the authors. Licensee MDPI, Basel, Switzerland. This article is an open access article distributed under the terms and conditions of the Creative Commons Attribution (CC BY) license (https:// creativecommons.org/licenses/by/ 4.0/).

1. Introduction

Selenium (Se), an essential micronutrient [1,2], is a critical component of Glutathione Peroxidase (GSH-Px), which has an irreplaceable effect on human health [3]. People usually absorb Se from the diet [4,5], which is rapidly excreted from the body mainly through urine after being metabolized [6]. Reactive oxygen species (ROS) produced by the placenta during pregnancy significantly impact placental function. As an essential trace element, Se has an irreplaceable role in antioxidants during pregnancy because of the antioxidant properties of selenoproteins [7]. The recommended Se intake is 55 μg/day [8,9], and its safe upper limit is 400 μg/day. Intake of more than 800 μg/day may lead to Se toxicity [9]: loss of hair and nails, poor neurological, skin, and dental health, garlic odor on the breath, and even paralysis [10]. Low Se status or Se deficiency has been found to be associated with adverse pregnancy outcomes such as preterm birth [11], pre-eclampsia, and hypertension during pregnancy [12]. In addition to blood (including blood, plasma, and serum), toenail, and hair [13], urinary Se is considered to be a valid biomarker for assessing Se status in humans [14]. Previous studies have shown that the time point of Se level assessment affects the accuracy of data, and pregnant women with adequate Se levels in the first trimester might be Se deficient in the third trimester. Hence, repeated measurements of urinary Se during a broader window are necessary [7,15].

Our body derives vitamin D from ultraviolet B (UV-B) radiation exposure to the skin, dietary intake, and dietary supplements [16]. Vitamin D_3, which was produced from the skin, and vitamin D_2 and D_3 from the diet are hydroxylated in the liver to produce 25-hydroxyvitamin D_2 [25(OH)D_2] and 25-hydroxyvitamin D_3 [25(OH)D_3]. Serum 25(OH)D is the key circulating metabolite of vitamin D, which has a two-week biological half-life and is a clinical measure of vitamin D status, although it will continue to undergo hydroxylation in the kidney to its active form: 1,25-hydroxyvitamin D [1,25(OH)$_2$D] [17]. The impact of a newborn's vitamin D deficiency is receiving increasing attention. Previous studies have shown that vitamin D levels in cord blood are associated with childhood diseases, such as asthma, wheezing, respiratory infections [18], and type 1 diabetes [19]. Many factors influence cord serum vitamin D levels, such as age, genetics, vitamin D intake, and outdoor activities [20]. In our previous study, a negative correlation was observed between repeatedly measured urinary cobalt (Co), vanadium (V), and thallium (Tl) concentrations during pregnancy and cord serum vitamin D status [21]. A positive correlation between serum Se concentration and vitamin D levels in humans was found in China [22]. However, the factors associated with vitamin D levels have not been thoroughly investigated. Therefore, we aimed to explore whether there is an association between Se concentrations in pregnant women and cord serum 25(OH)D levels in newborns.

Given the above, this study was based on a prospective birth cohort to assess maternal physical Se status. It used repeatedly measured Se levels to estimate the association between prenatal Se concentrations and cord serum 25(OH)D levels to provide epidemiological evidence for health care during pregnancy.

2. Materials and Methods

2.1. Study Population

Our participants were from a prospective cohort study in Wuhan, China. The pregnant women were enrolled who were: (1) <16 weeks of pregnancy with a singleton gestation at first prenatal care; (2) residents in Wuhan and willing to have prenatal visits and delivery at the target hospital; (3) willing to provide urine samples and cord blood samples and cooperate with questionnaires. From September 2013 to June 2015, a total of 3198 pregnant women entered our cohort, and 2564 provided at least one urine sample. Among them, we selected 1698 pregnant women who provided cord blood samples during delivery, excluding two pregnant women with missing prepregnancy body mass index (BMI) data and one pregnant woman with missing multivitamin D dietary supplement data, leaving 1695 pairs of mothers and infants enrolled in our study for analysis. Pregnant women in the first trimester (13.1 ± 1.1 weeks, $n = 1579$), second trimester (24.1 ± 3.4 weeks, $n = 979$), and third trimester (35.0 ± 3.1 weeks, $n = 924$) were included, and 570 participants provided urine samples in all three trimesters. Our study was approved by the Ethics Committee of Tongji Medical College of Huazhong University of Science and Technology.

2.2. Covariates

Covariates were obtained through interviews and medical records. Interviews were conducted using questionnaires to investigate demographic and socioeconomic characteristics, including maternal age, height, prepregnancy weight, education level, lifestyle factors (smoking, alcohol consumption, passive smoking), and vitamin D supplementation. Date of last menstrual period (LMP), gestation, pregnancy complications [e.g., gestational diabetes (GDM), pregnancy-induced hypertension (PIH), and anemia], mode of delivery, date of delivery, gestational age, and sex of the newborns were obtained from medical records. The prepregnancy body mass index (BMI) of mothers was calculated based on prepregnancy weight and height. The gestational week was calculated using the time of urine sample collection minus LMP. Weight gain during pregnancy was calculated based on prepregnancy weight versus predelivery weight. Passive smoking was defined as exposure to secondhand smoking in the home or workplace during pregnancy [23]. We divided the delivery season into Cold (December–May) and Warm (June–November) according to the climatic features of Wuhan, China: long winter and summer, short spring and autumn [21,24].

2.3. Urine Collection and Se Measurement

The urine samples were collected at the first, second, and third trimester of gestation in polypropylene cups and stored in sterile 5 mL pp tubes in refrigerators at −20 °C. Urinary Se, V, Co, and Tl concentrations were detected using an inductively coupled plasma mass spectrometry (ICP-MS), and the details of the method can be found in our previously published articles [25]. Urine samples were taken out of the −20 °C refrigerators and brought to room temperature before determination. After being mixed thoroughly with a turbine, urine samples were added to 1.2% (v/v) nitric acid overnight, sonicated at 40 °C for 1 h before formal detection on the machine, and finally analyzed in helium mode. Human urine specimens (SRM2670a) were used as external quality controls to evaluate the accuracy of ICP-MS in each batch of experiments. A blank sample (1.2% (v/v) HNO_3) was added after each batch of urine samples was analyzed, and the line was flushed to control potential contamination. The limit of detections (LODs) for urinary Se, V, Co, and Tl were 0.224, 0.002, 0.010, and 0.020 µg/L, respectively, and the intraday variability of Se, V, Co, and Tl detected in urine samples was 0.553%−1.118%. Se level for one urine sample was below the LOD of Se. The interday variability was 0.272%−0.816%. Concentrations of Se, V, Co, and Tl were adjusted for variation in dilution by urinary specific gravity (SG) through the following equation: $P_c = P_i [(SG_m − 1)/(SG_i − 1)]$, P_c is the SG-adjusted urinary Se, V, Co, and Tl concentration (ng/mL), P_i is the observed urinary Se, V, Co, and Tl concentrations (µg/L), SG_m is the median SG for the urine samples of each trimester, and SG is the specific gravity of each urine sample. SG was by a pocket refractometer while preparing urinary samples for analysis (Atago PAL-10S;Atago, Tokyo, Japan). In our study, 11 pregnant women had missing urinary specific gravity data in the first trimester, 10 in the second trimester, and six in the third trimester.

2.4. Cord Serum Collection and 25(OH)D Analyses

Details on the processing of cord blood samples and the detection of cord serum vitamin D were described in our previous article [21]. Cord blood samples are obtained immediately after delivery, centrifuged to extract cord serum, and stored in a −80 °C refrigerator prior to the determination. Liquid chromatography and triple quadrupole mass spectrometry couples (LC-MS/MS) were used to determine the levels of $25(OH)D_2$ and $25(OH)D_3$ in cord serum. The intrabatch and interbatch coefficients of variation were less than 15%. The detection limits (LODs) for $25(OH)D_2$ and $25(OH)D_3$ were 0.5 and 1.0 ng/mL, respectively. The concentrations of 25(OH)D were equated to the sum of $25(OH)D_2$ and $25(OH)D_3$.

2.5. Statistical Analysis

Urinary Se was replaced as LOD/2 if the concentration was below the value of LOD. Median, upper quartile, lower quartile, 25th percentile, and 75th percentile were used to describe the distributions of urinary Se concentrations at the first, second, and third trimester of gestation and whole pregnancy (averaged SG-adjusted concentrations across three trimesters) were also analyzed. The concentrations of urinary Se and cord serum 25(OH)D were naturally ln-transformed because the distributions were right-skewed. Intraclass correlation coefficient (ICC) was calculated using a linear mixed model to examine the reproducibility of participants' SG-adjusted urinary Se levels in the first, second, and third trimesters.

We explored the association between the whole pregnancy (averaged SG-adjusted concentrations across three trimesters) urinary Se levels of pregnant women and cord serum 25(OH)D by fitting a generalized linear model (GLM). Furthermore, generalized estimating equations models (GEE) were used to investigate associations between repeatedly measured urinary Se levels and cord serum 25(OH)D. We also assessed the association between categorical variables based on tertile distribution of average SG-adjusted urinary Se levels in all three trimesters with newborn's vitamin D deficiency using a GLM model (cord serum total 25(OH)D concentration < 20 ng/mL was considered vitamin D deficiency) [26]. We calculated the percent change of cord serum vitamin D for per doubling maternal urinary Se concentrations increase using the formula: percent change (%Δ) = $[e^{(\ln 2 \times \beta)} - 1]$, where β was the coefficient from GLM and GEE models [27].

Confounders were introduced based on biological and statistical considerations. Bivariate summary analyses ($p < 0.1$) were applied to all variables. Urinary metals (V, Co, TL) concentrations were added to the model as covariates. Only one pregnant woman smoked during pregnancy, and no one reported drinking, so smoking and drinking during pregnancy were not added to the model as covariates. The final covariates included in the model were: maternal age, prepregnancy BMI, season of birth, mode of delivery, gestational weight gain, passive smoking before or during pregnancy, and multivitamin supplement use during pregnancy.

Season of birth has been considered to be associated with cord serum 25(OH)D levels in previous studies [21,28]. Therefore, our analyses were stratified by infant birth season (warm or cold) and performed separately.

Many previous studies have linked cord serum 25(OH)D levels to pregnancy complications such as gestational diabetes mellitus (GDM), pregnancy-induced hypertension (PIH), and anemia [20]. Therefore, a sensitivity analysis was carried out among pregnant women without these diseases to validate the robustness of our results.

This study performed data analyses with version 9.4 Statistical Analysis System (SAS; SAS Institute Inc., Cary, NC, USA; version 9.4). All tests were bilateral, and p values < 0.05 were defined as statistically significant.

3. Results

3.1. Characteristics of the Study Population

Table 1 lists the main characteristics of our participants. The average age of the 1695 pregnant women in this study was 28.37. Most of the pregnant women were primigravida (86.49%). About half of the women had an education level above high school (48.26%). Mothers who took multivitamin supplements during pregnancy were almost ten times more than those who did not take them. Thirteen pregnant women drank alcohol before pregnancy, and none of them continued during pregnancy. Thirteen pregnant women smoked before pregnancy, one woman continued to smoke during pregnancy, and 32.04% smoked passively before six months of pregnancy or during pregnancy. As for health status during pregnancy, 35 mothers had pregnancy-induced hypertension (PIH), 102 pregnant women had gestational diabetes mellitus (GDM), and 68 pregnant women had anemia. Of the newborns, 55.69% were born in the warm season, 53.81% were male, and 53.22% were delivered by cesarean section.

3.2. Distributions and Variability of Maternal Urinary Se and Cord Serum 25(OH)D Concentrations

The urinary Se concentrations of pregnant women are shown in Table 2. The concentrations (median (5th percentile, 95th percentile)) of urinary Se adjusted by SG in pregnant women was 17.82 (8.48, 51.58) μg/L for the first trimester, 10.39 (5.08, 26.18) μg/L for the second trimester, 11.51 (5.33, 35.18) μg/L for the third trimester, and 12.63 (7.44, 22.54) μg/L for whole pregnancy (average concentrations across three trimesters). The median value (5th percentile, 95th percentile) of 25(OH)D concentrations was 21.10 (5.53, 49.98) ng/mL. The concentration distribution of other urinary metals (V, Co, Tl) can be seen in Supplementary Material Table S2. The intraclass correlation coefficients (ICC) (Supplementary Material Table S1) of SG-adjusted urinary Se, V, Co, and Tl were 0.48 (95% CI: 0.44, 0.52), 0.40 (95% CI: 0.36, 0.45), 0.24 (95% CI: 0.20, 0.29), and 0.41 (95% CI: 0.37, 0.45), ranged from 0.24 to 0.48, which indicated poor to fair reproducibility.

Table 1. Characteristics of mother-infant pairs (n = 1695).

Characteristics	n	Mean ± SD or Percent
Age (years)		28.37 ± 3.29
≤24	150	8.85
25–29	1036	61.12
30–34	420	24.78
≥35	89	5.25
Prepregnancy BMI (kg/m^2)		20.76 ± 2.75
Underweight (<18.5)	336	19.82
Normal (18.5–23.9)	1151	67.91
Overweight (≥24)	208	12.27
Gestational weight gain (kg)		16.39 ± 4.78
Parity		
Multiparous	229	13.51
Nulliparous	1466	86.49
Educational level		
High school and below	877	51.74
More than high school	818	48.26
Multivitamin supplement use during pregnancy		
No	153	9.03
Yes	1542	90.97
Passive smoking before/during pregnancy		
No	1152	67.96
Yes	543	32.04
Drinking before pregnancy		
No	1682	99.23
Yes	13	0.77
Gestational age (week)		39.30 ± 1.20
Mode of delivery		
Vaginal delivery	793	46.78
Cesarean delivery	902	53.22
Season of birth		
Cold (December–May)	751	44.31
Warm (June–November)	944	55.69
Infant sex		
Male	912	53.81
Female	783	46.19
PIH		
No	1660	97.94
Yes	35	2.06
GDM		
No	1593	93.98
Yes	102	6.02
Anemia		
No	1627	95.99
Yes	68	4.01

3.3. Individual Urinary Se and Cord Serum 25(OH)D

Table 3 shows the association between repeated measurements of urinary Se and cord serum 25(OH)D concentrations. In model 1, we found a positive association between urinary Se and cord serum 25(OH)D concentrations in the second trimester, with per doubling of urinary Se concentration increasing cord serum 25(OH)D concentrations by 8.95% (95% confidence interval (CI): 3.20%, 15.04%). After concentrations of V, Co, and Tl during each trimester were included in model 2 simultaneously, urinary Se concentrations were associated with cord serum 25(OH)D concentrations in the first trimester, second trimester, and the third trimester with each twofold increase in urinary Se being associated with 8.76% (95% CI: 4.30%, 13.41%), 15.44% (95% CI: 9.18%, 22.06%), and 11.84% (95% CI:

6.09%, 17.89%) increase in cord serum 25(OH)D. A generalized linear model (GLM) was used to analyze the relationship between urinary Se concentrations in whole pregnancy and cord serum 25(OH)D concentrations. In model 1 and model 2, per doubling of average urinary Se levels increase were associated with 16.86% (95% CI: 5.33%, 29.67%), 21.14% (95% CI: 8.69%, 35.02%) increase in cord serum 25(OH)D.

Table 2. The distributions of maternal urinary Se and cord serum 25(OH)D concentrations during pregnancy.

Concentrations	n	Percentiles				
		5th	25th	50th	75th	95th
Urinary Se (μg/L)						
Unadjusted						
first trimester	1539	3.16	8.99	15.96	29.17	64.07
second trimester	979	2.72	6.13	10.36	17.54	36.47
third trimester	924	3.00	6.37	10.63	18.66	42.65
Whole pregnancy *	570	4.79	8.30	12.30	17.81	27.36
SG-adjusted						
first trimester	1528	8.48	13.27	17.82	26.52	51.58
second trimester	969	5.08	7.79	10.39	14.14	26.18
third trimester	918	5.33	8.50	11.51	16.01	35.18
Whole pregnancy *	570	7.44	10.09	12.63	15.38	22.54
Cord serum 25(OH)D (ng/mL)						
25(OH)D$_2$	1695	0.25	0.96	1.15	1.47	2.51
25(OH)D$_3$	1695	4.29	11.27	19.79	31.09	48.53
Total 25(OH)D	1695	5.53	12.39	21.10	32.47	49.98

* Average concentrations across three trimesters.

Table 3. Associations of maternal urinary Se concentrations and cord serum 25(OH)D level.

Variable	Model 1		Model 2	
	%Δ (95%CI)	p-Value	%Δ (95%CI)	p-Value
Selenium				
1st trimester [a]	0.79 (−2.94, 4.67)	0.683	8.76 (4.30, 13.41)	<0.0001
2nd trimester [a]	8.95 (3.20, 15.04)	0.002	15.44 (9.18, 22.06)	<0.0001
3rd trimester [a]	3.18 (−1.82, 8.42)	0.217	11.84 (6.09, 17.89)	<0.0001
Whole pregnancy [b]	16.86 (5.33, 29.67)	0.003	21.14 (8.69, 35.02)	0.0005

CI, confidence interval. [a] Generalized estimating equation model, model 1 adjusted for maternal age, prepregnancy BMI, season of birth, mode of delivery, gestational weight gain, passive smoking before/during pregnancy, and multivitamin supplement use during pregnancy. Model 2 adjusted for covariates in model 1 and SG-adjusted metals levels (Vanadium, Cobalt, Thallium). [b] Generalized linear model, model 2 adjusted for covariates in model 1 and additionally adjusted average SG-adjusted concentrations of each metal (Vanadium, Cobalt, Thallium) across different trimesters.

3.4. Association between Urinary Se Levels and Newborns' Vitamin D Deficiency

As shown in Table 4 in the analysis of prenatal Se levels and newborns' vitamin D deficiency, among all mother-infant pairs, vitamin D deficiency risk increased 59% in the low [0.59 (95% CI: 0.12, 1.06)] and 52% in the medium [0.52 (95%CI: 0.06, 0.97)] tertiles of urinary Se concentrations vs. the high group (p for trend = 0.01). After stratified by the season of birth, a significant association between urinary Se levels and vitamin D deficiency was observed among newborns who were born in the cold season [0.91 (95% CI: 0.19, 1.64) in the low group and 1.02 (95% CI: 0.28, 1.77) in medium group vs. high group, p for trend = 0.02], but not in the warm season ($p > 0.05$).

Table 4. Association between urinary Se levels and newborns' vitamin D deficiency.

Se Concentrations (μg/L SG)	All [a] β (95%CI)	p-Value	Cold Season [b] β (95%CI)	p-Value	Warm Season [c] β (95%CI)	p-Value
Low (<10.92)	0.59 (0.12, 1.06)	0.014	0.91 (0.19, 1.64)	0.013	0.52 (−0.12, 1.17)	0.111
Medium (10.92–14.34)	0.52 (0.06, 0.97)	0.026	1.02 (0.28, 1.77)	0.007	0.30 (−0.31, 0.91)	0.334
High (>14.34)	Reference		Reference		Reference	
p for trend		0.015		0.018		0.109

[a] Generalized linear model, adjusted for maternal age, prepregnancy BMI, season of birth, mode of delivery, gestational weight gain, multivitamin supplements use during pregnancy, passive smoking before/during pregnancy, and SG-adjusted metals levels (Vanadium, Cobalt, Thallium). [b] Infants born in the cold season (Dec–May), adjusted for covariates except season of birth in a. [c] Infants born in the warm season (June–November), adjusted for covariates except season of birth in a.

3.5. Sensitive Analysis

After excluding pregnant women with GDM, PIH, or anemia, the results were almost unchanged (Table S3), indicating that the association between urinary Se concentrations and cord serum 25(OH)D would not be influenced by these diseases.

4. Discussion

Based on a prospective cohort study design, we included 1695 pregnant women in Wuhan to investigate the specific trimester Se levels in urine during pregnancy and explore the association between urinary Se level and cord serum 25(OH)D status. For our participants, low levels of mothers' urinary Se were observed to be a risk factor for newborns' vitamin D deficiency (<20 ng/mL), and the negative effect seems to be more prominent in newborns who were born during the cold season.

The urinary Se concentration adjusted by urinary specific gravity (median) of the participants in our study (Wuhan, Central China) was 17.82 μg/L for the first trimester (n = 1528), 10.9 μg/L for the second trimester (n = 969), 11.51 μg/L for the third trimester (n = 918), and 12.63 μg/L for whole pregnancy (average SG-adjusted concentrations across three trimesters) (n = 570). The median value of unadjusted urinary Se concentration in the general population of northeastern China was 17 μg/L, while our data for pregnant women were lower (median = 10.36–15.96 μg/L) [29]. The data we obtained were lower than in Mexico (third trimester: 35.8 μg/L, n = 132), Greece (second trimester: 22.8 μg/L (unadjusted), n = 176 [30]; 22 μg/L, n = 575 [31]), but higher than in Bangladesh (first trimester: 9.0 μg/L, n = 74; 6.7, n = 152) [32].

Only one paper from China showed a positive association between serum Se and vitamin D in menopausal women with osteoporosis [22]. As far as we know, our study is the first epidemiological study to investigate the association of maternal urinary Se concentrations with cord serum 25(OH)D levels. Our previous study suggested the potential effects of prenatal exposure to metals (V, Co, and Tl) on decreased cord serum 25(OH)D concentrations [21]. After controlling for the above three urinary metals concentrations, the effect of urinary Se on cord serum 25(OH)D was increased, indicating a potential additive effect of prenatal exposure to V, Co, and Tl, and Se status during pregnancy, so it is required to adjust the metal concentration. Our finding suggests robust relationships between pregnant Se levels and cord serum 25(OH)D status, which are unlikely to be false positives.

We also performed a sensitivity analysis, and the association remained significant after excluding pregnant women diagnosed with GDM, PIH, and anemia during pregnancy. The results were similar to the main analyses, indicating the results were independent of these diseases.

When we stratified the analysis according to the delivery season, we observed that a low level of urinary Se status during the cold season was associated with a newborn's vitamin D deficiency. The potential mechanism is unknown, but a possible reason is that mothers who give birth during the warm season have more exposure to the sun's ultraviolet (UV) rays. The 7-dehydrocholesterol in the skin is converted to previtamin D_3 upon penetration by solar UV-B radiation (wavelength: 290–315 nm) and then rapidly converted to vitamin D_3 [16]. Consequently, pregnant women who give birth in the warm season (Jun–Nov) are less likely to be vitamin D deficient than in the cold season (Dec–May), and the excessive vitamin D produced in the body is broken down by UV-B exposure. Therefore, Se is more protective of vitamin D in mothers who give birth in the cold season.

In our study, we found a positive association between Se levels during pregnancy and cord serum 25(OH)D levels. We assumed the potential mechanism for this effect might be the protective effect of Se on the liver, which is known to be a protective factor against liver necrosis [33]. The liver is the site of vitamin D hydroxylation [17]. Se is considered to have an excellent antioxidant capacity and protects intracellular structures from oxidative damage. Selenoprotein is also involved in synthesizing mitochondria, stabilizing the endoplasmic reticulum, and plays a role in preventing oxidative stress in the placenta [2,34].

Our study has some advantages. The first strength relies on its prospective cohort design and the repeated measurements of urinary Se concentrations in the first, second, and third trimesters during pregnancy, which allowed us to explore the trimester-specific effects of Se levels and cord serum 25(OH)D and identify the critical windows of Se supplement. Additionally, to the best of our knowledge, it is the first time to explore the association between urinary Se levels and cord serum 25(OH)D. Then we had a large sample size for the analysis; we had 1695 pregnant women added to the research.

Nevertheless, some limitations should be acknowledged. First, we measured Se levels in urinary samples; however, blood Se is considered the best biomarker for measuring Se status in humans [13,35]. However, it has also been suggested that urinary Se is a valid biomarker for assessing Se status in humans [14]. Secondly, only an epidemiological association was observed, and we were unable to provide a mechanistic aspect to the study. Third, vitamin D intake in the daily diet of pregnant mothers was missing in our study, but previous studies have suggested that there is no association between dietary vitamin D intake and cord blood vitamin D levels, possibly due to low dietary intake of vitamin D [28,36]. In addition, the previous studies found that 25(OH)D concentrations increased from the first trimester to the third trimester [37]. However, in our study, urinary selenium levels were lowest in mid-pregnancy and highest in early pregnancy. In our study, we only focused on cord serum vitamin D levels and did not test serum vitamin D in early, mid, and late pregnancy, so this point is also a drawback of our study. The prevalence of GDM in the entire population of our cohort was approximately 9.8%, which can be found in our previously published article [25]. However, our outcome indicator in this study was cord serum vitamin D. Therefore, our study population was pregnant women who provided at least one urine as well as cord blood sample during pregnancy, and we hypothesized that people in this population are more focused on lifestyle and health care during pregnancy. Conditions such as GDM are widely noted pregnancy complications, which may explain the low prevalence of these three pregnancy complications in our population. Future research is warranted to explore the underlying mechanisms.

5. Conclusions

In summary, our study shows that urinary Se concentration during pregnancy is a protective factor on cord serum 25(OH)D level. A low level of urinary Se is a risk factor for vitamin D deficiency in newborns.

Supplementary Materials: The following supporting information can be downloaded at: https://www.mdpi.com/article/10.3390/nu14091715/s1, Table S1: Intraclass correlation coefficients (ICC) of SG-adjusted urinary metals concentrations in different trimesters, Table S2. The distributions of metal concentrations during pregnancy, Table S3. Sensitive analysis.

Author Contributions: H.G., conceptualization, methodology, software, formal analysis, writing—original draft preparation; H.Z., investigation, validation; T.Z., investigation; W.X., data curation, writing—review and editing, supervision; S.X., resources, project administration, funding acquisition; Y.L., conceptualization, writing—review and editing, resources, project administration, funding acquisition. All authors have read and agreed to the published version of the manuscript.

Funding: This research was supported by the National Natural Science Foundation of China (42077398), Program for Huazhong University of Science and Technology (HUST) Academic Frontier Youth Team (2018QYTD12), and the National Institutes of Health R01ES029082.

Institutional Review Board Statement: The study was conducted according to the guidelines of the Declaration of Helsinki, and approved by the ethics committee of Tongji Medical College, Huazhong University of Science and Technology (No. [2014] 14#), and the study hospital (No.2010009).

Informed Consent Statement: Informed consent was obtained from all subjects involved in the study. Written informed consent has been obtained from the patient(s) to publish this paper.

Data Availability Statement: The data presented in this study are available upon request from the corresponding author.

Acknowledgments: We thank all Wuhan Children's Hospital staff and participants.

Conflicts of Interest: The authors declare no conflict of interest.

References

1. Rayman, M.P. The importance of selenium to human health. *Lancet* **2000**, *356*, 233–241. [CrossRef]
2. Labunskyy, V.M.; Hatfield, D.L.; Gladyshev, V.N. Selenoproteins: Molecular pathways and physiological roles. *Physiol. Rev.* **2014**, *94*, 739–777. [CrossRef] [PubMed]
3. Avissar, N.; Whitin, J.C.; Allen, P.Z.; Palmer, I.S.; Cohen, H.J. Antihuman plasma glutathione peroxidase antibodies: Immunologic investigations to determine plasma glutathione peroxidase protein and selenium content in plasma. *Blood* **1989**, *73*, 318–323. [CrossRef] [PubMed]
4. Rayman, M.P. Selenium and human health. *Lancet* **2012**, *379*, 1256–1268. [CrossRef]
5. Combs, G.F., Jr. Biomarkers of selenium status. *Nutrients* **2015**, *7*, 2209–2236. [CrossRef]
6. Kang, D.; Lee, J.; Wu, C.; Guo, X.; Lee, B.J.; Chun, J.S.; Kim, J.H. The role of selenium metabolism and selenoproteins in cartilage homeostasis and arthropathies. *Exp. Mol. Med.* **2020**, *52*, 1198–1208. [CrossRef]
7. Habibi, N.; Grieger, J.A.; Bianco-Miotto, T. A Review of the Potential Interaction of Selenium and Iodine on Placental and Child Health. *Nutrients* **2020**, *12*, 2678. [CrossRef]
8. Wesselink, E.; Koekkoek, W.A.C.; Grefte, S.; Witkamp, R.F.; van Zanten, A.R.H. Feeding mitochondria: Potential role of nutritional components to improve critical illness convalescence. *Clin. Nutr.* **2019**, *38*, 982–995. [CrossRef]
9. Institute of Medicine (US) National Academies Press (US). *Dietary Reference Intakes for Vitamin C, Vitamin E, Selenium, and Carotenoids*; Institute of Medicine: Washington, DC, USA, 2000. [CrossRef]
10. Johnson, C.C.; Fordyce, F.M.; Rayman, M.P. Symposium on 'Geographical and geological influences on nutrition': Factors controlling the distribution of selenium in the environment and their impact on health and nutrition. *Proc. Nutr. Soc.* **2010**, *69*, 119–132. [CrossRef]
11. Rayman, M.P.; Wijnen, H.; Vader, H.; Kooistra, L.; Pop, V. Maternal selenium status during early gestation and risk for preterm birth. *CMAJ* **2011**, *183*, 549–555. [CrossRef]
12. Rayman, M.P.; Bath, S.C.; Westaway, J.; Williams, P.; Mao, J.; Vanderlelie, J.J.; Perkins, A.V.; Redman, C.W. Selenium status in U.K. pregnant women and its relationship with hypertensive conditions of pregnancy. *Br. J. Nutr.* **2015**, *113*, 249–258. [CrossRef] [PubMed]
13. Longnecker, M.P.; Stram, D.O.; Taylor, P.R.; Levander, O.A.; Howe, M.; Veillon, C.; McAdam, P.A.; Patterson, K.Y.; Holden, J.M.; Morris, J.S.; et al. Use of selenium concentration in whole blood, serum, toenails, or urine as a surrogate measure of selenium intake. *Epidemiology* **1996**, *7*, 384–390. [CrossRef] [PubMed]
14. Phiri, F.P.; Ander, E.L.; Lark, R.M.; Bailey, E.H.; Chilima, B.; Gondwe, J.; Joy, E.J.M.; Kalimbira, A.A.; Phuka, J.C.; Suchdev, P.S.; et al. Urine selenium concentration is a useful biomarker for assessing population level selenium status. *Environ. Int.* **2020**, *134*, 105218. [CrossRef] [PubMed]
15. Ambroziak, U.; Hybsier, S.; Shahnazaryan, U.; Krasnodebska-Kiljanska, M.; Rijntjes, E.; Bartoszewicz, Z.; Bednarczuk, T.; Schomburg, L. Severe selenium deficits in pregnant women irrespective of autoimmune thyroid disease in an area with marginal selenium intake. *J. Trace Elem. Med. Biol.* **2017**, *44*, 186–191. [CrossRef]
16. Holick, M.F. Vitamin D deficiency. *N. Engl. J. Med.* **2007**, *357*, 266–281. [CrossRef]
17. Holick, M.F. High prevalence of vitamin D inadequacy and implications for health. *Mayo Clin. Proc.* **2006**, *81*, 353–373. [CrossRef]

18. Feng, H.; Xun, P.; Pike, K.; Wills, A.K.; Chawes, B.L.; Bisgaard, H.; Cai, W.; Wan, Y.; He, K. In utero exposure to 25-hydroxyvitamin D and risk of childhood asthma, wheeze, and respiratory tract infections: A meta-analysis of birth cohort studies. *J. Allergy Clin. Immunol.* **2017**, *139*, 1508–1517. [CrossRef]
19. Tapia, G.; Marild, K.; Dahl, S.R.; Lund-Blix, N.A.; Viken, M.K.; Lie, B.A.; Njolstad, P.R.; Joner, G.; Skrivarhaug, T.; Cohen, A.S.; et al. Maternal and Newborn Vitamin D-Binding Protein, Vitamin D Levels, Vitamin D Receptor Genotype, and Childhood Type 1 Diabetes. *Diabetes Care* **2019**, *42*, 553–559. [CrossRef]
20. Tsiaras, W.G.; Weinstock, M.A. Factors influencing vitamin D status. *Acta Derm. Venereol.* **2011**, *91*, 115–124. [CrossRef]
21. Fang, X.; Qu, J.; Huan, S.; Sun, X.; Li, J.; Liu, Q.; Jin, S.; Xia, W.; Xu, S.; Wu, Y.; et al. Associations of urine metals and metal mixtures during pregnancy with cord serum vitamin D Levels: A prospective cohort study with repeated measurements of maternal urinary metal concentrations. *Environ. Int.* **2021**, *155*, 106660. [CrossRef]
22. Yixin, H.; Xiaobing, S.; Runqi, X.; Yu, B.; Xiang, G. Relationship between serum selenium level and bone mineral density and bone metabolism indexes in postmenopausal women. *Chin. J. Osteoporos.* **2021**, *27*, 1329–1332. (In Chinese)
23. Vardavas, C.I.; Hohmann, C.; Patelarou, E.; Martinez, D.; Henderson, A.J.; Granell, R.; Sunyer, J.; Torrent, M.; Fantini, M.P.; Gori, D.; et al. The independent role of prenatal and postnatal exposure to active and passive smoking on the development of early wheeze in children. *Eur. Respir. J.* **2016**, *48*, 115–124. [CrossRef]
24. Weather, C. Introduction of Wuhan City. Available online: http://www.weather.com.cn/cityintro/101200101.shtml (accessed on 15 April 2022). (In Chinese).
25. Liu, W.; Zhang, B.; Huang, Z.; Pan, X.; Chen, X.; Hu, C.; Liu, H.; Jiang, Y.; Sun, X.; Peng, Y.; et al. Cadmium Body Burden and Gestational Diabetes Mellitus: A Prospective Study. *Environ. Health Perspect.* **2018**, *126*, 027006. [CrossRef] [PubMed]
26. Holick, M.F.; Binkley, N.C.; Bischoff-Ferrari, H.A.; Gordon, C.M.; Hanley, D.A.; Heaney, R.P.; Murad, M.H.; Weaver, C.M.; Endocrine, S. Evaluation, treatment, and prevention of vitamin D deficiency: An Endocrine Society clinical practice guideline. *J. Clin. Endocrinol. Metab.* **2011**, *96*, 1911–1930. [CrossRef] [PubMed]
27. Barrera-Gomez, J.; Basagana, X. Models with transformed variables: Interpretation and software. *Epidemiology* **2015**, *26*, e16–e17. [CrossRef] [PubMed]
28. Baiz, N.; Dargent-Molina, P.; Wark, J.D.; Souberbielle, J.C.; Slama, R.; Annesi-Maesano, I.; Group, E.M.-C.C.S. Gestational exposure to urban air pollution related to a decrease in cord blood vitamin d levels. *J. Clin. Endocrinol. Metab.* **2012**, *97*, 4087–4095. [CrossRef] [PubMed]
29. Zhou, Q.; Guo, W.; Jia, Y.; Xu, J. Serum and Urinary Selenium Status in Patients with the Pre-diabetes and Diabetes in Northeast China. *Biol. Trace Elem. Res.* **2019**, *191*, 61–69. [CrossRef] [PubMed]
30. Howe, C.G.; Margetaki, K.; Vafeiadi, M.; Roumeliotaki, T.; Karachaliou, M.; Kogevinas, M.; McConnell, R.; Eckel, S.P.; Conti, D.V.; Kippler, M.; et al. Prenatal metal mixtures and child blood pressure in the Rhea mother-child cohort in Greece. *Environ. Health* **2021**, *20*, 1. [CrossRef]
31. Kippler, M.; Bottai, M.; Georgiou, V.; Koutra, K.; Chalkiadaki, G.; Kampouri, M.; Kyriklaki, A.; Vafeiadi, M.; Fthenou, E.; Vassilaki, M.; et al. Impact of prenatal exposure to cadmium on cognitive development at preschool age and the importance of selenium and iodine. *Eur. J. Epidemiol.* **2016**, *31*, 1123–1134. [CrossRef]
32. Skroder, H.; Engstrom, K.; Kuehnert, D.; Kippler, M.; Francesconi, K.; Nermell, B.; Tofail, F.; Broberg, K.; Vahter, M. Associations between Methylated Metabolites of Arsenic and Selenium in Urine of Pregnant Bangladeshi Women and Interactions between the Main Genes Involved. *Environ. Health Perspect.* **2018**, *126*, 027001. [CrossRef]
33. Liu, W.; Li, X.; Wong, Y.S.; Zheng, W.; Zhang, Y.; Cao, W.; Chen, T. Selenium nanoparticles as a carrier of 5-fluorouracil to achieve anticancer synergism. *ACS Nano* **2012**, *6*, 6578–6591. [CrossRef]
34. Shchedrina, V.A.; Zhang, Y.; Labunskyy, V.M.; Hatfield, D.L.; Gladyshev, V.N. Structure-function relations, physiological roles, and evolution of mammalian ER-resident selenoproteins. *Antioxid. Redox Signal.* **2010**, *12*, 839–849. [CrossRef] [PubMed]
35. Fairweather-Tait, S.J.; Bao, Y.; Broadley, M.R.; Collings, R.; Ford, D.; Hesketh, J.E.; Hurst, R. Selenium in human health and disease. *Antioxid. Redox Signal.* **2011**, *14*, 1337–1383. [CrossRef] [PubMed]
36. Jones, A.P.; Palmer, D.; Zhang, G.; Prescott, S.L. Cord blood 25-hydroxyvitamin D3 and allergic disease during infancy. *Pediatrics* **2012**, *130*, e1128–e1135. [CrossRef] [PubMed]
37. Wang, X.; Jiao, X.; Tian, Y.; Zhang, J.; Zhang, Y.; Li, J.; Yang, F.; Xu, M.; Yu, X.; Shanghai Birth Cohort, S. Associations between maternal vitamin D status during three trimesters and cord blood 25(OH)D concentrations in newborns: A prospective Shanghai birth cohort study. *Eur. J. Nutr.* **2021**, *60*, 3473–3483. [CrossRef] [PubMed]

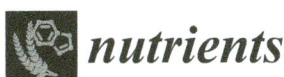

Article

The Influence of Maternal Vitamin E Concentrations in Different Trimesters on Gestational Diabetes and Large-for-Gestational-Age: A Retrospective Study in China

Qianling Zhou [1,*], Mingyuan Jiao [2], Na Han [2], Wangxing Yang [1], Heling Bao [1] and Zhenghong Ren [1]

1. Department of Maternal and Child Health, School of Public Health, Peking University, Beijing 100191, China; sibulanliqi@pku.edu.cn (W.Y.); baohl@bjmu.edu.cn (H.B.); rzhong65@126.com (Z.R.)
2. Tongzhou Maternal and Child Health Care Hospital of Beijing, Beijing 101101, China; 13522833318@163.com (M.J.); hanna_7656@163.com (N.H.)
* Correspondence: qianling.zhou@bjmu.edu.cn; Tel.: +86-(10)-828-0122-2105

Abstract: Vitamin E can protect pregnant women from oxidative stress and further affect pregnancy outcomes. This study aimed to investigate maternal vitamin E concentration in each trimester and its associations with gestational diabetes (GDM) and large-for-gestational-age (LGA). The data were derived from Peking University Retrospective Birth Cohort in Tongzhou, collected from 2015 to 2018 (n = 19,647). Maternal serum vitamin E were measured from blood samples collected in each trimester. Logistic regressions were performed to analyze the association between maternal vitamin E levels and outcomes. The median levels of maternal vitamin E increased from the first (10.00 mg/L) to the third (16.00 mg/L) trimester. Among mothers who had inadequate vitamin E levels, most of them had excessive amounts. Excessive vitamin E level in the second trimester was a risk factor for GDM (aOR = 1.640, 95% CI: 1.316–2.044) and LGA (aOR = 1.334, 95% CI: 1.022–1.742). Maternal vitamin E concentrations in the first and second trimesters were positively associated with GDM (first: aOR = 1.056, 95% CI: 1.038–1.073; second: aOR = 1.062, 95% CI: 1.043–1.082) and LGA (first: aOR = 1.030, 95% CI: 1.009–1.051; second: aOR = 1.040, 95% CI: 1.017–1.064). Avoiding an excess of vitamin E during pregnancy might be an effective measure to reduce GDM and LGA. Studies to explore the potential mechanisms are warranted.

Keywords: vitamin E; gestational diabetes mellitus (GDM); large-for-gestational-age (LGA)

1. Introduction

Vitamin E is a lipid-soluble antioxidant that corrects oxidative imbalance and protects tissue from damage [1,2]. For pregnant women, oxidative stress is associated with poor perinatal outcomes. Maternal vitamin E levels during pregnancy have been found to have a significant impact on pregnancy and birth outcomes [3,4]. For instance, maternal plasma concentrations of α-tocopherol at 16 and at 28 weeks of gestation were positively related to fetal growth and associated with an increased risk of delivering large-for-gestational-age (LGA) infants [5]. However, excessive vitamin E may lead to abortion and interfere with fetal development [6]. The majority of the existing evidence examined maternal vitamin E at one or two time points. It is important to detect the association between maternal vitamin E at different trimesters and pregnancy outcomes in order to identify sensitive time period for monitoring and intervention.

Gestational diabetes mellitus (GDM) is one of the most common medical complications in pregnancy and is greatly impacted by maternal nutrition status. GDM is a risk factor for many adverse pregnancy outcomes, such as maternal preeclampsia, stillbirth, fetal intrauterine growth retardation, and macrosomia [7]. GDM affects 2% to 25% of pregnancies globally [8]. According to a recent meta-analysis involving 79,064 Chinese participants from 25 papers, the total incidence of GDM in mainland China was 14.8% (95% confidence

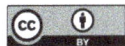

interval 12.8–16.7%) [9]. Studies have not yet reached a consensus on the influence of maternal vitamin E concentration on the occurrence of GDM. A meta-analysis found that the level of vitamin E was significantly lower in GDM women compared to healthy pregnant women [10]. However, two recent studies found opposite results and reported that serum vitamin E levels of GDM patients were excessive in mid- and late pregnancy [11,12]. Notably, the majority of previous studies examined vitamin E levels at late pregnancy (after the diagnosis of GDM); therefore, the influence of maternal vitamin E on the occurrence of GDM could not be determined.

Infant birth weight is an important indicator of fetal growth. LGA refers to babies whose birth weight is above the 90th percentile of the average weight of the same gestational age. The global incidence of LGA was 9.4%–18.01% in recent years [13–15]. A review of the literature published between 1989 and 2019 found that the prevalence of LGA ranged from 4.3% (Korea) to 22.1% (China) in Asia, while different growth charts were used to define LGA [16]. According to the study "The Chinese Collaborative Study Group for Etiologies of NICU Deaths", the risk of neonatal death with LGA at an early stage was 1.94 times higher than that of normal newborns (OR = 2.938, 95% CI: 1.346–6.416) [17]. Gadhok et al. [18] found that low levels of vitamin E of pregnant women who admitted in hospital for delivery were associated with fetal intrauterine growth restriction. Maternal vitamin E deficiency was associated with low birth weight [19]. In contrast, a high serum vitamin E concentration in pregnant women could lead to macrosomia [20]. However, according to the current literature, the association between maternal vitamin E and LGA has not been explored.

The existing evidence was limited by its relatively small sample size, the examination of vitamin E in only one or two trimesters, the absence of some important confounding factors, and a lack of details in the study design. The present study was conducted to examine maternal vitamin E concentrations in different trimesters and to explore their associations with adverse pregnancy outcomes, including GDM and LGA. The present study was improved by using a retrospective study design with a relatively large sample size and would demonstrate the importance of adequate vitamin E levels during pregnancy in the prevention of adverse pregnancy and birth outcomes.

2. Materials and Methods

2.1. Study Design and Setting

The data was derived from Peking University Retrospective Birth Cohort in Tongzhou based on the hospital information system. This study conducted from July 2015 to January 2018 in the Tongzhou Maternal and Child Health Care Hospital of Beijing. Tongzhou, located in southeastern Beijing, is the city's deputy administrative center. The district emphasizes the development of culture, education, science, and tourism. At the end of 2018, there were a total of 1.58 million residents in Tongzhou district.

2.2. Study Population

Participants were pregnant women who had a maternity check-up at the Tongzhou Maternal and Child Health Care Hospital of Beijing between July 2015 and December 2017 (n = 57,332), had their vitamin E measured in any trimester during pregnancy, delivered at the hospital, and whose complete background information was available. Some values that were considered as abnormal were recorded as a missing value in the analyses, including infant birth weight < 354 g, maternal height < 110 cm or >200 cm, pre-pregnancy weight > 130 kg or <30 kg, delivery gestational age > 43 weeks, and parity > gravidity. Alongside this, women with stillbirth and multiple pregnancies were excluded from the analyses and women with other pregnancy complications and pregnancy risk factors (i.e., thyroid disease, tumor, hypertensive disorder complicating pregnancy, asthma, ovarian cyst, acute fatty liver of pregnancy, taking drugs contraindicated during pregnancy, etc.) were excluded in the study of GDM. All pregnant women in this study agreed to provide their information to the hospital.

2.3. Vitamin E Measurement

Participants had vitamin E measurements in each trimester after the collection of blood samples. The first step was to collect venous blood samples from the participants and store the serum at −80 degrees Celsius in a light-proof place. This was followed by pretreatment with centrifugation and extraction to ensure that impurities and proteins were discarded and that the vitamins were completely separated. The high-performance liquid chromatography method was conducted to measure vitamin E concentrations, in which α-Tocpherol was used as the standard, and 1290 Infinity high-performance liquid chromatography (Agilent) and C18 chromatographic column were applied. A flow rate of 1.0 mL/min was adopted in the measurement. Vitamin E concentrations of the testing and quality control samples were calculated from the standard curve equation, which was established by measuring standard substances. The criterion for determining that a batch was within the control was that the concentrations of the quality control samples were all in the range of mean ± 2 S.D.

2.4. Data Collection

Data were obtained from the hospital's electronic information system. Data used in this analysis included maternal vitamin E concentration in each trimester, participants' sociodemographic characteristics, parity, maternal pre-pregnancy BMI, gestational weeks at the time of vitamin E tests, folic acid usage (between 1 to 3 months pre-pregnancy and 3 months post-conception), maternal and neonatal outcomes, including GDM, multiple pregnancy, infant birth weight, and preterm birth.

Ethics approval was obtained from the Institutional Review Board (IRB 00001052-19006) of the Peking University Health Science Centre before the implementation of the research. All data used for analysis were anonymous.

2.5. Variables and Definitions

The outcome variables of this study included GDM and LGA. GDM was a condition in which women without previously diagnosed diabetes exhibited high blood glucose levels during pregnancy. In the second trimester, all pregnant women routinely took the Oral Glucose Tolerance Test (OGTT) in a morning after eight hours' fasting. According to the standard set by the International Association of Diabetes and Pregnancy Study Groups, GDM was diagnosed if there was one or more abnormal values for the following: fasting blood glucose level ≥ 5.1 mmol/L, blood glucose level ≥ 10.0 mmol/L one hour after the consumption of glucose, and blood glucose level ≥ 8.5 mmol/L two hours after the consumption of glucose [21]. LGA is defined as the birth weight of infants above the 90th percentile of the average weight of the same gestational age, according to the international anthropometric standards [22]. Infant birth weight was measured immediately after delivery by midwives.

Serum vitamin E was an independent variable. According to the WHO, vitamin E concentrations were classified into three groups: deficient (<5.0 mg/L), adequate (5.0–20.0 mg/L), and excessive (≥ 20.0 mg/L) [23]. Weight and height self-reported by the participants in the first antenatal examination were used to calculate pre-pregnancy BMI, which was further divided into four groups (<18.50, 18.50–23.99, 24.00–27.99, ≥ 28.00 kg/m^2). Preterm birth referred to live births with <37 gestational weeks [24]. A multiple pregnancy occurred when more than one fetus was delivered in a single pregnancy. The first, second, and third trimesters were indicated as a gestational week of ≤ 13 weeks, between 14 and 27 weeks, and of ≥ 28 weeks, respectively.

2.6. Statistically Analyses

Vitamin E levels during each trimester were assessed for normality by the Kolmogorov-Smirnov test. The median (IQR) was used to describe the central and dispersion tendency of vitamin E concentrations in each trimester. Categorical variables were described by frequencies and percentages. Differences between outcomes (GDM and LGA) in different maternal characteristics and maternal concentrations were explored by χ^2 tests, Fisher's exact tests, or Mann-Whitney U-test. Multivariate logistic regression analyses were further performed to examine the independent effect of vitamin E concentration/status in each trimester on the outcomes. Variables having a $p < 0.1$ in the univariate analyses were adjusted in the multivariate analyses as potential confounders. The association was presented using the odds ratio (OR) and its 95% confidence interval (CI). Data analyses were performed by SPSS version 20, and a $p < 0.05$ was considered statistically significant. In addition, restricted cubic splines (RCS) were performed to explore the dose-response relationships of maternal vitamin E levels and the risks of GDM and LGA, with the use of 20.0 mg/L as the reference value. RCS was performed using R 4.1.3.

3. Results

3.1. General Characteristics of the Participants

A total of 19,647 women were included in this study. The majority of them were between 21 and 30 years old (64.9%), were primiparous (60.3%), were of Han ethnicity (94.0%), had a high school education level and/or above (78.7%), had a normal pre-pregnancy BMI (63.1%), and had used folic acid between 1–3 months pre-pregnancy and 3 months post-conception (91.2%). In this study population, the prevalence of preterm birth was 3.9% (Table 1).

Table 1. Maternal characteristics and birth outcomes (n = 19,647).

	N	%
Maternal age		
≤20	137	0.7
21–30	12,752	64.9
>30	6758	34.4
Parity		
Primiparous	11,851	60.3
Multiparous	7796	39.7
Maternal ethnicity		
Han	18,472	94.0
Ethnic minorities	1174	6.0
Maternal education		
Below high school	4114	21.4
High school or college	7651	39.8
University or higher	7475	38.9
Maternal pre-pregnancy BMI		
<18.50	2123	11.0
18.5–23.99	12,144	63.1
24.00–27.99	3753	19.5
≥28.00	1236	6.4
Folic acid usage		
Yes	17,911	91.2
No	1736	8.8
Preterm birth		
Yes	771	3.9
No	18,827	96.1

3.2. Maternal Vitamin E Status during Three Trimesters

There were 16,705, 5520 and 2190 women taking vitamin E measurements in the first, second and third trimesters, respectively. Table 2 shows an increasing trend of the mean vitamin E concentrations (10.00 mg/L, 14.60 mg/L, 16.00 mg/L) and the proportion of excessive vitamin E concentrations (0.2%, 9.0%, 13.6%) from the first to the third trimester. However, vitamin E concentrations were adequate for the majority of participants in all trimesters (>86%). Only in the first trimester was there a deficient concentration of vitamin E (0.1%) (Table 2).

Table 2. Vitamin E levels during pregnancy.

	1st Trimester Median (IQR) or N (%)	2nd Trimester Median (IQR) or N (%)	3rd Trimester Median (IQR) or N (%)
Vitamin E	n = 16,705	n = 5520	n = 2190
Median, mg/L	10.00	14.60	16.00
Q1, Q3, mg/L	8.70, 11.50	12.30, 17.20	14.10, 18.40
Deficient	14 (0.1)	0 (0.0)	0 (0.0)
Adequate	16,650 (99.7)	5028 (91.1)	1892 (86.4)
Excessive	41 (0.2)	492 (8.9)	298 (13.6)

3.3. The Association between Maternal Vitamin E Status/Concentration and Outcomes (GDM and LGA), Univariate Analyses

Supplementary Tables S1 and S2 show the univariate associations between maternal characteristics and outcomes (including GDM and LGA). When looking at the univariate association between maternal vitamin E status/concentration and outcomes, an excessive level of vitamin E was associated with the occurrences of GDM ($p < 0.001$) and LGA ($p = 0.004$) in the second trimester (Table 3). Pregnant women who suffered from GDM had higher vitamin E concentrations in all trimesters than women without GDM. Women who gave birth to LGA infants had a higher serum vitamin E concentration in the first and second trimesters than women who gave birth to non-LGA infants (Table 4).

Table 3. The association between vitamin E status and GDM and large for gestational age (LGA), by univariate analyses.

	Vitamin E Status	GDM	Non-GDM	p [a]	LGA	Non LGA	p [b]
		n (%)			n (%)		
First trimester	Not excessive	4026 (29.6)	9595 (70.4)	0.898	2814 (17.7)	13,100 (82.3)	0.333
	Excessive	10 (28.6)	25 (71.4)		9 (23.7)	29 (76.3)	
Second trimester	Not excessive	1095 (26.8)	2987 (73.2)	<0.001	887 (18.5)	3906 (81.5)	0.004
	Excessive	156 (39.5)	239 (60.5)		114 (23.9)	362 (76.1)	
Third trimester	Not excessive	330 (22.2)	1154 (77.8)	0.060	258 (14.7)	1494 (85.3)	0.415
	Excessive	66 (28.2)	168 (71.8)		46 (16.6)	231 (83.4)	

[a] The p value is reported from Chi-square test; [b] The p value is reported from Fisher's exact test.

Table 4. The association between vitamin E concentration (continuous variable) and GDM and large for gestational age (LGA), by univariate analyses.

	GDM	Non-GDM	p [a]	LGA	Non LGA	p [a]
	Median (IQR)			Median (IQR)		
First trimester	10.20 (8.90, 11.80)	9.90 (8.60, 11.30)	<0.001	10.30 (8.90, 11.80)	9.90 (8.70, 11.40)	<0.001
Second trimester	15.20 (13.00, 17.90)	14.30 (11.90, 16.80)	<0.001	15.20 (12.90, 17.70)	14.60 (12.30, 17.10)	<0.001
Third trimester	16.50 (14.50, 18.90)	15.95 (13.90, 18.20)	0.002	16.55 (14.45, 18.70)	16.00 (14.10, 18.40)	0.046

[a] The p value is reported from Mann–Whitney U-test.

3.4. The Adjusted Association between Maternal Vitamin E Status/Concentration and Outcomes (GDM and LGA)

After controlling for potential confounders, multivariate analyses revealed that excessive vitamin E in the second trimester was a risk factor for the occurrence of GDM (OR = 1.640, 95% CI: 1.316–2.044) and LGA (OR = 1.334, 95% CI: 1.022–1.742) (Table 5). Restricted cubic spline analyses demonstrated that there were linear relationships between vitamin E and the outcomes (p-non-linear $\geq$ 0.05, Supplementary Figures S1 and S2). Vitamin E concentrations in the first and second trimesters were positively associated with GDM (first: OR = 1.056, 95% CI: 1.038–1.073; second: OR = 1.062, 95% CI: 1.043–1.082) and LGA births (first: OR = 1.030, 95% CI: 1.009–1.051; second: OR = 1.040, 95% CI: 1.017–1.064) (Table 6).

Table 5. The association between vitamin E status and GDM and large for gestational age (LGA), by multivariate logistic regressions.

	GDM [a]		LGA [b]	
	OR (95% CI)	p	OR (95% CI)	p
First trimester vitamin E status (excessive)	0.691 (0.325–1.469)	0.336	1.312 (0.573–3.008)	0.521
Second trimester vitamin E status (excessive)	1.640 (1.316–2.044)	<0.001	1.334 (1.022–1.742)	0.034
Third trimester vitamin E status (excessive)	-	-	1.160 (0.773–1.742)	0.473

[a] Maternal age, parity, maternal pre-pregnancy BMI, and folic acid usage were adjusted; [b] Maternal age, parity, maternal education, maternal pre-pregnancy BMI and gestational weight gain were adjusted.

Table 6. The association between vitamin E concentration (continuous variable) and GDM and large for gestational age (LGA), by multivariate logistic regressions.

	GDM [a]		LGA [b]	
	OR (95% CI)	p	OR (95% CI)	p
First trimester vitamin E concentration	1.056 (1.038–1.073)	<0.001	1.030 (1.009–1.051)	0.005
Second trimester vitamin E concentration	1.062 (1.043–1.082)	<0.001	1.040 (1.017–1.064)	0.001
Third trimester vitamin E concentration	-	-	1.026 (0.983–1.071)	0.233

[a] Maternal age, parity, maternal pre-pregnancy BMI, and folic acid usage were adjusted; [b] Maternal age, parity, maternal education, maternal pre-pregnancy BMI and gestational weight gain were adjusted.

4. Discussion

The present study found that maternal vitamin E levels increased from the first to the third trimester among our study participants. For mothers who had inadequate vitamin E levels, the majority had excessive levels in the second and third trimesters. After controlling for potential confounders, excessive vitamin E in the second trimester was a risk factor for GDM and LGA. Maternal vitamin E concentrations in the first and second trimesters were positively associated with the occurrence of GDM and LGA.

The maternal serum vitamin E levels in different trimesters demonstrated in our study were consistent with a number of studies in different areas of China, which reflected an increasing trend of vitamin E concentrations from the first to the third trimester [25–29] and a much larger proportion of excessive vitamin E cases than deficient cases [30–32]. For instance, a study among 12,340 pregnant women was recruited between 2013 and 2014 in the prenatal clinics of hospitals in seven districts (Haidian, Huairou, Dongcheng, Mentougou, Pinggu, Tongzhou, and Xicheng districts) of Beijing, China. That multidistrict study found that maternal serum vitamin E concentrations in the first, second and third trimesters were 9.10 ± 2.47, 14.24 ± 3.66 and 15.80 ± 5.01 mg/L, respectively. There were 5.6% women had abnormal vitamin E concentrations, and 5.37% had excessive levels [33]. Excessive vitamin E concentration during pregnancy may cause abortion and interfere with fetal development [6]. Owing to the vitamin E status of pregnant women in China, over-consumption or supplementation with vitamin E during pregnancy should be cautious.

The relationship between maternal vitamin E levels during pregnancy and GDM was not consistent in the literature. A meta-analysis of 11 studies reported that the level of vitamin E was significantly lower in the third trimester of pregnancy in GDM women in comparison to the healthy pregnant women [10]. However, the studies included were dominated by cross-sectional and case-control studies with small sample sizes (n < 100). In contrast, Song et al. selected 1000 pregnant women with GDM and 1000 pregnant women without GDM who were admitted to a hospital in Dalian, China from January 2017 to June 2018 and found that the serum vitamin E level of GDM pregnant women (21.34 ± 4.93 mg/mL) was significantly higher than that of non-GDM pregnant women (16.25 ± 5.49 mg/L) in late pregnancy [12]. Our results were similar to Song et al. [12], and we found that maternal vitamin E concentration in the second trimester was positively associated with the risk of GDM. Our results contributed to the literature in revealing the influence of maternal vitamin E during early and mid-pregnancy on the development of GDM. Further experimental studies to explore the related mechanism and prospective studies to confirm our results are warranted.

The association between maternal vitamin E and LGA in our study was consistent with a cohort study among 1231 pregnant women in the US. This US study measured maternal α-tocopherol levels at entry (16.0 ± 0.15 weeks) and at 28 weeks of gestation and found that each unit increase in α-tocopherol concentration increased the odds of delivering LGA babies by 8.8% at entry and 6.7% at week 28 [5]. Likewise, a prospective cohort study in South Korea found that birth weight was the highest when the concentrations of both vitamins C and E in the second trimester were high [34]. Besides, our result was similar to our previous exploration of the associations between maternal vitamin E and macrosomia [20]. The above evidence contributed vitamin E to be an antioxidant, which defensed against oxidative stress and impairment to fetal growth. Moreover, maternal GDM is a risk factor for LGA. It is likely that maternal vitamin E affects the development of GDM, and further influences the occurrence of LGA. It might be interesting to further explore the mediation or moderation role of GDM on the association between maternal vitamin E and LGA.

Our study has some strengths. First, unlike the majority of studies focusing on vitamin E status in a single trimester, our study explored the association between maternal vitamin E in every trimester and pregnancy outcomes. Changes in vitamin E levels from the first to the third trimester were also illustrated. Second, the sample size of this study was relatively large, and the potential confounders were adjusted in multivariate analyses. The accuracy of the results was thus enhanced. Limitations of our study should also be acknowledged. First, we were unable to collect blood samples in all trimesters for every participant; therefore, missing data in the exposure variables existed. Second, the generalizability of our findings was not confirmed because our study was conducted in a maternal and child hospital in a district of Beijing. Third, since it was a retrospective study using data from the hospital's medical records, some potential confounders were not collected and analyzed, such as dietary intake and vitamin E supplementation. Finally, in our study, urine sample was not collected, and biomarkers of vitamin E were not examined. As a result, we were not able to study the metabolism of vitamin E [35] and understand the reasons for the excess of vitamin E among some present women. Further studies to address this aspect are warranted.

5. Conclusions

Vitamin E excess among pregnant women appears to be a public health issue in China. Our study demonstrated a positive association between excessive vitamin E in the second trimester and the risks of GDM and LGA. Further experimental studies are necessary to explore the mechanism between maternal vitamin E and the above pregnancy outcomes.

Supplementary Materials: The following supporting information can be downloaded at: https://www.mdpi.com/article/10.3390/nu14081629/s1, Table S1: The association between maternal characteristics and GDM, by univariate analyses (n = 16,243); Table S2: The association between maternal characteristics and large for gestational age (LGA), by univariate analyses (n = 18,699). Figure S1: The relationship of (a) first trimester and (b) second trimester vitamin E levels and 8 GDM (reference is 20.0 mL/L). Maternal age, parity, maternal pre-pregnancy BMI, folic acid usage were adjusted. Figure S2: The relationship of (a) first trimester, (b) second trimester and (c) third trimester 12 vitamin E levels and 13 LGA (reference is 20.0 mL/L). Maternal age, parity, maternal education, maternal pre-pregnancy BMI and gestational weight gain 14 were adjusted

Author Contributions: Q.Z. conceptualized the study, analyzed the data and drafted the manuscript. W.Y. assisted in data analyses. Z.R. assisted in data analyses and provided critical comments on this paper. H.B. was responsible for data management, data cleaning, and assisted in drafting the manuscript. N.H. and M.J. were responsible for data collection, and assisted in drafting the manuscript. All authors have read and agreed to the published version of the manuscript.

Funding: This research was funded by the Peking University Research Initiation Fund (BMU2018YJ005) and National Natural Science Foundation of China (81973053).

Institutional Review Board Statement: The study was conducted according to the guidelines of the Declaration of Helsinki, and all procedures involving human subjects were approved by the Institutional Review Board (IRB 00001052-19005) of the Peking University Health Science Centre.

Informed Consent Statement: Informed consent was obtained from all subjects involved in the study.

Data Availability Statement: The data presented in this study are available on request from the corresponding author. The data are not publicly available due to privacy.

Acknowledgments: We sincerely thank the research group of Peking University Retrospective Birth Cohort in Tongzhou based on the hospital information system. We appreciated the health professionals in Tongzhou Maternal and Child Health Care Hospital of Beijing for data collection and management.

Conflicts of Interest: The authors declare no conflict of interest. The funders had no role in the design of the study; in the collection, analyses, or interpretation of data; in the writing of the manuscript, or in the decision to publish the results.

References

1. Erdemli, M.E.; Aksungur, Z.; Gul, M.; Yigitcan, B.; Bag, H.G.; Altinoz, E.; Turkoz, Y. The effects of acrylamide and vitamin E on kidneys in pregnancy: An experimental study. *J. Matern. Fetal Neonatal Med.* **2019**, *32*, 3747–3756. [CrossRef] [PubMed]
2. Traber, M.G. Vitamin E. *Adv. Nutr.* **2021**, *12*, 1047–1048. [CrossRef] [PubMed]
3. Cave, C.; Hanson, C.; Schumacher, M.; Lyden, E.; Furtado, J.; Obaro, S.; Delair, S.; Kocmich, N.; Rezac, A.; Izevbigie, N.; et al. A Comparison of Vitamin E Status and Associated Pregnancy Outcomes in Maternal–Infant Dyads between a Nigerian and a United States Population. *Nutrients* **2018**, *10*, 1300. [CrossRef] [PubMed]
4. Niki, E.; Traber, M.G. A history of vitamin E. *Ann. Nutr. Metab.* **2012**, *61*, 207–212. [CrossRef]
5. Scholl, T.O.; Chen, X.; Sims, M.; Stein, T.P. Vitamin E: Maternal concentrations are associated with fetal growth. *Am. J. Clin. Nutr.* **2006**, *84*, 1442–1448. [CrossRef]
6. Burton, G.J.; Jauniaux, E. Placental Oxidative Stress: From Miscarriage to Preeclampsia. *J. Soc. Gynecol. Investig.* **2004**, *11*, 342–352. [CrossRef]
7. Lei, Q.; Niu, J.; Lv, L.; Dua, D.; Wen, J.; Lin, X.; Mai, C.; Zhou, Y. Clustering of metabolic risk factors and adverse pregnancy outcomes: A prospective cohort study. *Diabetes/Metab. Res. Rev.* **2016**, *32*, 835–842. [CrossRef]
8. Zhu, Y.; Zhang, C. Prevalence of Gestational Diabetes and Risk of Progression to Type 2 Diabetes: A Global Perspective. *Curr. Diabetes Rep.* **2016**, *16*, 7. [CrossRef]
9. Gao, C.; Sun, X.; Lu, L.; Liu, F.; Yuan, J. Prevalence of gestational diabetes mellitus in mainland China: A systematic review and meta-analysis. *J. Diabetes Investig.* **2019**, *10*, 154–162. [CrossRef]
10. Foruzan, S.; Parvin, A.; Faal, C.S.; Shayesteh, J.; Zeynab, M.; Maryam, Z. Serum vitamin E level and gestational diabetes mellitus: A systematic review and meta-analysis. *J. Diabetes Metab. Disord.* **2020**, *19*, 1787–1795.
11. Zhu, L.; Hu, J.; Guo, L.; Yuan, N.; Yang, X. Levels of serum vitamin A and vitamin E in late pregnant women with gestational diabetes mellitus. *Matern. Child Health Care China* **2021**, *36*, 1471–1473. (In Chinese) [CrossRef]
12. Song, D.; Lu, X.; Hu, X.; Feng, A.; Liu, C.; Lv, W.; Li, C. Correlative analysis between Fat-soluble vitamins A, D and E and Gestational Diabetes. *Prog. Mod. Biomed.* **2020**, *20*, 115–117, 139. (In Chinese) [CrossRef]
13. Chiavaroli, V.; Castorani, V.; Guidone, P.; Derraik, J.G.; Liberati, M.; Chiarelli, F.; Mohn, A. Incidence of infants born small-and large-for-gestational-age in an Italian cohort over a 20-year period and associated risk factors. *Ital. J. Pediatr.* **2016**, *42*, 42. [CrossRef] [PubMed]
14. Hua, X.-G.; Jiang, W.; Hu, R.; Hu, C.-Y.; Huang, K.; Li, F.-L.; Zhang, X.-J.J. Large for gestational age and macrosomia in pregnancies without gestational diabetes mellitus. *J. Matern. Fetal Neonatal Med.* **2020**, *33*, 3549–3558. [CrossRef] [PubMed]
15. Jeyaseelan, L.; Yadav, B.; Silambarasan, V.; Vijayaselvi, R.; Jose, R. Large for gestational age births among south Indian women: Temporal trend and risk factors from 1996 to 2010. *J. Obstet. Gynaecol. India* **2016**, *66*, 42–50. [CrossRef]
16. Harvey, L.; van Elburg, R.; van der Beek, E.M. Macrosomia and large for gestational age in Asia: One size does not fit all. *J. Obstet. Gynaecol. Res.* **2021**, *47*, 1929–1945. [CrossRef]
17. The Chinese Collaborative Study Group for Etiologies of NICU Deaths. Death causes and mortality risks of large for gestational age infants: A multi-center case—Control study. *Chin. J. Evid. Based Pediatrics* **2019**, *14*, 401–405. (In Chinese)
18. Gadhok, K.A.; Sharma, K.T.; Maheep, S.; Rakesh, K.; Vardey, K.S.; Poonam, S.; Manisha, S. Natural Antioxidant Vitamins Status in Pregnancies Complicated with Intrauterine Growth Restriction. *Clin. Lab.* **2017**, *63*, 941–945. [CrossRef]
19. Russell, S. 'The role of nutritional and environmental health in' preventing birth defects. *J. Aust. Tradit. Med. Soc.* **2018**, *24*, 155–160.
20. Yang, W.; Jiao, M.; Xi, L.; Han, N.; Luo, S.; Xu, X.; Zhou, Q.; Wang, H. The association between maternal fat-soluble vitamin concentrations during pregnancy and infant birth weight in China. *Br. J. Nutr.* **2021**, *125*, 1058–1066. [CrossRef]

21. Metzger, B.E.; Gabbe, S.G.; Persson, B.; Buchanan, T.A.; Catalano, P.A.; Damm, P.; Dyer, A.R.; Leiva, A.; Hod, M.; Kitzmiler, J.L.; et al. International association of diabetes and pregnancy study groups recommendations on the diagnosis and classification of hyperglycemia in pregnancy. *Diabetes Care* **2010**, *33*, 676–682. [CrossRef] [PubMed]
22. Villar, J.; Ismail, L.C.; Victora, C.G.; Ohuma, E.O.; Bertino, E.; Altman, D.G.; Lambert, A.; Papageorghiou, A.T.; Carvalho, M.; Jaffer, Y.A.; et al. International standards for newborn weight, length, and head circumference by gestational age and sex: The Newborn Cross-Sectional Study of the INTERGROWTH-21st Project. *Lancet* **2014**, *384*, 857–868. [CrossRef]
23. Institute of Medicine (US.). Panel on Dietary Antioxidants and Related Compounds. In *Dietary Reference Intakes for Vitamin C, Vitamin E, Selenium, and Carotenoids: A Report of the Panel on Dietary Antioxidants and Related Compounds, Subcommittees on Upper Reference Levels of Nutrients and of Interpretation and Use of Dietary Reference Intakes, and the Standing Committee on the Scientific Evaluation of Dietary Reference Intakes, Food and Nutrition Board, Institute of Medicine*; National Academy Press: Washington, DC, USA, 2000; 506p.
24. Goldenberg, R.L.; Culhane, J.F.; Iams, J.D.; Romero, R. Preterm birth 1—Epidemiology and causes of preterm birth. *Lancet* **2008**, *371*, 75–84. [CrossRef]
25. Liang, L.; Ye, Y.; Yang, Z.; Huang, H.; Zheng, X. Study of the relationship between serum vitamin A and vitamin E levels in pregnant women and risk factors of the pregnancy cycle and maternal age. *J. Pract. Med. Tech.* **2021**, *28*, 191–193. (In Chinese)
26. Xue, J.; Chen, Y.; Cui, L.; Peng, Z.; Li, J. Study on the relationship between vitamin A, D, E content in blood during pregnancy and pregnancy-related diseases. *Chin. J. Fam. Plan. Gynecotokology* **2020**, *12*, 81–84. (In Chinese)
27. Wu, J. Analysis of the results of serum vitamin A and E levels in pregnant women during pregnancy. *J. Med. Forum.* **2018**, *39*, 93–95. (In Chinese)
28. Ren, H.; Lin, L. Analysis of nutritional status and related factors of seven vitamins in serum of pregnant women at different stages of pregnancy. *Chin. Remedies Clin.* **2020**, *20*, 1312–1314. (In Chinese)
29. Jiang, Y.; Feng, J.; Yang, P. Analysis of the results of serum vitamin A and E levels in pregnant women during pregnancy. *China Pr. Med* **2020**, *15*, 72–73. (In Chinese)
30. Wang, Y.; Zhao, W.; Yao, W.; Zhou, Q.; Wu, N.; Wang, R. Analysis of Serum Vitamin A and E Levels and the Influencing Factors in Full-term Pregnant Women. *Shenzhen J. Integr. Tradit. Chin. West. Med.* **2020**, *30*, 1–4. (In Chinese)
31. Du, M.; Yu, Y.; Huang, J.; Duan, G.; Zhu, J.; Yang, S.; Lu, Y.; Tang, P. Survey on the levels of serum vitamin A and vitamin E in the women during the first trimester of pregnancy in Dali. *Matern. Child Health Care China* **2020**, *35*, 909–911. (In Chinese) [CrossRef]
32. Niu, H.; Xue, X.; Zhong, X. Serum vitamin A and E levels in pregnant women in Huai'an region from 2017 to 2018. *J. Hyg. Res.* **2020**, *49*, 41–43. [CrossRef]
33. Han, C.; Qian, N.; Yan, L.; Jiang, H. Role of serum vitamin A and E in pregnancy. *Exp. Ther. Med.* **2018**, *16*, 5185–5189.
34. Lee, B.E.; Hong, Y.C.; Lee, K.H.; Kim, Y.J.; Kim, W.K.; Chang, N.S.; Park, E.A.; Park, H.S.; Hann, H.J. Influence of maternal serum levels of vitamins C and E during the second trimester on birth weight and length. *Eur. J. Clin. Nutr.* **2004**, *58*, 1365–1371. [CrossRef] [PubMed]
35. Bartolini, D.; Marinelli, R.; Giusepponi, D.; Galarini, R.; Barola, C.; Stabile, A.M.; Sebastiani, B.; Paoletti, F.; Betti, M.; Rende, M.; et al. Alpha-Tocopherol Metabolites (the Vitamin E Metabolome) and Their Interindividual Variability during Supplementation. *Antioxidants* **2021**, *10*, 173. [CrossRef]

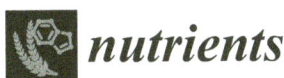

Article

Maternal Zinc, Copper, and Selenium Intakes during Pregnancy and Congenital Heart Defects

Jiaomei Yang [1], Yijun Kang [1], Qianqian Chang [1], Binyan Zhang [1], Xin Liu [1], Lingxia Zeng [1], Hong Yan [1,2,3] and Shaonong Dang [1,2,*]

[1] Department of Epidemiology and Health Statistics, School of Public Health, Xi'an Jiaotong University Health Science Center, Xi'an 710061, China; violetyjm18@xjtu.edu.cn (J.Y.); tjkyj@xjtu.edu.cn (Y.K.); cqq20160820@stu.xjtu.edu.cn (Q.C.); zhangbinyan@stu.xjtu.edu.cn (B.Z.); xinliu@xjtu.edu.cn (X.L.); tjzlx@xjtu.edu.cn (L.Z.); yanghonge@xjtu.edu.cn (H.Y.)

[2] Key Laboratory of Environment and Genes Related to Diseases, Xi'an Jiaotong University, Ministry of Education, Xi'an 710061, China

[3] Nutrition and Food Safety Engineering Research Center of Shaanxi Province, Xi'an 710061, China

* Correspondence: tjdshn@xjtu.edu.cn; Tel.: +86-029-8265-5104

Abstract: The effects of zinc, copper, and selenium on human congenital heart defects (CHDs) remain unclear. This study aimed to investigate the associations of the maternal total, dietary, and supplemental intakes of zinc, copper, and selenium during pregnancy with CHDs. A hospital-based case-control study was performed, including 474 cases and 948 controls in Northwest China. Eligible participants waiting for delivery were interviewed to report their diets and characteristics in pregnancy. Mixed logistic regression was adopted to examine associations and interactions between maternal intakes and CHDs. Higher total intakes of zinc, selenium, zinc to copper ratio, and selenium to copper ratio during pregnancy were associated with lower risks of total CHDs and the subtypes, and the tests for trend were significant (all $p < 0.05$). The significantly inverse associations with CHDs were also observed for dietary intakes of zinc, selenium, zinc to copper ratio, selenium to copper ratio, and zinc and selenium supplements use during pregnancy and in the first trimester. Moreover, high zinc and high selenium, even with low or high copper, showed a significantly reduced risk of total CHDs. Efforts to promote zinc and selenium intakes during pregnancy need to be strengthened to reduce the incidence of CHDs in the Chinese population.

Keywords: zinc; copper; selenium; congenital heart defects; pregnancy

Citation: Yang, J.; Kang, Y.; Chang, Q.; Zhang, B.; Liu, X.; Zeng, L.; Yan, H.; Dang, S. Maternal Zinc, Copper, and Selenium Intakes during Pregnancy and Congenital Heart Defects. *Nutrients* **2022**, *14*, 1055. https://doi.org/10.3390/nu14051055

Academic Editor: Yunxian Yu

Received: 24 December 2021
Accepted: 8 February 2022
Published: 2 March 2022

Publisher's Note: MDPI stays neutral with regard to jurisdictional claims in published maps and institutional affiliations.

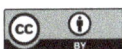

Copyright: © 2022 by the authors. Licensee MDPI, Basel, Switzerland. This article is an open access article distributed under the terms and conditions of the Creative Commons Attribution (CC BY) license (https://creativecommons.org/licenses/by/4.0/).

1. Introduction

Congenital heart defects (CHDs) are the most common birth defects in the world, with an estimated birth prevalence of 9.4‰ [1]. CHDs remain the leading cause of morbidity, mortality, and disability in infancy and childhood [2] and can cause lifelong physical and mental comorbidities, imposing huge burdens on the family and society [2]. The estimated CHDs prevalence among live births is 9.0‰ in China, with more than 150,000 incident cases each year [3]. However, the potential mechanisms for most CHDs remain to be unclear. Therefore, it is important to identify modifiable risk factors to provide evidence for the primary prevention of CHDs.

Maternal nutrition during pregnancy, as an important modifiable factor, is critical for fetal development [4]. Animal studies have shown that prenatal zinc deficiency during gestation led to heart malformations in offspring [5]. Copper deficiency induced heart anomalies in rats [6], and copper excess induced high mortality and morphological malformations in the embryos and larvae of Pagrus major [7]. Maternal selenium deficiency was reported to relate to miscarriages, premature births, and intrauterine growth retardation [8–10]. However, there is little evidence from human studies about the effects of zinc, copper, and selenium on CHDs [11–16], and the results were not consistent [11–16]. One study reported an inverse association between zinc level and ventricular septal defects (VSD) [16], while another study found no associations of zinc level with CHDs and the subtypes [13]. There was even one study reporting higher zinc levels in the CHDs cases than in the healthy controls [11]. Two studies showed a positive association between copper level and CHDs [13,15], while the other two studies reported no association [14,16]. One study found an inverse association between selenium level and CHDs [12], while another study showed a positive association [14]. Thus, it is warranted to further conduct studies among humans to elucidate the effects of zinc, copper, and selenium on CHDs.

Diet and dietary supplements are the main sources of body zinc, copper, and selenium among pregnant women. As there are no reliable biological markers for zinc, copper, and selenium status, estimated usual intakes from the diet and supplements may be the optimal indicators of maternal zinc, copper, and selenium status for epidemiologic studies [17]. However, to our knowledge, there has been no available human study specifically exploring the associations between maternal intakes of zinc, copper, and selenium during pregnancy and CHDs. Moreover, complex antagonistic interactions among zinc, copper, and selenium have been reported in previous studies [18–20]. However, to our knowledge, there is only one published study involving the interactions of zinc and copper levels on CHDs [13]. Therefore, the current study aimed to investigate the relationships between maternal total, dietary, and supplemental intakes of zinc, copper, and selenium during pregnancy and CHDs among humans in Northwest China. The interactions among maternal intakes of zinc, copper, and selenium during pregnancy on CHDs were also explored in this study.

2. Materials and Methods

2.1. Study Design and Participants

Between August 2014 and August 2016, we performed a case-control study in six tertiary comprehensive hospitals in Xi'an City, Northwest China. The study design was previously published in detail [21,22]. Briefly, participants were enrolled among the pregnant women who were waiting for delivery in the obstetrics departments. These participants were all inhabitants of Northwest China and resided in Shaanxi, China, during pregnancy, where the trace element concentrations are not considerably different [23]. Mothers whose fetuses were diagnosed with isolated CHDs and had no chromosomal abnormalities or gene disorders were included in the cases, and mothers whose fetuses were diagnosed with no congenital malformations were included in the controls. Mothers with gestational diabetes or multiple gestations were excluded from this study because of potentially different etiologies. Because of the low birth incidence of CHDs, any eligible case mothers were included in the study without sampling methods. Specialists from the ultrasound, pediatrics, and obstetrics departments conducted the diagnoses of the cases and controls. The diagnostic criteria were standard and strictly enforced by these qualified specialists in each hospital. A telephone follow-up was also undertaken within one year after birth to confirm the diagnoses. All the CHDs diagnoses were ascertained by echocardiography and/or cardiac catheterization and/or surgery. The controls were randomly selected each month in each hospital, and the ratio of the number of cases to controls included in the same month in the same hospital was 1:2. On the assumptions of the estimated percentages of pregnant women taking foods rich in nutrients more than three times a week in cases and controls being 37.2% and 45.0%, respectively, the correlation of exposure between cases and controls being zero, the type I error rate 0.05, and the power of the test 80%, the sample sizes of cases and controls were 474 and 948, respectively.

This study was approved by the Xi'an Jiaotong University Health Science Center on March 2012 (No.2012008). Participants provided written informed consents.

2.2. Dietary Assessment

Eligible women waiting for delivery in the hospital were interviewed to recall diets in the entire pregnancy through a 111-item semi-quantitative food frequency questionnaire (FFQ). The median time between interview completion and date of delivery was two days for both the cases and controls. Maternal dietary patterns and nutrient intakes tend to be stable across pregnancy [24,25]; thus, maternal dietary intakes during the whole pregnancy are comparable with those during the critical period of cardiac development in the 3rd-8th week of gestation [21,22,26]. The FFQ was established according to a validated FFQ used for pregnant women in Northwest China [27]. Pearson's correlation coefficients for zinc, copper, and selenium between the FFQ and the average of six 24 h recalls were 0.67, 0.54, and 0.59, respectively, and for other nutrients, they ranged from 0.53 to 0.70 [27]. Women recalled consumption frequency according to eight predefined categories and reported portion sizes with the assistance of food portion images [28]. Participants also reported the type/brand and the number of dietary supplements taken and the number of days taking dietary supplements in each trimester of pregnancy. Daily nutrient intakes were derived by the Chinese Food Composition Tables [29,30]. The total intake of one nutrient was calculated as the sum of dietary and supplemental intakes.

2.3. Covariates

General information of the participants was collected face-to-face by a standard questionnaire. The study covariates included (1) socio-demographic characteristics: maternal age ($\geq$30 years/<30 years), residence (urban/rural), maternal education (senior high school or above/junior high school or below), maternal work (farmers/others), and parity ($\geq$1/0); (2) maternal health-related factors in the first trimester: folate/iron supplements use (no/yes), passive smoking (no/yes), medication use (no/yes), and anemia (no/yes); and (3) dietary diversity score: the sum of ten food groups scores according to the FAO Minimum Dietary Diversity for Women guideline [31], with each group assigned a score of 1 if consumed and 0 if not consumed [26]. The ten food groups consist of starchy staple foods, pulse, nuts and seeds, dairy products, flesh foods, eggs, dark green leafy vegetables, vitamin A-rich fruits and vegetables, other vegetables, and other fruits [31]. Women having no paid employment outside their homes were classified as farmers. Passive smoking was defined as exposure to another person's tobacco smoke for more than 15 min/d. Anemia during the first trimester was diagnosed by the physicians using the criteria of hemoglobin concentration lower than 110 g/L.

2.4. Statistical Analysis

In univariate comparisons, categorical variables were compared between groups using the χ^2 test, and continuous variables were compared between groups using Mann–Whitney U test because of the non-normal distributions observed according to the Shapiro–Wilk test. Considering the clustering in the design through hospitals, we used mixed logistic regression models to estimate ORs (95%CIs) for total CHDs and CHDs subtypes associated with total and dietary intakes of zinc, copper, selenium, zinc to copper ratios, selenium to copper ratios, and zinc to selenium ratios and maternal zinc, copper, and selenium supplements use during pregnancy. Total and dietary intakes were divided into four categories according to the quartiles of the control distribution. Total and dietary zinc, copper, and selenium intakes were also categorized by the recommended nutrient intakes (RNIs) for Chinese pregnant women, which were 9.5 mg/d, 0.9 mg/d, and 65 mg/d, respectively [32]. Maternal zinc, copper, and selenium supplements uses were considered as binary categories (yes/no) because of the low amount of intake. The socio-demographic characteristics (maternal age, residence, education, work, and parity), maternal health-related factors in the first trimester (folate/iron supplements use, passive smoking, medication use, and anemia), and dietary diversity score were chosen as confounders in the models because they were reported to be associated with CHDs [26,33,34] and changed the estimates by more than 10% [35]. Since the intake of each mineral was highly correlated to the others, we did not mutually adjust for the intake of each mineral to avoid multicollinearity in the models [36]. Maternal supplements use and dietary intake of specific minerals were additionally mutually adjusted. P for trend was calculated by including quartile specific median intake in the model. To further explore the shape of the significant associations of total and dietary intakes with total CHDs, we used restricted cubic splines with three knots in the fully adjusted models. Moreover, we evaluated the interactions by introducing cross-product terms into regression models to assess whether the associations were modified by maternal age, residence, education, work, and folate/iron supplements use during the first trimester.

We evaluated the interactions between zinc and copper, selenium and copper, and zinc and selenium by introducing cross-product terms into regression models. We also re-categorized total zinc, copper, and selenium intakes as "low" and "high" according to the medians in the controls and evaluated the risk of total CHDs associated with high or low intakes of total zinc, copper, and selenium by mixed logistic regression using the combination of low intake as the reference.

The statistical analyses were performed using the Stata software (version 15.0; StataCorp, College Station, TX, USA). All tests were two-tailed with $p < 0.05$ considered statistically significant.

3. Results

3.1. Basic Characteristics of the Study Sample

Case mothers were less likely to reside in urban areas, have higher educational levels, work outside, and be nulliparity compared to the controls (Table 1). Folate/iron supplements use in the first trimester was more common in the controls than in the cases, while passive smoking, medication use, and anemia in the first trimester were more common in the cases than in the controls. Case mothers had lower dietary diversity scores and total energy intake in pregnancy than the controls. Moreover, case mothers had significantly lower total and dietary intakes of zinc, copper, selenium, zinc to copper ratios, and selenium to copper ratios during pregnancy than the controls. There were no differences in maternal age, neonatal gender, and total and dietary zinc to selenium ratios between the two groups. The percentages of case mothers having total zinc, copper, and selenium intakes below the RNIs for Chinese pregnant women were 85.7%, 15.2%, and 97.1%, respectively, which were all higher than those in control mothers (67.4%, 8.4%, and 88.3%, respectively).

Table 1. Basic characteristics of the study participants.

	Cases ($N = 474$)	Controls ($N = 948$)	p
Socio-demographic characteristics, %			
Maternal age ≥ 30 years	33.5	34.2	0.812
Urban residence	66.0	71.6	0.030
Maternal education, senior high school or above	58.9	80.7	<0.001
Maternal work, farmers	49.5	21.0	<0.001
Nulliparity	57.8	80.3	<0.001
Maternal health-related factors in the first trimester, %			
Folate/iron supplements use	76.6	89.2	<0.001
Passive smoking	33.5	9.3	<0.001
Medication use	41.6	30.4	<0.001
Anemia	16.9	10.9	<0.001
Neonatal gender, male, %	52.3	49.7	0.348
Dietary diversity score, median (25th percentile, 75th percentile)	5.0 (3.0, 6.0)	6.0 (4.0, 8.0)	<0.001
Daily components intake during pregnancy, median (25th percentile, 75th percentile)			
Total energy, kcal	1753.2 (1452.4, 2086.1)	1907.1 (1563.3, 2415.9)	0.001
Total zinc, mg	5.1 (3.2, 7.3)	7.2 (5.1, 10.9)	<0.001
Dietary zinc, mg	4.7 (3.1, 6.8)	6.4 (4.6, 9.1)	<0.001
Total copper, mg	1.6 (1.1, 2.1)	2.0 (1.4, 2.7)	<0.001
Dietary copper, mg	1.6 (1.1, 2.1)	1.9 (1.2, 2.5)	<0.001
Total selenium, mg	23.2 (15.4, 32.8)	32.5 (22.7, 46.6)	<0.001
Dietary selenium, mg	22.7 (15.1, 32.6)	30.9 (21.9, 43.7)	<0.001
Total zinc to copper ratio	3.2 (2.4, 4.4)	3.8 (3.1, 4.8)	<0.001

Table 1. Cont.

	Cases (N = 474)	Controls (N = 948)	p
Dietary zinc to copper ratio	3.1 (2.4, 4.2)	3.6 (3.0, 4.5)	<0.001
Total selenium to copper ratio	14.7 (10.8, 20.7)	16.7 (13.5, 21.6)	<0.001
Dietary selenium to copper ratio	14.7 (10.8, 20.9)	17.2 (13.7, 22.7)	<0.001
Total zinc to selenium ratio	0.21 (0.18, 0.25)	0.22 (0.19, 0.27)	0.280
Dietary zinc to selenium ratio	0.21 (0.18, 0.25)	0.21 (0.18, 0.23)	0.270

Categorical variables are compared between groups by χ^2 test, and continuous variables are compared between groups by Mann–Whitney U test.

3.2. Maternal Total and Dietary Zinc, Copper, and Selenium Intakes during Pregnancy and CHDs

When comparing the quartile 4 (highest), quartile 3, and quartile 2 to the quartile 1 (lowest) of total zinc intake, the fully adjusted ORs (95%CIs) for total CHDs were 0.22 (0.12–0.42), 0.57 (0.36–0.91), and 0.65 (0.45–0.94), respectively, and the test for trend was significant ($p < 0.001$) (Table 2). When comparing the quartile 4, quartile 3, and quartile 2 to the quartile 1 of total selenium intake, the fully adjusted ORs (95%CIs) for total CHDs were 0.29 (0.15–0.54), 0.52 (0.33–0.81), and 0.70 (0.50–0.99), respectively, and the test for trend was significant ($p = 0.009$). Moreover, quartile 4 and quartile 3 of total zinc and selenium intakes showed significantly lower risks of VSD and atrial septal defects (ASD) compared to the lowest quartile, and the tests for trend were significant (all $p < 0.004$). Total zinc to copper ratio and total selenium to copper ratio were inversely associated with the risks of total CHDs, VSD, and ASD (all P for trend <0.02). However, we observed no significant associations of total copper intake and total zinc to selenium ratio with total CHDs, VSD, and ASD. Similarly, dietary intakes of zinc, selenium, zinc to copper ratio, and selenium to copper ratio during pregnancy were inversely associated with the risks of total CHDs, VSD, and ASD, while no significant associations of dietary copper intake and dietary zinc to selenium ratio with the risks of total CHDs, VSD, and ASD were found (Table S1).

Table 2. Quartiles of maternal total zinc, copper, and selenium intakes during pregnancy and congenital heart defects.

	Cutoffs	Cases/Controls	Total CHDs (N_{cases} = 474)		VSD (N_{cases} = 223)	ASD (N_{cases} = 218)
			Unadjusted OR (95%CI)	Adjusted OR (95%CI) [1]	Adjusted OR (95%CI) [1]	Adjusted OR (95%CI) [1]
Total zinc intake (mg/d)						
Quartile 1	<5.09	241/236	1	1	1	1
Quartile 2	5.09–7.21	110/238	0.45 (0.34, 0.60)	0.65 (0.45, 0.94)	0.71 (0.39, 1.27)	0.61 (0.36, 1.03)
Quartile 3	7.21–10.86	82/237	0.34 (0.25, 0.46)	0.57 (0.36, 0.91)	0.53 (0.32, 0.86)	0.55 (0.32, 0.96)
Quartile 4	≥10.86	41/237	0.17 (0.12, 0.25)	0.22 (0.12, 0.42)	0.14 (0.05, 0.35)	0.21 (0.09, 0.48)
p for trend [2]			<0.001	<0.001	0.002	0.001
Total copper intake (mg/d)						
Quartile 1	<1.37	153/237	1	1	1	1
Quartile 2	1.37–1.95	167/237	1.10 (0.82, 1.46)	1.26 (0.90, 1.77)	1.30 (0.84, 2.03)	1.19 (0.77, 1.85)
Quartile 3	1.95–2.70	103/237	0.66 (0.48, 0.90)	1.24 (0.82, 1.85)	1.37 (0.81, 2.31)	1.13 (0.68, 1.88)
Quartile 4	≥2.70	51/237	0.33 (0.23, 0.47)	0.66 (0.38, 1.16)	0.77 (0.37, 1.64)	0.54 (0.26, 1.14)
p for trend [2]			<0.001	0.534	0.943	0.344
Total selenium intake (mg/d)						
Quartile 1	<22.68	227/237	1	1	1	1
Quartile 2	22.68–32.45	124/237	0.55 (0.41, 0.73)	0.70 (0.50, 0.99)	0.64 (0.40, 1.01)	0.71 (0.45, 1.13)
Quartile 3	32.45–46.61	76/237	0.33 (0.24, 0.46)	0.52 (0.33, 0.81)	0.47 (0.26, 0.85)	0.55 (0.31, 0.98)
Quartile 4	≥46.51	47/237	0.21 (0.14, 0.30)	0.29 (0.15, 0.54)	0.13 (0.05, 0.34)	0.25 (0.11, 0.59)
P for trend [2]			<0.001	0.009	<0.001	0.003

Table 2. Cont.

	Cutoffs	Cases/Controls	Total CHDs (N_{cases} = 474)		VSD (N_{cases} = 223)	ASD (N_{cases} = 218)
			Unadjusted OR (95%CI)	Adjusted OR (95%CI) [1]	Adjusted OR (95%CI) [1]	Adjusted OR (95%CI) [1]
Total zinc to copper ratio						
Quartile 1	<3.10	225/237	1	1	1	1
Quartile 2	3.10–3.84	92/237	0.41 (0.30, 0.55)	0.59 (0.41, 0.84)	0.64 (0.41, 1.00)	0.67 (0.43, 1.05)
Quartile 3	3.84–4.81	69/237	0.31 (0.22, 0.42)	0.43 (0.29, 0.63)	0.42 (0.26, 0.70)	0.40 (0.24, 0.67)
Quartile 4	≥4.81	88/237	0.39 (0.29, 0.53)	0.58 (0.41, 0.82)	0.49 (0.30, 0.78)	0.66 (0.44, 0.98)
p for trend [2]			<0.001	<0.001	<0.001	0.017
Total selenium to copper ratio						
Quartile 1	<13.48	197/237	1	1	1	1
Quartile 2	13.48–16.68	101/237	0.51 (0.38, 0.69)	0.65 (0.46, 0.92)	0.58 (0.37, 0.91)	0.96 (0.62, 1.48)
Quartile 3	16.68–21.61	75/237	0.38 (0.28, 0.52)	0.45 (0.31, 0.65)	0.36 (0.22, 0.59)	0.48 (0.29, 0.78)
Quartile 4	≥21.61	101/237	0.51 (0.38, 0.69)	0.65 (0.46, 0.93)	0.48 (0.30, 0.77)	0.70 (0.44, 1.10)
p for trend [2]			<0.001	0.002	<0.001	0.019
Total zinc to selenium ratio						
Quartile 1	<0.19	139/237	1	1	1	1
Quartile 2	0.19–0.22	127/237	0.91 (0.68, 1.23)	0.86 (0.60, 1.22)	0.94 (0.59, 1.50)	0.88 (0.56, 1.38)
Quartile 3	0.22–0.27	119/237	0.86 (0.63, 1.16)	1.02 (0.71, 1.45)	1.34 (0.84, 2.14)	0.99 (0.63, 1.56)
Quartile 4	≥0.27	89/237	0.64 (0.46, 0.88)	0.84 (0.58, 1.23)	1.07 (0.65, 1.76)	0.94 (0.59, 1.50)
p for trend [2]			0.008	0.588	0.451	0.925

ASD—atrial septal defects; CHDs—congenital heart defects; VSD—ventricular septal defects. [1] Adjusted for total energy intake in pregnancy, socio-demographic characteristics (maternal age, residence, education, work, and parity), maternal health-related factors in the first trimester (folate/iron supplements use, passive smoking, medication use, and anemia), and dietary diversity score. [2] p for trend across quartiles is calculated using the median for each quartile as a continuous variable.

Mothers whose total zinc and selenium intakes met the RNIs had significantly lower risks of total CHDs (total zinc: OR = 0.56, 95%CI = 0.37–0.84; total selenium: OR = 0.23, 95%CI = 0.11–0.49), VSD, and ASD (Table 3). However, the fully adjusted ORs were not significant for total CHDs, VSD, and ASD associated with total copper intake meeting the RNI. Similarly, mothers whose dietary zinc and selenium intakes met the RNIs had lower risks of total CHDs, while no significant associations of dietary copper intake meeting the RNI with total CHDs, VSD, and ASD were observed (Table S2).

Figure 1 depicts the restricted cubic spline curves for the associations between total intakes of zinc, selenium, zinc to copper ratio, and selenium to copper ratio in pregnancy and total CHDs. The risk for total CHDs decreased with increasing intakes of total zinc and selenium in pregnancy and reached a plateau of total zinc and selenium above 15.1 mg/d and 61.7 mg/d, respectively. The risk for total CHDs decreased with increasing total zinc to copper ratio when the ratio was below 6.0 and then slightly increased when the ratio above 6.0. The risk for total CHDs decreased with increasing the total selenium to copper ratio when the ratio was below 28.4 and then slightly increased when the ratio was above 28.4. The restricted cubic spline curves for the relationships between dietary intakes of zinc, selenium, zinc to copper ratio, and selenium to copper ratio during pregnancy and total CHDs showed similar shapes as to the corresponding total intakes (Figure S1).

When introducing interaction terms into the regression models, the associations of maternal total and dietary intakes of zinc, copper, selenium, zinc to copper ratios, selenium to copper ratios, and zinc to selenium ratios with CHDs did not meaningfully vary by maternal age, residence, education, work, and folate/iron supplements use in the first trimester, and the tests for interactions were not significant (all $p > 0.05$).

Table 3. Maternal total zinc, copper, and selenium intakes categorized by the recommended nutrient intakes (RNIs) during pregnancy and congenital heart defects.

		Total CHDs (N_{cases} = 474)		VSD (N_{cases} = 223)	ASD (N_{cases} = 218)
	Cases/Controls	Unadjusted OR (95%CI)	Adjusted OR (95%CI) [1]	Adjusted OR (95%CI) [1]	Adjusted OR (95%CI) [1]
Total zinc intake					
Below the RNI	406/639	1	1	1	1
Met the RNI	68/309	0.35 (0.26, 0.46)	0.56 (0.37, 0.84)	0.46 (0.26, 0.82)	0.53 (0.31, 0.91)
p		<0.001	0.006	0.009	0.021
Total copper intake					
Below the RNI	72/80	1	1	1	1
Met the RNI	402/868	0.51 (0.37, 0.72)	0.96 (0.63, 1.47)	0.91 (0.53, 1.55)	0.85 (0.50, 1.44)
p		<0.001	0.860	0.728	0.540
Total selenium intake					
Below the RNI	460/837	1	1	1	1
Met the RNI	14/111	0.23 (0.13, 0.40)	0.23 (0.11, 0.49)	0.17 (0.05, 0.51)	0.18 (0.07, 0.47)
p		<0.001	<0.001	0.002	<0.001

ASD—atrial septal defects; CHDs—congenital heart defects; VSD—ventricular septal defects; RNI—recommended nutrients intake. [1] Adjusted for total energy intake in pregnancy, socio-demographic characteristics (maternal age, residence, education, work, and parity), maternal health-related factors in the first trimester (folate/iron supplements use, passive smoking, medication use, and anemia), and dietary diversity score.

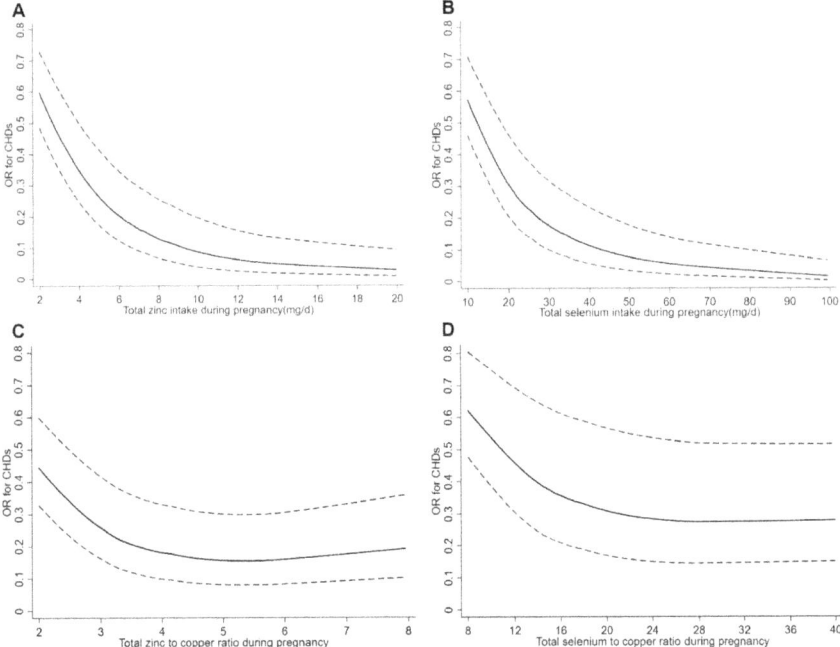

Figure 1. Restricted cubic spline models of total congenital heart defects (CHDs) risk associated with (A) total zinc intake, (B) total selenium intake, (C) total zinc to copper ratio, and (D) total selenium to copper ratio during pregnancy. Adjusted for total energy intake in pregnancy, socio-demographic characteristics (maternal age, residence, education, work, and parity), maternal health-related factors in the first trimester (folate/iron supplements use, passive smoking, medication use, and anemia), and dietary diversity score.

Although there were no significant multiplicative interactions among total zinc and copper, selenium and copper, or zinc and selenium in the regression models (all $p > 0.05$), some significant results were derived from the categorical variables as shown in Figure 2. High zinc, even with low or high copper intake, showed a lower risk for total CHDs than that of low zinc and low copper. Similarly, high selenium, even with low or high copper intake, showed a lower risk for total CHDs than that of low selenium and low copper. Compared with low zinc and low selenium, high zinc and high selenium intakes reduced the risk of total CHDs (OR = 0.51, 95%CI = 0.33–0.79). Moreover, using low zinc, low copper, and low selenium intakes as the reference, high zinc, low copper, and high selenium intakes (OR = 0.55, 95%CI = 0.33–0.97) and high zinc, high copper, and high selenium intakes (OR = 0.53, 95%CI = 0.32–0.96) showed a significantly lower risk of total CHDs.

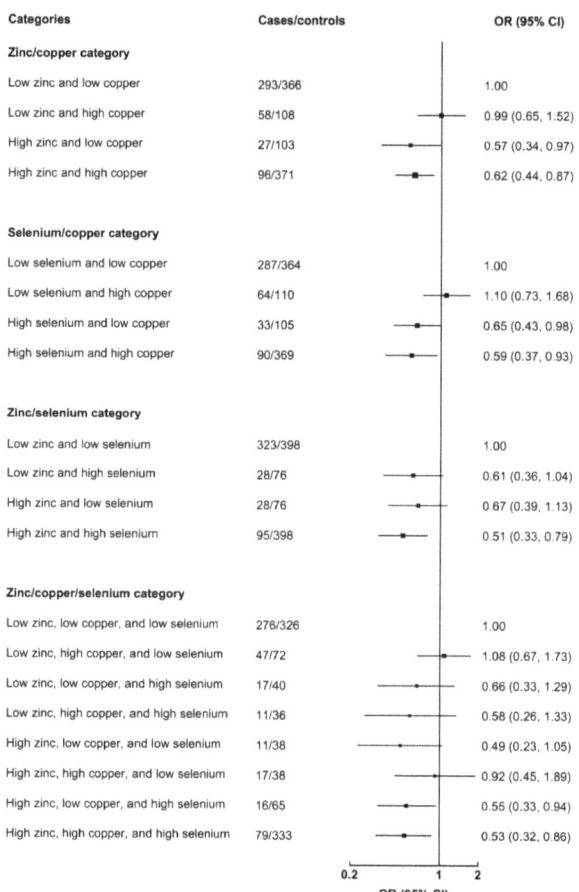

Figure 2. Interaction effects among total zinc, copper, and selenium intakes in pregnancy on total congenital heart defects. Adjusted for total energy intake in pregnancy, socio-demographic characteristics (maternal age, residence, education, work, and parity), maternal health-related factors in the first trimester (folate/iron supplements use, passive smoking, medication use, and anemia), and dietary diversity score. Low zinc, low copper, and low selenium indicate the intakes below medians of the control distribution, and high zinc, high copper, and high selenium indicate the intakes equal or above medians of the control distribution. The black boxes represent odds ratios, and the horizontal lines represent 95%CIs.

3.3. Maternal Zinc, Copper, and Selenium Supplements Uses during Pregnancy and CHDs

Maternal zinc and selenium supplements uses during pregnancy were associated with reduced risks of total CHDs (zinc supplements use: OR = 0.53, 95%CI = 0.37–0.76; selenium supplements use: OR = 0.45, 95%CI = 0.30–0.68), VSD, and ASD (Table S3). Maternal zinc supplements use during the first trimester was associated with reduced risks of total CHDs (OR = 0.58, 95%CI = 0.38–0.91) and ASD, and maternal selenium supplements use during the first trimester was associated with a lower risk of total CHDs (OR = 0.52, 95%CI = 0.31–0.85). However, we observed no significant associations of maternal copper supplements use in pregnancy and in the first trimester with CHDs.

4. Discussion

In the present case-control study, we observed that higher total intakes of zinc, selenium, zinc to copper ratio, and selenium to copper ratio during pregnancy were associated with reduced risks of total CHDs and the subtypes. The significantly inverse associations with CHDs were also observed for dietary intakes of zinc, selenium, zinc to copper ratio, and selenium to copper ratio during pregnancy, and maternal zinc and selenium supplements use during pregnancy and in the first trimester. Moreover, high zinc and high selenium, even with low or high copper, showed a significantly lower risk of total CHDs. To our knowledge, this is the first human study to specifically explore the relationships between maternal total, dietary, and supplemental intakes of zinc, copper, and selenium during pregnancy and CHDs.

4.1. Comparisons with Other Studies

To date, few human studies have explored the effects of zinc, copper, and selenium on CHDs [11–16]. The related human studies involved zinc, copper, and selenium status in blood, hair, and teeth samples among mothers, neonates, and children [11–16]. However, the results remained controversial [11–16]. One study reported an inverse association between zinc level in children's blood and VSD [16], while another study found no associations of zinc level in maternal hair with CHDs and the subtypes [13]. There was even one study reporting higher zinc levels in maternal and neonatal blood in the CHDs cases than in the healthy controls [11]. Two studies showed positive associations of copper levels in maternal hair and children's teeth with CHDs [13,15], while the other two studies reported no associations of copper levels in maternal and children's blood with CHDs and VSD [14,16]. One study observed an inverse association between selenium level in maternal hair and CHDs [12], while another study showed a positive association in maternal blood [14]. The present study focused on maternal intakes of zinc, copper, and selenium during pregnancy and found significant inverse associations of zinc and selenium intakes with CHDs but no significant association for copper intake. These inconsistent results may be partially due to the differences in exposure measurement methods, sample size, study population, and genetic backgrounds. Moreover, the selenium status of an individual was largely determined by not only food sources but also the soil selenium concentration [37]. The selenium concentration in soil is generally influenced by geographical location, seasonal changes, protein content, and food processing [38]. People from different regions may have different baseline selenium statuses due to the soil selenium status, further leading to different health outcomes. Previous studies have reported that some dietary factors, such as cereal-based diets and fiber-rich foods, may inhibit zinc absorption [39] and further influence the association between zinc intake and health outcomes. Future studies integrating maternal minerals intakes and biological markers with genetic and soil factors are warranted to explore these relationships.

To our knowledge, there is only one published study involving the interactions of zinc and copper on CHDs [13]. This previous study did not observe a significant interaction between copper and zinc levels on CHDs [13], which was consistent with the finding in the present study. To our knowledge, there have been no previous studies of selenium–copper and zinc–selenium interactions on CHDs. Although no multiplicative interactions among zinc, copper, and selenium intakes during pregnancy on CHDs were observed in our study, the results of categorical variables suggested that high zinc and high selenium intakes, even with low or high copper, reduced the risk of CHDs. It seems that the simultaneous high intakes of zinc and selenium during pregnancy might have an additive effect on the association with CHDs. Given the rarity of research on the joint effects of zinc, copper, and selenium for fetal cardiovascular development, further studies are warranted to confirm and interpret these findings.

4.2. Possible Mechanisms

Zinc is involved in the synthesis of many lipids, nucleic acids, and proteins. Zinc deficiency could induce alterations in the distribution of connexin-43 and HNK-1 in fetal hearts and result in the occurrence of heart anomalies [5]. Zinc deficiency could also activate apoptotic and inflammatory processes and decrease TGF-β1 expression and nitric oxide synthase activity in cardiac tissue [40]. Zinc supplementation was reported to significantly downregulate protein and mRNA expression of metallothionein in the developing heart of embryos and decreased apoptosis and reduced levels of reactive oxygen species, regarded as a potential therapy for diabetic cardiac embryopathy [41].

Copper ions serve as an important catalytic cofactor in the redox chemistry of proteins exerting fundamental biological functions, such as cytochrome C oxidase, Cu/Zn superoxide dismutase, and ceruloplasmin. With a relatively high DNA binding affinity, copper may displace zinc ions in zinc-finger transcription factors and interfere with their functions in fetuses [42]. Inhibition of zinc-finger transcription factors, such as GATA4 and Zac1, could lead to embryonic lethality, thin ventricular walls, or abnormal looping morphogenesis of the primary heart tube [43,44]. However, no significant results were found on the associations of dietary and supplemental copper intakes with CHDs in the present study. The reason may come from the fact that few pregnant women have copper deficiency and excess in our study population. In fact, the percentages of participants with total copper intake below the RNI (0.9 mg/d) were 15.2% in the cases and 8.4% in the controls, and no participants had a total copper intake above the tolerable upper intake level (8 mg/d) in the two groups.

Selenium is essential for antioxidant enzyme activities and normal fetal development [45]. Selenium deficiency in pregnancy might contribute to congenital anomalies, including neural tube defects and orofacial clefts [46–48]. Selenium exposure was reported to be associated with the changes in epigenetic patterning in both human and animal studies [49,50], which may exert effects on fetal cardiovascular development. It is noteworthy to mention that the study area in Northwest China is a relatively selenium deficient area, in which pregnant women tend to have low selenium status at baseline and can benefit more from the increased intake of selenium from diet and supplements.

Antagonisms between zinc, copper, and selenium have been shown in previous studies [18–20]. High zinc levels reduced the transport of copper into the blood, whereas high copper reduced zinc transport into the blood [19]. Copper was reported to negatively affect selenoprotein expression and activity via limiting UGA recoding [20]. Selenium had an antagonistic effect on zinc absorption by zinc-depleted rats, and zinc had an antagonistic effect on selenium absorption by zinc-adequate rats [18]. Given the rarity of research on the interactions of zinc, copper, and selenium on CHDs, the potential mechanisms involved need to be further explored.

4.3. Strengths and Limitations

The present study provides valuable evidence on the relationships between maternal total, dietary, and supplemental intakes of zinc, copper, and selenium during pregnancy and CHDs among humans. However, some limitations should be acknowledged. First, selection bias cannot be excluded because of the fact that pregnant women with CHDs fetuses tend to choose comprehensive hospitals for delivery, including the six selected hospitals in our study. Selection bias may also come from the fact that CHDs fetuses that did not survive were not included in the current study. If low maternal intakes of zinc and selenium in pregnancy increased CHDs risk and caused spontaneous and elective abortions, the relationships would be underestimated. Second, recall bias cannot be excluded because maternal information in pregnancy was recalled by participants waiting for delivery in the obstetrics departments. However, previous studies have suggested that nutrient intakes and events during pregnancy could be recalled well even after years [51,52]. To minimize bias, we made efforts to help participants recall accurately in the survey. For one thing, standard questionnaires and supporting materials such as food portion images and calendars were applied to collect information. For another, the survey was tested in a pilot study, and interviewers were rigorously trained according to the standard guides before the formal survey. Third, exposure misclassification may cause because we collected dietary information during the whole pregnancy rather than in the 3rd–8th week of gestation, the critical period of cardiac development. However, previous studies have reported that maternal dietary patterns and nutrient intakes were stable across pregnancy [24,25]. Fourth, we cannot separately assess the associations between maternal zinc, copper, and selenium intakes and other CHDs subtypes because of the limited sample size. Finally, we cannot fully exclude all other unobserved and unknown confounders and cannot reveal a real causal association.

5. Conclusions

The current study suggests that higher intakes of zinc and selenium from diet and supplements during pregnancy may reduce CHDs risk. This study also suggests that high intakes of zinc and selenium during pregnancy seem to have an additive effect on the association with CHDs. These findings imply the importance of promoting zinc and selenium intakes in pregnancy to reduce the incidence of CHDs in Northwest China. Future human studies with data on maternal minerals intakes, biological markers, and genetic and soil factors are warranted to confirm these findings and to elucidate underlying mechanisms.

Supplementary Materials: The following supporting information can be downloaded at https://www.mdpi.com/article/10.3390/nu14051055/s1, Figure S1: Restricted cubic spline models of total congenital heart defects (CHDs) risk associated with (A) dietary zinc intake, (B) dietary selenium intake, (C) dietary zinc to copper ratio, and (D) dietary selenium to copper ratio during pregnancy. Models are adjusted for total energy intake in pregnancy, socio-demographic characteristics (maternal age, residence, education, work, and parity), maternal health-related factors in the first trimester (folate/iron supplements use, passive smoking, medication use, and anemia), and dietary diversity score. Models are additionally adjusted for maternal supplements uses of zinc, copper, and selenium in the associations between dietary intakes of corresponding minerals and CHDs; Table S1: Quartiles of maternal dietary zinc, copper, and selenium intakes during pregnancy and congenital heart defects; Table S2: Maternal dietary zinc, copper, and selenium intakes categorized by the recommended nutrient intakes (RNIs) during pregnancy and congenital heart defects; Table S3: Maternal zinc, copper, and selenium supplements use during pregnancy and congenital heart defects.

Author Contributions: Conceptualization, J.Y., S.D. and H.Y.; methodology, J.Y., S.D. and L.Z.; formal analysis, J.Y., Y.K., Q.C., B.Z. and X.L.; investigation, J.Y., Y.K., Q.C., B.Z. and X.L.; data curation, L.Z., S.D. and H.Y.; writing—original draft preparation, J.Y.; writing—review and editing, S.D. and H.Y.; supervision, S.D. and H.Y.; project administration, S.D. and L.Z.; funding acquisition, J.Y., S.D. and H.Y. All authors have read and agreed to the published version of the manuscript.

Funding: This research was funded by the National Natural Science Foundation of China (82103852), China Postdoctoral Science Foundation (2019M663751), National Natural Science Foundation of China (81230016), Shaanxi Health and Family Planning Commission (Sxwsjswzfcght2016-013), and National Key R&D Program of China (2017YFC0907200, 2017YFC0907201).

Institutional Review Board Statement: The study was conducted according to the guidelines of the Declaration of Helsinki and approved by the Xi'an Jiaotong University Health Science Center on March 2012 (No.2012008).

Informed Consent Statement: Informed consent was obtained from all subjects involved in the study.

Data Availability Statement: The data present in this study are available on request from the corresponding authors.

Acknowledgments: The authors thank all medical staff involved in the study for recruiting the participants. The authors also thank all mothers and infants who participated in the study and all investigators who contributed to data collection.

Conflicts of Interest: The authors declare no conflict of interest.

References

1. Liu, Y.; Chen, S.; Zuhlke, L.; Black, G.C.; Choy, M.K.; Li, N.; Keavney, B.D. Global birth prevalence of congenital heart defects 1970–2017, updated systematic review and meta-analysis of 260 studies. *Int. J. Epidemiol.* **2019**, *48*, 455–463. [CrossRef] [PubMed]
2. Donofrio, M.T.; Moon-Grady, A.J.; Hornberger, L.K.; Copel, J.A.; Sklansky, M.S.; Abuhamad, A.; Cuneo, B.F.; Huhta, J.C.; Jonas, R.A.; Krishnan, A.; et al. Diagnosis and treatment of fetal cardiac disease: A scientific statement from the American Heart Association. *Circulation* **2014**, *129*, 2183–2242. [CrossRef] [PubMed]
3. Zhao, Q.M.; Liu, F.; Wu, L.; Ma, X.J.; Niu, C.; Huang, G.Y. Prevalence of congenital heart disease at live birth in China. *J. Pediatr.* **2019**, *204*, 53–58. [CrossRef]
4. Mousa, A.; Naqash, A.; Lim, S. Macronutrient and micronutrient intake during pregnancy: An overview of recent evidence. *Nutrients* **2019**, *11*, 443. [CrossRef] [PubMed]
5. Lopez, V.; Keen, C.L.; Lanoue, L. Prenatal zinc deficiency: Influence on heart morphology and distribution of key heart proteins in a rat model. *Biol. Trace Elem. Res.* **2008**, *122*, 238–255. [CrossRef] [PubMed]
6. Beckers-Trapp, M.E.; Lanoue, L.; Keen, C.L.; Rucker, R.B.; Uriu-Adams, J.Y. Abnormal development and increased 3-nitrotyrosine in copper-deficient mouse embryos. *Free Radic. Biol. Med.* **2006**, *40*, 35–44. [CrossRef] [PubMed]
7. Cao, L.; Huang, W.; Liu, J.; Ye, Z.; Dou, S. Toxicity of short-term copper exposure to early life stages of red sea bream, *Pagrus major*. *Environ. Toxicol. Chem.* **2010**, *29*, 2044–2052. [CrossRef] [PubMed]
8. Ojeda, M.L.; Nogales, F.; Romero-Herrera, I.; Carreras, O. Fetal programming is deeply related to maternal selenium status and oxidative balance; Experimental offspring health repercussions. *Nutrients* **2021**, *13*, 2085. [CrossRef] [PubMed]
9. Rayman, M.P.; Wijnen, H.; Vader, H.; Kooistra, L.; Pop, V. Maternal selenium status during early gestation and risk for preterm birth. *Cmaj* **2011**, *183*, 549–555. [CrossRef]
10. Zachara, B.A. Selenium in complicated pregnancy. A review. *Adv. Clin. Chem.* **2018**, *86*, 157–178. [PubMed]
11. Dilli, D.; Doğan, N.N.; Örün, U.A.; Koç, M.; Zenciroğlu, A.; Karademir, S.; Akduman, H. Maternal and neonatal micronutrient levels in newborns with CHD. *Cardiol. Young.* **2018**, *28*, 523–529. [CrossRef] [PubMed]
12. Guo, Y.; Yu, P.; Zhu, J.; Yang, S.; Yu, J.; Deng, Y.; Li, N.; Liu, Z. High maternal selenium levels are associated with increased risk of congenital heart defects in the offspring. *Prenat. Diagn.* **2019**, *39*, 1107–1114. [CrossRef] [PubMed]
13. Hu, H.; Liu, Z.; Li, J.; Li, S.; Tian, X.; Lin, Y.; Chen, X.; Yang, J.; Deng, Y.; Li, N.; et al. Correlation between congenital heart defects and maternal copper and zinc concentrations. *Birth Defects Res. A Clin. Mol. Teratol.* **2014**, *100*, 965–972. [CrossRef] [PubMed]
14. Ou, Y.; Bloom, M.S.; Nie, Z.; Han, F.; Mai, J.; Chen, J.; Lin, S.; Liu, X.; Zhuang, J. Associations between toxic and essential trace elements in maternal blood and fetal congenital heart defects. *Env. Int.* **2017**, *106*, 127–134. [CrossRef] [PubMed]
15. Yalçin, S.S.; Dönmez, Y.; Aypar, E.; Yalçin, S. Element profiles in blood and teeth samples of children with congenital heart diseases in comparison with healthy ones. *J. Trace Elem. Med. Biol.* **2021**, *63*, 126662. [CrossRef] [PubMed]
16. Zhu, Y.; Xu, C.; Zhang, Y.; Xie, Z.; Shu, Y.; Lu, C.; Mo, X. Associations of trace elements in blood with the risk of isolated ventricular septum defects and abnormal cardiac structure in children. *Env. Sci. Pollut. Res. Int.* **2019**, *26*, 10037–10043. [CrossRef] [PubMed]
17. Mares-Perlman, J.A.; Subar, A.F.; Block, G.; Greger, J.L.; Luby, M.H. Zinc intake and sources in the US adult population: 1976–1980. *J. Am. Coll. Nutr.* **1995**, *14*, 349–357. [CrossRef]
18. House, W.A.; Welch, R.M. Bioavailability of and interactions between zinc and selenium in rats fed wheat grain intrinsically labeled with 65Zn and 75Se. *J. Nutr.* **1989**, *119*, 916–921. [CrossRef] [PubMed]
19. Ojo, A.A.; Nadella, S.R.; Wood, C.M. In vitro examination of interactions between copper and zinc uptake via the gastrointestinal tract of the rainbow trout (Oncorhynchus mykiss). *Arch. Env. Contam. Toxicol.* **2009**, *56*, 244–252. [CrossRef]
20. Schwarz, M.; Lossow, K.; Schirl, K.; Hackler, J.; Renko, K.; Kopp, J.F.; Schwerdtle, T.; Schomburg, L.; Kipp, A.P. Copper interferes with selenoprotein synthesis and activity. *Redox. Biol.* **2020**, *37*, 101746. [CrossRef]
21. Yang, J.; Kang, Y.; Cheng, Y.; Zeng, L.; Shen, Y.; Shi, G.; Liu, Y.; Qu, P.; Zhang, R.; Yan, H.; et al. Iron intake and iron status during pregnancy and risk of congenital heart defects: A case-control study. *Int. J. Cardiol.* **2020**, *301*, 74–79. [CrossRef] [PubMed]
22. Yang, J.; Kang, Y.; Cheng, Y.; Zeng, L.; Yan, H.; Dang, S. Maternal dietary patterns during pregnancy and congenital heart defects: A case-control study. *Int. J. Env. Res. Public Health* **2019**, *16*, 2957. [CrossRef] [PubMed]
23. Zheng, L. *Soil Trace Elements in China*; Phoenix Science Press: Nanjing, China, 1996.
24. Crozier, S.R.; Robinson, S.M.; Godfrey, K.M.; Cooper, C.; Inskip, H.M. Women's dietary patterns change little from before to during pregnancy. *J. Nutr.* **2009**, *139*, 1956–1963. [CrossRef] [PubMed]
25. Rifas-Shiman, S.L.; Rich-Edwards, J.W.; Willett, W.C.; Kleinman, K.P.; Oken, E.; Gillman, M.W. Changes in dietary intake from the first to the second trimester of pregnancy. *Paediatr. Perinat. Epidemiol.* **2006**, *20*, 35–42. [CrossRef] [PubMed]

26. Yang, J.; Cheng, Y.; Zeng, L.; Dang, S.; Yan, H. Maternal dietary diversity during pregnancy and congenital heart defects: A case-control study. *Eur. J. Clin. Nutr.* **2021**, *75*, 355–363. [CrossRef] [PubMed]
27. Cheng, Y.; Yan, H.; Dibley, M.J.; Shen, Y.; Li, Q.; Zeng, L. Validity and reproducibility of a semi-quantitative food frequency questionnaire for use among pregnant women in rural China. *Asia Pac. J. Clin. Nutr.* **2008**, *17*, 166–177. [PubMed]
28. Yang, J.; Dang, S.; Cheng, Y.; Qiu, H.; Mi, B.; Jiang, Y.; Qu, P.; Zeng, L.; Wang, Q.; Li, Q.; et al. Dietary intakes and dietary patterns among pregnant women in Northwest China. *Public Health Nutr.* **2017**, *20*, 282–293. [CrossRef] [PubMed]
29. Institute of Nutrition and Food Safety, China Center for Disease Control. *China Food Composition Book 2*; Peking University Medical Press: Beijing, China, 2005.
30. Institute of Nutrition and Food Safety, China Center for Disease Control. *China Food Composition Book 1*, 2nd ed.; Peking University Medical Press: Beijing, China, 2009.
31. FAO; FHI 360. *Minimum Dietary Dieversity for Women: A Guide for Measurement*; FAO: Rome, Italy, 2016.
32. Chinese Nutrition Society. *Chinese Dietary Guideline*; People's Medical Publishing House: Beijing, China, 2016.
33. Feng, Y.; Cai, J.; Tong, X.; Chen, R.; Zhu, Y.; Xu, B.; Mo, X. Non-inheritable risk factors during pregnancy for congenital heart defects in offspring: A matched case-control study. *Int. J. Cardiol.* **2018**, *264*, 45–52. [CrossRef] [PubMed]
34. Pei, L.; Kang, Y.; Zhao, Y.; Yan, H. Prevalence and risk factors of congenital heart defects among live births: A population-based cross-sectional survey in Shaanxi province, Northwestern China. *BMC Pediatr.* **2017**, *17*, 18. [CrossRef] [PubMed]
35. Mickey, R.M.; Greenland, S. The impact of confounder selection criteria on effect estimation. *Am. J. Epidemiol.* **1989**, *129*, 125–137. [CrossRef]
36. Nakamura, M.; Miura, A.; Nagahata, T.; Shibata, Y.; Okada, E.; Ojima, T. Low Zinc, Copper, and manganese intake is associated with depression and anxiety symptoms in the Japanese working population: Findings from the eating habit and well-being study. *Nutrients* **2019**, *11*, 847. [CrossRef]
37. Iqbal, S.; Ali, I.; Rust, P.; Kundi, M.; Ekmekcioglu, C. Selenium, zinc, and manganese status in pregnant women and its relation to maternal and child complications. *Nutrients* **2020**, *12*, 725. [CrossRef] [PubMed]
38. Mehdi, Y.; Hornick, J.L.; Istasse, L.; Dufrasne, I. Selenium in the environment, metabolism and involvement in body functions. *Molecules* **2013**, *18*, 3292–3311. [CrossRef] [PubMed]
39. Shah, D.; Sachdev, H.P. Zinc deficiency in pregnancy and fetal outcome. *Nutr. Rev.* **2006**, *64*, 15–30. [CrossRef]
40. Juriol, L.V.; Gobetto, M.N.; Mendes Garrido Abregú, F.; Dasso, M.E.; Pineda, G.; Güttlein, L.; Carranza, A.; Podhajcer, O.; Toblli, J.E.; Elesgaray, R.; et al. Cardiac changes in apoptosis, inflammation, oxidative stress, and nitric oxide system induced by prenatal and postnatal zinc deficiency in male and female rats. *Eur. J. Nutr.* **2018**, *57*, 569–583. [CrossRef] [PubMed]
41. Kumar, S.D.; Vijaya, M.; Samy, R.P.; Dheen, S.T.; Ren, M.; Watt, F.; Kang, Y.J.; Bay, B.H.; Tay, S.S. Zinc supplementation prevents cardiomyocyte apoptosis and congenital heart defects in embryos of diabetic mice. *Free Radic. Biol. Med.* **2012**, *53*, 1595–1606. [CrossRef] [PubMed]
42. Peña, M.M.; Lee, J.; Thiele, D.J. A delicate balance: Homeostatic control of copper uptake and distribution. *J. Nutr.* **1999**, *129*, 1251–1260. [CrossRef] [PubMed]
43. Duffy, J.Y.; Overmann, G.J.; Keen, C.L.; Clegg, M.S.; Daston, G.P. Cardiac abnormalities induced by zinc deficiency are associated with alterations in the expression of genes regulated by the zinc-finger transcription factor GATA-4. *Birth Defects Res. B Dev. Reprod. Toxicol.* **2004**, *71*, 102–109. [CrossRef]
44. Yuasa, S.; Onizuka, T.; Shimoji, K.; Ohno, Y.; Kageyama, T.; Yoon, S.H.; Egashira, T.; Seki, T.; Hashimoto, H.; Nishiyama, T.; et al. Zac1 is an essential transcription factor for cardiac morphogenesis. *Circ. Res.* **2010**, *106*, 1083–1091. [CrossRef] [PubMed]
45. Martín, I.; Gibert, M.J.; Pintos, C.; Noguera, A.; Besalduch, A.; Obrador, A. Oxidative stress in mothers who have conceived fetus with neural tube defects: The role of aminothiols and selenium. *Clin. Nutr.* **2004**, *23*, 507–514. [CrossRef]
46. Cengiz, B.; Söylemez, F.; Oztürk, E.; Cavdar, A.O. Serum zinc, selenium, copper, and lead levels in women with second-trimester induced abortion resulting from neural tube defects: A preliminary study. *Biol. Trace. Elem. Res.* **2004**, *97*, 225–235. [CrossRef]
47. Hammouda, S.A.; Abd Al-Halim, O.A.; Mohamadin, A.M. Serum levels of some micronutrients and congenital malformations: A prospective cohort study in healthy saudi-arabian first-trimester pregnant women. *Int. J. Vitam. Nutr. Res.* **2013**, *83*, 346–354. [CrossRef] [PubMed]
48. Pi, X.; Wei, Y.; Li, Z.; Jin, L.; Liu, J.; Zhang, Y.; Wang, L.; Ren, A. Higher concentration of selenium in placental tissues is associated with reduced risk for orofacial clefts. *Clin. Nutr.* **2019**, *38*, 2442–2448. [CrossRef] [PubMed]
49. Davis, C.D.; Uthus, E.O.; Finley, J.W. Dietary selenium and arsenic affect DNA methylation in vitro in Caco-2 cells and in vivo in rat liver and colon. *J. Nutr.* **2000**, *130*, 2903–2909. [CrossRef] [PubMed]
50. Pilsner, J.R.; Hall, M.N.; Liu, X.; Ahsan, H.; Ilievski, V.; Slavkovich, V.; Levy, D.; Factor-Litvak, P.; Graziano, J.H.; Gamble, M.V. Associations of plasma selenium with arsenic and genomic methylation of leukocyte DNA in Bangladesh. *Environ. Health Perspect.* **2011**, *119*, 113–118. [CrossRef] [PubMed]
51. Bosco, J.L.; Tseng, M.; Spector, L.G.; Olshan, A.F.; Bunin, G.R. Reproducibility of reported nutrient intake and supplement use during a past pregnancy: A report from the Children's Oncology Group. *Paediatr. Perinat. Epidemiol.* **2010**, *24*, 93–101. [CrossRef] [PubMed]
52. Bunin, G.R.; Gyllstrom, M.E.; Brown, J.E.; Kahn, E.B.; Kushi, L.H. Recall of diet during a past pregnancy. *Am. J. Epidemiol.* **2001**, *154*, 1136–1142. [CrossRef] [PubMed]

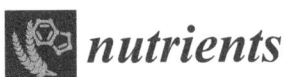

Article

Maternal Hemoglobin Concentrations and Birth Weight, Low Birth Weight (LBW), and Small for Gestational Age (SGA): Findings from a Prospective Study in Northwest China

Danmeng Liu [1,†], Shanshan Li [2,†], Binyan Zhang [1], Yijun Kang [1], Yue Cheng [3], Lingxia Zeng [1], Fangyao Chen [1], Baibing Mi [1], Pengfei Qu [4], Doudou Zhao [4], Zhonghai Zhu [1], Hong Yan [1,5,6], Duolao Wang [7] and Shaonong Dang [1,*]

1. Department of Epidemiology and Health Statistics, School of Public Health, Health Science Center, Xi'an Jiaotong University, Xi'an 710061, China; liudanmeng1214@stu.xjtu.edu.cn (D.L.); zhangbinyan@stu.xjtu.edu.cn (B.Z.); tjkyj@xjtu.edu.cn (Y.K.); tjzlx@mail.xjtu.edu.cn (L.Z.); chenfy@xjtu.edu.cn (F.C.); xjtu.mi@xjtu.edu.cn (B.M.); zhonghai_zhu@mail.xjtu.edu.cn (Z.Z.); yanhonge@xjtu.edu.cn (H.Y.)
2. School of Public Health, Shandong First Medical University & Shandong Academy of Medical Sciences, Taian 271016, China; lishanshan@sdfmu.edu.cn
3. Department of Nutrition, School of Public Health, Health Science Center, Xi'an Jiaotong University, Xi'an 710061, China; chengy@mail.xjtu.edu.cn
4. Translational Medicine Center, Northwest Women's and Children's Hospital, Xi'an 710061, China; xinxi3057@stu.xjtu.edu.cn (P.Q.); zhaodoudou1223@stu.xjtu.edu.cn (D.Z.)
5. Nutrition and Food Safety Engineering Research Center of Shaanxi Province, Xi'an 710061, China
6. Key Laboratory of Environment and Gene-Related Diseases, Xi'an Jiaotong University, Ministry of Education, Xi'an 710061, China
7. Department of Clinical Sciences, Liverpool School of Tropical Medicine, Liverpool L3 5QA, UK; duolao.wang@lstmed.ac.uk

* Correspondence: tjdshn@xjtu.edu.cn
† These authors contributed equally to this work.

Abstract: Birth weight and related outcomes have profound influences on life cycle health, but the effect of maternal hemoglobin concentration during pregnancy on birth weight is still unclear. This study aims to reveal the associations between maternal hemoglobin concentrations in different trimesters of pregnancy and neonatal birth weight, LBW, and SGA. This was a prospective study based on a cluster-randomized controlled trial conducted from July 2015 to December 2019 in rural areas of Northwest China. Information on maternal socio-demographic status, health-related factors, antenatal visits, and neonatal birth outcomes were collected. A total of 3748 women and their babies were included in the final analysis. A total of 65.1% and 46.3% of the participants had anemia or hemoglobin ≥ 130 g/L during pregnancy. In the third trimester, maternal hemoglobin concentration was associated with birth weight in an inverted U-shaped curve and with the risks of LBW and SGA in extended U-shaped curves. The relatively higher birth weight and lower risks for LBW and SGA were observed when hemoglobin concentration was 100–110 g/L. When maternal hemoglobin was <70 g/L or >130 g/L, the neonatal birth weight was more than 100 g lower than that when the maternal hemoglobin was 100 g/L. In conclusion, both low and high hemoglobin concentrations in the third trimester could be adverse to fetal weight growth and increase the risks of LBW and SGA, respectively. In addition to severe anemia, maternal hemoglobin >130 g/L in the third trimester should be paid great attention to in the practice of maternal and child health care.

Keywords: maternal hemoglobin concentration; neonatal birth weight; LBW; SGA; nonlinear association; prospective study

1. Introduction

Birth weight is critical for the evaluation of fetal growth and the prediction of neonatal mortality and morbidity [1]. The poor birth weight caused by limited intrauterine growth and development could further result in adverse birth outcomes including low birth weight (LBW) and small for gestational age (SGA). According to the WHO criteria, LBW infants are those born weighing < 2500 g [2], and infants born SGA are defined as those weighing below the 10th centile of birth weight by sex for a specific completed gestational age of a given reference population [3]. The prevalence of LBW/SGA is relatively high in the middle- and low-income countries, especially in economically undeveloped regions [3,4]. Both LBW and SGA are the main causes of neonatal mortality and morbidity. Infants with LBW/SGA have a considerably higher risk of short-term morbidities, including infections, respiratory depression, jaundice, hypoglycemia, hypothermia, and so on. In the long-term, LBW/SGA are related to many health issues, including cognitive deficiencies, mental retardation, cerebral palsy, gastrointestinal morbidity, and metabolic disorders such as obesity, diabetes, and cardiovascular diseases [2,4–6]. Therefore, poor fetal weight growth harms life cycle health, and identifying its potential influencing factors is of great significance for the prevention of short- and long-term diseases.

Maternal nutrition during pregnancy critically determines fetal nutrition and has a significant contribution to fetal and neonatal health. Maternal intakes of micronutrients such as folic acid and iron are crucial for fetal growth and development [7]. Hemoglobin concentration is a key indicator reflecting the maternal nutrition status during pregnancy, especially the iron status [8]. Previous studies reported that maternal hemoglobin concentration was associated with neonatal birth weight as well as LBW and SGA, but there is no consistent conclusion. Rasmussen et al. found a strong independent inverse correlation between the lowest second-trimester hemoglobin and birth weight, but no relationship was observed in the first trimester [9]. Haider et al. reported that neonatal birth weight increased by 14 g for every 1 g/L increase in average hemoglobin in the third trimester. Steer et al. observed that the maximum mean birth weight was achieved with a lowest hemoglobin concentration in pregnancy of 85–95 g/L, which indicated a nonlinear relationship between maternal hemoglobin during pregnancy and birth weight [10]. A recent meta-analysis revealed a U-shaped curve association between maternal hemoglobin concentration and adverse birth outcomes, which suggested that both low and high hemoglobin concentrations might be risk factors for fetal growth [11].

Pregnant women have a high prevalence of anemia [12]. Lots of studies have reported that maternal anemia during pregnancy is associated with risks of intrauterine growth restriction, preterm birth, LBW, and SGA [13–15]. However, the associations were diverse in different gestational trimesters. The associations between maternal anemia and the increased risks of preterm birth, LBW, and SGA were strong in the first trimester [16–19], but were weak in the second or third trimester [16,18,20–23]. Additionally, maternal anemia in the third trimester may reduce the risks of adverse birth outcomes [21]. As for the associations between high hemoglobin concentration and birth outcomes, the results in the existing literature are controversial. Some studies showed that high hemoglobin concentration significantly reduced the risks of LBW or preterm birth [23,24]. However, several studies indicated that maternal higher hemoglobin concentrations during pregnancy were associated with increased risks of adverse birth outcomes [18,22,25].

Accordingly, the relationships between maternal hemoglobin concentration and birth outcomes reported in previous studies are complicated and have been disputed. The inconsistencies of the findings were mainly attributed to the differences in research design, sample size, time of hemoglobin measurement, hemoglobin classification cut-offs, race, and region of investigation [20,23]. Additionally, most of the previous studies focused on the effect of maternal anemia, and the relatively fewer studies that reported the association of maternal high hemoglobin concentrations with birth outcomes were conducted mainly in developed countries [26]. Evidence from the Chinese population, especially those in the underdeveloped regions, is lacking. Therefore, the present study aims to reveal the associations between maternal hemoglobin concentrations (within the entire hemoglobin range) in different trimesters of pregnancy and neonatal birth weight, LBW, and SGA, through a prospective study in Northwest China.

2. Materials and Methods

2.1. Study Design and Participants

The data was from a cluster-randomized controlled trial (registration number in ClinicalTrials.gov: NCT02537392) which was conducted from July 2015 to December 2019 in rural areas of Northwest China. The original trial aimed to evaluate the effect of micronutrient supplementation during pregnancy on congenital heart disease (primary outcome) and other birth outcomes. Detailed design and methods of this trial have been described elsewhere [27]. A brief introduction is as follows. A cluster randomization method was used to randomize the townships (the unit of randomization) of the study region to the intervention groups (the folic acid group (the control group), folic acid + iron group, and folic acid + vitamin B complex group) with a 1:1:1 ratio before enrolment. Women aged 15–49 years and with less than 20 weeks gestational age were invited to participate, and the exclusion criteria at recruitment included (1) use of supplements containing iron or vitamin B complex for more than 2 weeks, (2) having given birth to children with congenital heart disease or other birth defects, and (3) having severe liver or kidney disease. In each township, eligible women with informed written consent were enrolled at the township-level health center, administered by a trained township maternal and child healthcare professional. Participants in each intervention group were required to use the corresponding nutrient supplements daily until delivery and were followed up from the time of enrolment to delivery. Information on maternal socio-demographic status, health-related factors, antenatal visits, and neonatal birth outcomes was collected. The participants received routine treatment and health care according to the Chinese clinical guidelines for the diagnosis and treatment of maternal anemia if they developed this during pregnancy [28].

Based on the original trial, the present study was conducted to investigate the associations between maternal hemoglobin during pregnancy and birth weight, LBW, and SGA. A total of 4383 eligible pregnant women enrolled in the original trial from December 2016 to December 2019 were included in the present study. Women who were lost to follow-up (n 205), withdrew (n 29), had spontaneous/induced abortion (n 147), had a stillbirth (n 5) or twin births (n 36) were excluded. In addition, since we focused on the maternal hemoglobin during pregnancy according to the study objective, a total of 3748 women who had hemoglobin records in each of the gestational trimesters (including the first, second, and third trimester) were finally included in the study (Figure 1). Women included in the final analysis had no significant difference in maternal socio-demographic characteristics and parity compared to those excluded from the study (Table S1).

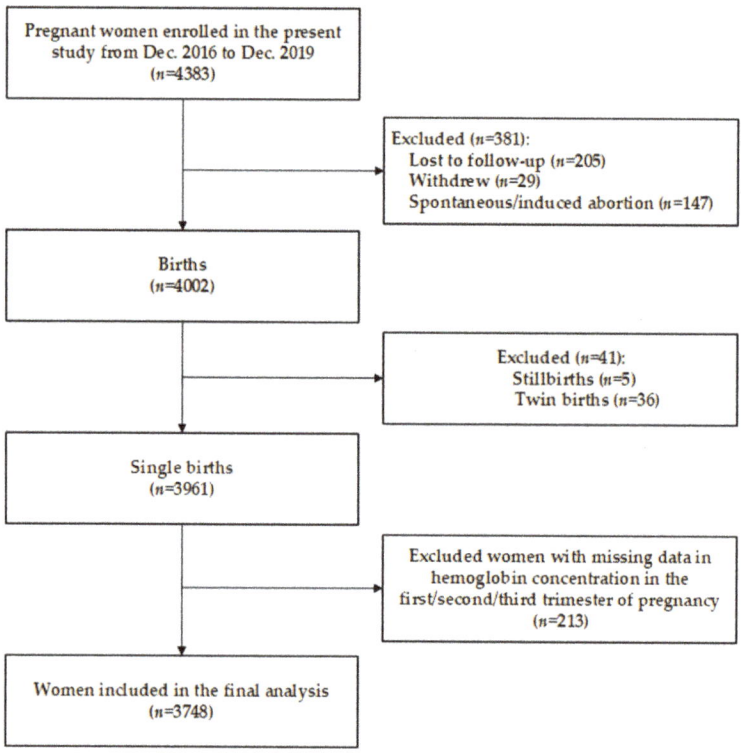

Figure 1. Study flowchart.

2.2. Sample Size

The sample size was calculated based on the main outcome (birth weight) of the study. Estimating the mean and standard deviation of the neonatal birth weight of women with non-anemia during pregnancy was 3250 g and 440 g [29], assuming the mean neonatal birth weight of anemic mothers was 50 g lower than the nonanemic mothers, and using a two-sided significance level of 5% and a power of 80%, a minimum estimated sample size was 1216 in each group. Considering a 10% loss rate, a minimum total of 2676 (1338 in each group) pregnant women were required. Our study included 3748 women in the final analysis, which met the sample size requirement.

2.3. Data Collection

Participants enrolment and follow-ups were conducted in the township-level health centers, and deliveries were completed in the county-level hospitals. Data collection was carried out by trained township maternal and child healthcare professionals and was supervised by investigators from Xi'an Jiaotong University Health Science Center. At enrolment, maternal socio-demographic characteristics (including age, education, occupation, and income), reproductive history, and date of last menstrual period were collected via face-to-face interviews. Baseline height and weight were measured using unified facilities. During follow-ups, after women attended the antenatal visits at county-level hospitals, the township maternal and child healthcare professionals collected their anthropometric and hematological records from their antenatal visits and accounted the number of antenatal visits at the end of the follow-ups. Maternal uses of interventional micronutrient supplements were investigated every two months during follow-ups, and other maternal micronutrient supplementations during pregnancy were collected within one week after delivery. Neonatal birth outcomes, including birth date, birth weight, gestational age, and gender, were obtained according to medical records. All information was entered into a web-based surveillance system by trained township maternal and child healthcare professionals, and routine data quality monitoring was carried out by researchers from Xi'an Jiaotong University Health Science Center.

2.4. Hemoglobin Measurement

Maternal hemoglobin measurement was conducted during antenatal visits at the county-level hospitals by the clinical laboratory technician. Hemoglobin concentration in a unit of g/L was measured through routine blood tests which were completed using the automatic hematology analyzer with the venous blood samples of participants. The township maternal and child healthcare professionals recorded the hemoglobin concentration according to the test results after antenatal visits.

The gestational age at antenatal visits was calculated according to the last menstrual period. The period of pregnancy was divided into trimesters according to the gestational age, which included the first trimester (0–12 weeks of gestational age), the second trimester (13–27 weeks of gestational age), and the third trimester (28 weeks of gestational age to the time of delivery). The present study only included women with at least one hemoglobin record in each trimester, and for women who had more than one hemoglobin record in a certain trimester, the lowest was used for analysis [10,30].

Maternal hemoglobin concentration < 110 g/L can be diagnosed as gestational anemia according to the WHO standard, and the severity of anemia was defined as follows: 100–109 g/L is mild anemia, 70–99 g/L is moderate anemia, and <70 g/L is severe anemia [31]. Maternal hemoglobin ≥ 130 g/L referred to a relatively-high hemoglobin concentration during pregnancy [24,26,32].

2.5. Outcome Assessment

The primary outcome of this study was neonatal birth weight, and the secondary outcomes were LBW and SGA. Birth weight was measured to the nearest 10 g with a baby scale within one hour after delivery. Gender (male/female) was recorded after delivery. Gestational age at delivery was calculated according to the last menstrual period and was confirmed by ultrasound scans. LBW was defined as birth weight < 2500 g according to the WHO [2]. SGA was defined as birth weight below the 10th percentile for gestational age and sex according to the standards for fetal growth and development in China [33].

2.6. Covariate Assessment

Based on the existing literature [4,34], covariates considered in the study mainly included two parts: (1) socio-demographic characteristics, including maternal age at enrolment (<25/25–34/≥35 years), education level (junior high school or below/senior high school/college or above), occupation (farmers/others), per capita annual household income (<5000/5000–9999/≥10,000 Yuan, where 1 Yuan = 0.156 $US on 8 November 2021), and township (48 townships); (2) health-related characteristics, including parity (primipara/multipara), gestational age at enrolment (≤12 weeks/>12 weeks), body mass index (BMI) at enrolment (underweight < 18.5/normal weight 18.5–23.9/overweight 24.0–27.9/obesity ≥ 28.0 kg/m^2), the times of antenatal visits (≤5/>5), and micronutrient supplementations (folic acid/folic acid + iron/folic acid + vitamin B complex). Maternal age and gestational age at enrolment were respectively calculated according to birth date and the last menstrual period. Height was measured to the nearest 0.1 cm with a stadiometer, and weight was measured to the nearest 0.1 kg with an electronic scale. BMI at enrolment was calculated as weight at enrolment in kilograms divided by height in meters squared, and was classified according to the standards recommended in the "Guidelines for prevention and control of overweight and obesity in Chinese adults" [35]. Micronutrient supplementation was classified according to the intervention groups in the original trial.

2.7. Statistical Analysis

Continuous variables were expressed as mean ± SDs, and categorical variables were described as numbers (proportions). Since the sample of the present study was obtained based on a cluster-randomized controlled trial (the township is the unit of randomization), the data collected had a hierarchical structure. Accordingly, generalized estimating equation (GEE) models [36] were applied to evaluate the associations of maternal hemoglobin concentration during pregnancy with the outcomes. The GEE model is a population average model used to estimate the associations between neighborhood characteristics (this refers to the factors related to the neighborhood that the study individuals belong to, and possess both physical and social attributes that could plausibly affect the health of individuals [37]) and health outcomes in multilevel studies [36]. In this study, the variable of township had the random effect, and maternal hemoglobin concentration in different trimesters of pregnancy and covariates had the fixed effects in the GEE models. The unadjusted model and adjusted model were established to estimate the changes in birth weight (normal distribution and identity link function) and RR for LBW/SGA (binomial distribution and log link function), as well as their accompanying 95% CI. The adjusted model was adjusted for socio-demographic characteristics (including maternal age, education, occupation, and per capita annual household income) and health-related characteristics (including parity, BMI at enrolment, gestational age at enrolment, number of antenatal visits, and micronutrient supplementation). When estimating the associations between maternal hemoglobin and birth weight/LBW, models were additionally adjusted for neonatal gender and gestational age at delivery.

Restricted cubic spline (RCS) function was further used to estimate the dose–response relationship between maternal hemoglobin concentration in different trimesters of pregnancy and the birth outcomes [38]. According to the cut-offs of hemoglobin that were used to classify the severity of gestational anemia [31] and the cut-off that represents a relatively-high maternal hemoglobin concentration [20,24], maternal hemoglobin at 70, 100, 110, 130 g/L were selected as the four knots set into the RCS models. In these models, maternal hemoglobin in different trimesters was set as independent variable (x-axis), and birth weight/LBW/SGA was set as dependent variable (y-axis). Hemoglobin at 110 g/L or the minimum value of hemoglobin was set as the reference value. Models were adjusted for socio-demographic and health-related characteristics as described above. The p-value for the overall association was used to evaluate the overall association between maternal hemoglobin and birth outcomes, and the p-value for the nonlinear association was used to assess any nonlinear association between maternal hemoglobin and birth outcomes.

Based on the above analyses, subgroup analyses according to maternal hemoglobin concentration and maternal characteristics (age, education level, income level, parity, BMI at enrolment, times of antenatal visits, and micronutrient supplementation) were further conducted to estimate the associations between maternal hemoglobin during pregnancy and neonatal birth weight in different subgroups.

All analyses were performed using SAS version 9.4 (SAS Institute, Cary, NC, USA). All statistical tests were two-tailed, and statistical significance was set as $p < 0.05$. SAS code for GEE models could be accessed in "SAS System Documentation" and referred to the GEE syntax under "The GENMOD Procedure". The RCS curve fitting was realized by an SAS macro program written by Desquilbet [38].

3. Results

3.1. Maternal Baseline Characteristics and Neonatal Birth Outcomes

As shown in Table 1, higher proportions of participants were observed in women aged 25–34 years (59.6%), with junior high school or below educational level (54.4%), farmers (87.8%), medium per capita annual household income (40.5%), normal weight (71.0%), and having attended no more than five antenatal visits (67.2%).

Table 1. Maternal baseline characteristics and neonatal birth outcomes (N = 3748).

Characteristics	Mean ± SD or n (%)
Socio-demographic characteristics	
Age (years)	26.2 ± 4.1
<25	1369 (36.5)
25–34	2235 (59.6)
≥35	144 (3.8)
Education	
Junior high school or below	2040 (54.4)
Senior high school	1179 (31.5)
College or above	529 (14.1)
Farmers	3292 (87.8)
Per capita annual household income (RMB)	
Low (<5000)	872 (23.3)
Medium (5000–9999)	1519 (40.5)
High (≥10,000)	1357 (36.2)
Health-related characteristics	
Primipara	1914 (51.1)
Gestational age at enrolment (weeks)	14.4 ± 6.1
≤12	1580 (42.2)
>12	2168 (57.8)
Height (cm)	159.8 ± 4.8
Weight at enrolment (kg)	55.5 ± 8.11
BMI at enrolment (kg/m^2)	
Underweight (<18.5)	408 (10.9)
Normal weight (18.5–23.9)	2662 (71.0)
Overweight (24.0–27.9)	553 (14.8)
Obesity (≥28.0)	125 (3.3)
More than five antenatal visits	1229 (32.8)
Micronutrient supplementation	
Folic acid	1363 (36.3)
Folic acid + iron	1130 (30.1)
Folic acid + vitamin B complex	1255 (33.4)
Birth outcomes	
Birth weight (g)	3233.4 ± 418.3
Gestational age at delivery (weeks)	39.7 ± 1.3
Gender, male	1936 (51.7)
LBW	99 (2.6)
SGA	501 (13.4)

LBW, low birth weight; SGA, small for gestational age.

The average neonatal birth weight was 3233.4 ± 418.3 g, and the average gestational age at delivery was 39.7 ± 1.3 weeks. The proportions of LBW and SGA infants were 2.6%, and 13.4%, respectively.

3.2. Maternal Hemoglobin Status in Different Trimesters of Pregnancy

Maternal hemoglobin concentrations in the first, second, and third trimesters of pregnancy were tested averagely at 10.2 (SD 2.0), 19.4 (SD 3.2), and 36.1 (SD 2.7) weeks of gestation. As displayed in Table 2, in the first, second, and third trimester, the prevalence of maternal anemia was 16.6%, 30.9%, and 45.9%; the rates of hemoglobin ≥130 g/L were 33.1%, 14.7%, and 8.2%, respectively. A total of 65.1% and 46.3% of the participants have had anemia or hemoglobin ≥130 g/L during pregnancy.

Table 2. Maternal hemoglobin status in different trimesters of pregnancy.

Hemoglobin (g/L)	Mean ± SD or n (%)
First trimester	
Average hemoglobin concentration	123.2 ± 14.4
Anemia (<110)	624 (16.6)
Severe anemia (<70)	0 (0.0)
Moderate anemia (70–99)	203 (5.4)
Mild anemia (100–109)	421 (11.2)
Normal (110–129)	1883 (50.2)
Hemoglobin ≥ 130	1241 (33.1)
Second trimester	
Average hemoglobin concentration	115.6 ± 13.4
Anemia (<110)	1157 (30.9)
Severe anemia (<70)	0 (0.0)
Moderate anemia (70–99)	427 (11.4)
Mild anemia (100–109)	730 (19.5)
Normal (110–129)	2039 (54.4)
Hemoglobin ≥ 130	552 (14.7)
Third trimester	
Average hemoglobin concentration	110.8 ± 13.9
Anemia (<110)	1720 (45.9)
Severe anemia (<70)	12 (0.3)
Moderate anemia (70–99)	719 (19.2)
Mild anemia (100–109)	989 (26.4)
Normal (110–129)	1720 (45.9)
Hemoglobin ≥ 130	308 (8.2)

3.3. Associations between Maternal Hemoglobin Concentrations during Pregnancy and Birth Weight-Related Outcomes

Table 3 displays the associations between maternal hemoglobin concentrations in different trimesters and neonatal birth weight, LBW, and SGA. In the first trimester, compared to women with normal hemoglobin concentration (110–129 g/L), women with hemoglobin ≥ 130 g/L had a significant increase in neonatal birth weight (adjusted changes: 26.5 g, 95% CI: 0.2, 52.8); no association between maternal hemoglobin with LBW and SGA was observed. In the second trimester, no association was found between maternal hemoglobin and the outcomes. In the third trimester, compared to women with normal hemoglobin concentration (110–129 g/L), women with severe anemia (<70 g/L) had a significant decrease in neonatal birth weight (adjusted changes: −216.3 g, 95% CI: −426.7, −5.9), and had a significant increase in risk of LBW (adjusted RR: 7.47, 95% CI: 2.53, 22.08). Women with mild anemia (100–109 g/L) had a significant increase in neonatal birth weight (adjusted changes: 46.5 g, 95% CI: 7.6, 85.3), and had a 27% reduced risk of SGA (adjusted RR: 0.73, 95% CI: 0.61, 0.87). Women with hemoglobin ≥130 g/L had a trend of reduction in neonatal birth weight, but the result was not statistically significant (adjusted changes: −30.7 g, 95% CI: −76.1, 14.7).

Table 3. Associations between maternal hemoglobin concentrations during pregnancy with neonatal birth weight, LBW, and SGA [1].

Outcomes	Hemoglobin (g/L)	Mean (SD) or n (%)	Unadjusted Model	Adjusted Model [2]
		Mean (SD)	Changes (95% CI)	Changes (95% CI)
Birth weight	First trimester			
	<70	-	-	-
	70–99	3240.6 (415.7)	21.0 (−51.0, 92.9)	26.6 (−34.0, 87.2)
	100–109	3238.1 (418.0)	18.4 (−29.5, 66.2)	25.1 (−20.5, 70.7)
	110–129	3221.1 (410.1)	Ref.	Ref.
	≥130	3249.1 (430.8)	29.0 (1.7, 56.4)	26.5 (0.2, 52.8)

Table 3. Cont.

Outcomes	Hemoglobin (g/L)	Mean (SD) or n (%)	Unadjusted Model	Adjusted Model [2]
	Second trimester			
	<70	-	-	-
	70–99	3258.0 (426.1)	27.5 (−3.3, 58.3)	30.8 (−3.2, 64.8)
	100–109	3221.8 (412.1)	−9.3 (−47.9, 29.4)	−5.0 (−44.6, 34.7)
	110–129	3230.1 (424.8)	Ref.	Ref.
	≥130	3241.5 (395.4)	10.9 (−26.9, 48.6)	11.5 (−22.8, 45.7)
	Third trimester			
	<70	2988.3 (549.6)	−230.5 (−455.2, −5.7)	−216.3 (−426.7, −5.9)
	70–99	3253.3 (413.5)	35.9 (−0.2, 71.9)	45.8 (9.9, 81.7)
	100–109	3259.2 (440.5)	42.1 (5.4, 78.8)	46.5 (7.6, 85.3)
	110–129	3220.0 (409.0)	Ref.	Ref.
	≥130	3193.4 (419.7)	−29.2 (−72.5, 14.2)	−30.7 (−76.1, 14.7)
		n (%)	RR (95% CI)	RR (95% CI)
LBW	First trimester			
	<70	-	-	-
	70–99	4 (2.0)	0.67 (0.22, 2.06)	0.72 (0.24, 2.16)
	100–109	9 (2.1)	0.77 (0.39, 1.54)	0.80 (0.39, 1.63)
	110–129	54 (2.9)	Ref.	Ref.
	≥130	32 (2.6)	0.91 (0.61, 1.38)	0.85 (0.54, 1.33)
	Second trimester			
	<70	-	-	-
	70–99	12 (2.8)	0.95 (0.44, 2.02)	1.10 (0.52, 2.29)
	100–109	17 (2.3)	0.79 (0.47, 1.34)	0.90 (0.52, 1.55)
	110–129	59 (2.9)	Ref.	Ref.
	≥130	11 (2.0)	0.70 (0.35, 1.41)	0.53 (0.20, 1.37)
	Third trimester			
	<70	2 (16.7)	6.36 (2.07, 19.59)	7.47 (2.53, 22.08)
	70–99	21 (2.9)	1.10 (0.76, 1.61)	1.20 (0.76, 1.91)
	100–109	23 (2.3)	0.88 (0.57, 1.37)	0.94 (0.58, 1.51)
	110–129	42 (2.4)	Ref.	Ref.
	≥130	11 (3.6)	1.51 (0.64, 3.54)	1.41 (0.49, 4.03)
SGA	First trimester			
	<70	-	-	-
	70–99	27 (13.3)	0.97 (0.68, 1.39)	0.98 (0.67, 1.44)
	100–109	51 (12.2)	0.89 (0.65, 1.23)	0.91 (0.65, 1.29)
	110–129	256 (13.6)	Ref.	Ref.
	≥130	167 (13.5)	0.99 (0.82, 1.20)	0.99 (0.81, 1.21)
	Second trimester			
	<70	-	-	-
	70–99	56 (13.1)	0.94 (0.77, 1.16)	1.03 (0.83, 1.28)
	100–109	90 (12.4)	0.89 (0.75, 1.06)	0.91 (0.76, 1.09)
	110–129	285 (14.0)	Ref.	Ref.
	≥130	70 (12.7)	0.91 (0.74, 1.11)	0.95 (0.75, 1.20)
	Third trimester			
	<70	2 (16.7)	1.12 (0.31, 4.11)	1.32 (0.35, 4.98)
	70–99	91 (12.7)	0.86 (0.70, 1.05)	0.87 (0.70, 1.09)
	100–109	104 (10.5)	0.72 (0.61, 0.84)	0.73 (0.61, 0.87)
	110–129	252 (14.7)	Ref.	Ref.
	≥130	52 (16.9)	1.16 (0.88, 1.53)	1.16 (0.87, 1.55)

LBW, low birth weight; SGA, small for gestational age; Ref., reference, SD, standard deviation; RR, relative risk; CI, confident interval. [1] Generalized estimating equation models with random effect at the township level were used to estimate the changes (95% CI) for birth weight and RR (95% CI) for LBW/SGA according to maternal hemoglobin level during pregnancy. [2] The model was adjusted for socio-demographic characteristics (including maternal age, education, occupation, and per capita annual household income) and health-related characteristics (including parity, BMI at enrolment, gestational age at enrolment, number of antenatal visits, and micronutrient supplementation). When estimating the associations between maternal hemoglobin and birth weight/LBW, models were additionally adjusted for neonatal gender and gestational age at delivery.

3.4. Dose–Response Relationships between Maternal Hemoglobin Concentrations and Birth Weight-Related Outcomes

RCS functions with four knots (maternal hemoglobin at 70, 100, 110, 130 g/L) were further applied to estimate the dose–response relationships between maternal hemoglobin in different trimesters of pregnancy and birth outcomes. In the first and second trimester, no dose–response relationship was found (data was not shown). In the third trimester, dose–response relationships were observed between maternal hemoglobin concentration and neonatal birth weight, LBW, and SGA (Figure 2).

An inverted U–shaped curve was fitted between maternal hemoglobin concentration in the third trimester and neonatal birth weight (both *p*-values for overall and non-linear association were <0.001). The relatively-higher neonatal birth weight was obtained among women with a hemoglobin concentration of close to 100 g/L. When maternal hemoglobin was <70 g/L, neonatal birth weight significantly increased with the increase of hemoglobin; when maternal hemoglobin was 70–100 g/L, birth weight still showed an increasing trend when maternal hemoglobin was rising; when maternal hemoglobin was >100 g/L, neonatal birth weight significantly decreased with the increase of maternal hemoglobin; when maternal hemoglobin was >130 g/L, neonatal birth weight was more than 100 g lower than that when the maternal hemoglobin was 100 g/L (Figure 2a).

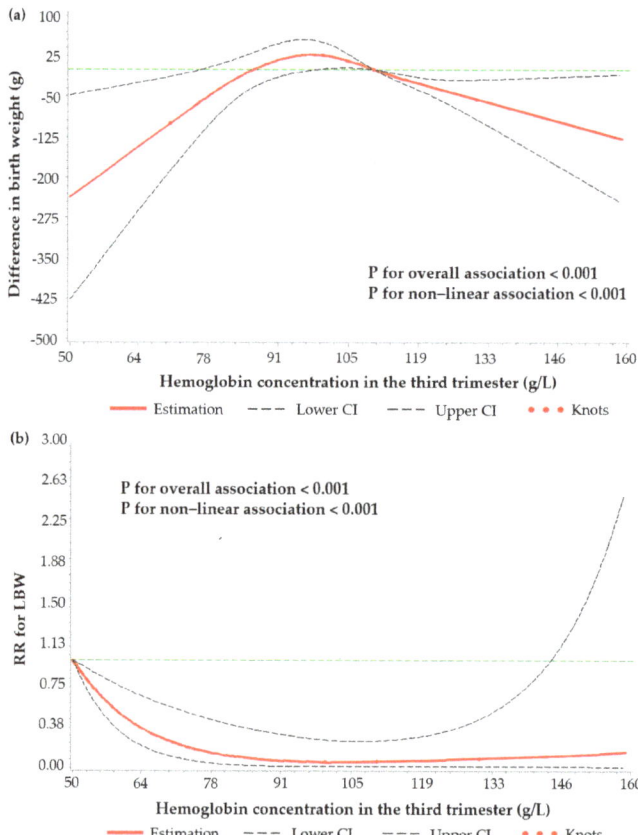

Figure 2. *Cont.*

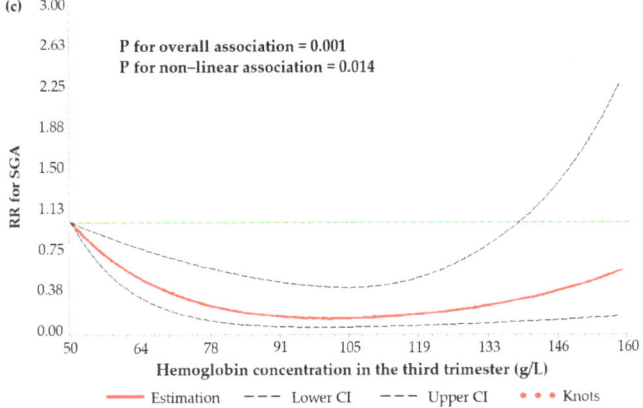

Figure 2. Dose-response relationships between maternal hemoglobin concentrations in the third trimester and (**a**) birth weight, (**b**) LBW, and (**c**) SGA. The associations were estimated using restricted cubic spline functions with four knots (including hemoglobin at 70, 100, 110, 130 g/L). Models were adjusted for socio-demographic characteristics (including maternal age, education, occupation, and per capita annual household income) and health-related characteristics (including parity, BMI at enrolment, gestational age at enrolment, number of antenatal visits, and micronutrient supplementation). When estimating the associations between maternal hemoglobin concentrations and birth weight/LBW, models were additionally adjusted for neonatal gender and gestational age at delivery. For birth weight, hemoglobin at 110 g/L was set as the reference value, and for LBW and SGA, the minimum value of hemoglobin was set as the reference value. Dashed lines represent the 95% CIs, and knots were displayed by dots. The horizontal dashed green line represents whether the difference in birth weight was 0 g or the RR for LBW/SGA was 1.00.

Extended U-shaped curves were obtained between maternal hemoglobin concentration in the third trimester with the risks of LBW and SGA (both *p*-values for overall and non-linear association were <0.05). Both the relatively lower risks for LBW and SGA were obtained among women with a hemoglobin concentration of 100–110 g/L. When maternal hemoglobin was <100 g/L, risks of both LBW and SGA were sharply increased with the decrease of hemoglobin; when maternal hemoglobin was >110 g/L, the risk of LBW was slightly increased with the rise of hemoglobin, and the risk of SGA was significantly increased with the increase of hemoglobin (Figure 2b,c).

3.5. Associations between Maternal Hemoglonbin in the Third Trimester and Birth Weight-Related Outcomes According to Hemoglobin Concentration and Maternal Characteristics

According to the above result, we used hemoglobin of 100 g/L in the third trimester as the cut-off to divide women into two groups and conducted the subgroup analyses according to maternal characteristics in each group. In the third trimester, among women with hemoglobin < 100 g/L, there is a positive but non-significant association between maternal hemoglobin and neonatal birth weight (adjusted changes: 2.4 g, 95% CI: −0.5, 5.4). Among women with hemoglobin ≥100 g/L, maternal hemoglobin was significantly negatively associated with neonatal birth weight (adjusted changes: −2.6 g, 95% CI: −4.1, −1.0). Similar associations were found in most of the subgroups according to maternal characteristics (Table S2).

In the third trimester, among women with hemoglobin <100 g/L, maternal hemoglobin was negatively associated with the risks of LBW/SGA (LBW: adjusted RR: 0.58, 95% CI: 0.42, 0.79; SGA: adjusted RR: 0.81, 95% CI: 0.67, 0.98). Among women with hemoglobin ≥100 g/L, maternal hemoglobin was positively associated with the risk of SGA (adjusted RR: 1.13, 95% CI: 1.04, 1.23). Similar associations were found in many subgroups according to maternal characteristics (Table S3).

4. Discussion

In the present prospective study, about two-thirds of the participants had anemia during pregnancy, and about half of the participants had hemoglobin ≥ 130 during gestation. We found that maternal hemoglobin concentration in the third trimester had an inverted U-shaped association with neonatal birth weight, and had extended U-shaped associations with the risks of LBW and SGA. The relatively higher birth weight and lower risks for LBW and SGA were observed when hemoglobin concentration was 100–110 g/L. Maternal hemoglobin < 70 g/L or >130 g/L was strongly related to the decreased birth weight and increased risks of LBW and SGA.

In our population from the rural areas of Northwest China, 65.1% of the participants had anemia during pregnancy. Our prevalence of gestational anemia was much higher than that of Western countries such as the United States (5.7%), Canada (11.5%), and Germany (12.3%), and it was also higher than that of Asian countries such as Japan (14.8%) and Singapore (23.8%) [39]. Additionally, the prevalence was higher than that of native cities such as Beijing (19.3%), Guangzhou (38.8%), and Chengdu (23.9%) [40]. The potential reason for the high prevalence of anemia in our population is that a large apart of the participants were farmers, lower educated, and at low/middle-income levels, who were less likely to achieve a balanced diet and adequate nutrition intake during pregnancy [41], which further contributed to the poor nutritional status, and induced maternal anemia. At the other end of the spectrum, it is worth noting that about half of the participants had hemoglobin ≥ 130 during pregnancy, which indicated that the problems of low and high hemoglobin levels during pregnancy coexisted in the study population.

In the present study, we found that maternal hemoglobin concentration in the third trimester was associated with neonatal birth weight in an inverted U-shaped curve and was associated with the risks of LBW and SGA in extended U-shaped curves. Women with severe anemia or hemoglobin > 130 g/L in the third trimester had significantly decreased neonatal birth weight and increased risks of LBW and SGA. Compared with previous studies [42,43], our results revealed a more complicated relationship between maternal hemoglobin and birth weight-related outcomes, in that both low and high hemoglobin concentration in the third trimester could have adverse effects on fetal weight growth. In our population, the relatively higher neonatal birth weight and lower risks of LBW and SGA were observed when hemoglobin concentration was in the range of 100 to 110 g/L, which implied that an appropriate hemoglobin level in the third trimester is beneficial to fetal weight growth, but the specific range still needs to be verified in future studies.

Similar nonlinear associations between maternal hemoglobin concentration and birth weight-related outcomes were shown in several previous studies [10,11,26,44]. In a retrospective analysis in the North-West Thames region, Steer et al. reported that the maximum mean birth weight was achieved with the lowest maternal hemoglobin concentration in pregnancy of 85–95 g/l and the lowest incidence of LBW occurred with the lowest hemoglobin of 95–105 g/l. The results displayed that the lowest maternal hemoglobin during pregnancy might have an inverted U-shaped relationship with neonatal birth weight and a U-shaped relationship with the risk of LBW [10]. In a prospective cohort study in two South Asian countries (Pakistan and India), Ali et al. found that the mean neonatal birth weight is higher when the maternal hemoglobin during pregnancy was 110–129 g/L and it decreased when the hemoglobin was <110 g/L or >130 g/L. The study also showed a U-shaped association between maternal hemoglobin and the risk of LBW [26]. Jung et al.'s systematic review and meta-analysis reported an extended U-shaped association between maternal hemoglobin and the risk of SGA [45].

The timing of maternal hemoglobin measurement varied in previous studies, which was one of the causes of inconsistent results. We measured maternal hemoglobin concentration in each trimester and the significant associations of maternal hemoglobin with risks of LBW and SGA were observed only in the third trimester, which was partially consistent with the results of Young et al.'s systematic review and meta-analysis in 2019 [24]. This review reported that low maternal hemoglobin concentration was significantly associated with an increased risk of LBW in the first and third trimester, but it was not significantly associated with SGA in any trimester. Our study did not observe any significant association in the first trimester, which might be due to the relatively lower prevalence of anemia in the first trimester in our population and the different severity of anemia from the populations in previous studies. In addition, this review showed that the evidence for high maternal hemoglobin concentrations across pregnancy and LBW/SGA was limited. Our study provided new evidence that both low and high maternal hemoglobin concentrations in the third trimester was associated with increased risks of LBW/SGA, and to some extent, it filled in the gap of related research. One potential explanation for our results is as follows. Fetal weight growth velocity reaches a peak in the third trimester (around 35 weeks of gestation) accompanied by a sharp increase in fetal nutritional demand [46]. Severe anemia or a relatively-high hemoglobin concentration in this period may lead to extremely inadequate maternal nutrient supply to the fetus, which seriously affects fetal weight growth and increases the risks of LBW and SGA [44,47].

The possible mechanisms involved in the relationship between low or high hemoglobin concentrations and fetal weight growth are as follows. Severe anemia in the third trimester leads to a decline in the body's oxygen supply capacity and poor placental development, which affects the maternal delivery of oxygen and nutrients to the fetus. These adverse effects further induce fetal chronic hypoxia and insufficient nutritional intake, which finally causes poor fetal weight growth and adverse birth outcomes such as LBW and SGA [26,47]. The harmful impacts of high maternal hemoglobin concentration on fetal growth may be attributed to the inadequate plasma volume expansion. A high hemoglobin concentration in the third trimester may indicate a failure in plasma volume expansion. Insufficient plasma volume expansion during pregnancy induces the increase of blood viscosity, and further leads to decrease in placental blood flow velocity and decline of placental nutrient delivery capacity, which finally affects fetal growth and development [18,44,48].

The plasma volume expansion is also an explanation for our results that better birth weight-related outcomes were obtained when maternal hemoglobin concentration in the third trimester was 100–110 g/L. The slightly lower hemoglobin concentrations in the third trimester may reflect an adequate plasma volume expansion and thus achieve the optimal nutrient transport from mother to fetus, which consequently promotes fetal growth and development [49]. Another possible explanation of the association of mild anemia and higher birth weight is that maternal absorbed iron may be preferentially transferred to the placenta and fetus during pregnancy, thus contributing to better fetal growth and development rather than to higher maternal iron stores, which may result in lower maternal hemoglobin concentration in the third trimester and higher neonatal birth weight [50].

To the best of our knowledge, the present study was the first prospective study that revealed nonlinear relationships between maternal hemoglobin concentration in the third trimester and birth weight-related outcomes in the Chinese population. We disclosed that both low and high hemoglobin concentrations could be harmful to fetal weight growth and increase the risks of LBW and SGA, and maternal hemoglobin > 130 g/L in the third trimester could be highly focused on, in addition to severe anemia, in maternal and child health care. Nonetheless, several limitations of the present study should be addressed. Firstly, this study was conducted in the rural areas of Northwest China, and thus the results mainly reflected the association between maternal hemoglobin during pregnancy and birth outcomes in women with disadvantaged socio-demographic conditions, which may limit the generalizability of the findings to other populations. However, it is noteworthy that, compared with women with disadvantaged socio-demographic status, those with advantaged socio-demographic status are more likely to have relatively higher hemoglobin concentrations during pregnancy, suggesting that the adverse impact of high hemoglobin in the third trimester on fetal weight growth should be paid more attention to in such populations. Secondly, although we carried out the analysis by controlling for some potential confounders, including socio-demographic and health-related factors, there were still some unobserved or unknown confounders that we could not fully investigate. For example, excessive maternal gestational weight gain was related to reduced risks of LBW and SGA [51]. Unfortunately, information about maternal weight gain during pregnancy was not available in the present study, and thus we could not control for its effect on the associations between maternal hemoglobin and birth weight-related outcomes. Finally, the present study only assessed the relationship between maternal hemoglobin and birth weight-related outcomes without evaluating the influences of maternal plasma volume expansion or iron status of mothers and infants, and thus the potential mechanisms involved could not be clarified. More in-depth and well-designed studies are recommended to explore the underlying mechanisms and to develop a more comprehensive and precise nutrition intervention strategy.

5. Conclusions

Maternal hemoglobin concentration in the third trimester had an inverted U-shaped association with neonatal birth weight, and had extended U-shaped associations with the risks of LBW and SGA. Both low and high hemoglobin concentrations in this period could be adverse to fetal weight growth and increase the risks of LBW and SGA, respectively. In addition to severe anemia, maternal hemoglobin > 130 g/L in the third trimester should be paid great attention to in the practice of maternal and child health care.

Supplementary Materials: The followings are available online at https://www.mdpi.com/article/10.3390/nu14040858/s1, Table S1: Comparison of maternal socio-demographic characteristics between women included and excluded in the study; Table S2: Associations between maternal hemoglobin concentration in the third trimester and neonatal birth weight in different subgroups; Table S3: Associations between maternal hemoglobin concentration in the third trimester and LBW/SGA in different subgroups.

Author Contributions: Conceptualization, S.D., L.Z. and H.Y.; Data curation, D.L. and S.D.; Formal analysis, D.L., S.L., B.M., D.W. and F.C.; Investigation, D.L., S.L., B.Z., Y.K., Y.C., B.M., P.Q., D.Z. and Z.Z.; Resources, H.Y., L.Z. and S.D.; Funding acquisition, S.D., H.Y. and Y.C.; Writing—original draft preparation, D.L. and S.L.; Writing—review and editing, D.L., S.L., B.Z., Y.K., Y.C., L.Z., F.C., B.M., P.Q., D.Z., Z.Z., H.Y., D.W. and S.D. All authors have read and agreed to the published version of the manuscript.

Funding: This research was funded by the Shaanxi Health and Family Planning Commission (grant number Sxwsjswzfcght2016–013), the National Natural Science Foundation of China (grant number 81230016 and 81202218), and the National Key Research and Development Program of China (grant number 2017YFC0907200 and 2017YFC0907201).

Institutional Review Board Statement: The study was conducted according to the guidelines of the Declaration of Helsinki, and approved by the Ethic Review Committee and Academic Committee of Xi'an Jiaotong University Health Science Center (approval no. 2012008).

Informed Consent Statement: Informed written consent was obtained from all subjects involved in the study.

Acknowledgments: The authors thank all participants and researchers who participated in this study. The authors are also grateful to the county hospitals and the county maternal and child health hospitals in study areas for their collaboration during the implementation of this study.

Conflicts of Interest: The authors declare no conflict of interest.

References

1. Dobbins, T.A.; Sullivan, E.A.; Roberts, C.L.; Simpson, J.M. Australian national birthweight percentiles by sex and gestational age, 1998–2007. *Med. J. Aust.* **2012**, *197*, 291–294. [CrossRef] [PubMed]
2. Goldenberg, R.L.; Culhane, J.F. Low birth weight in the United States. *Am. J. Clin. Nutr.* **2007**, *85*, 584s–590s. [CrossRef] [PubMed]
3. Lee, A.C.C.; Katz, J.; Blencowe, H.; Cousens, S.; Kozuki, N.; Vogel, J.P.; Adair, L.; Baqui, A.H.; Bhutta, Z.A.; Caulfield, L.E.; et al. National and regional estimates of term and preterm babies born small for gestational age in 138 low-income and middle-income countries in 2010. *Lancet Glob. Health* **2013**, *1*, e26–e36. [CrossRef]

4. Blencowe, H.; Krasevec, J.; de Onis, M.; Black, R.E.; An, X.; Stevens, G.A.; Borghi, E.; Hayashi, C.; Estevez, D.; Cegolon, L.; et al. National, regional, and worldwide estimates of low birthweight in 2015, with trends from 2000: A systematic analysis. *Lancet Glob. Health* **2019**, *7*, e849–e860. [CrossRef]
5. Lee, A.C.; Kozuki, N.; Cousens, S.; Stevens, G.A.; Blencowe, H.; Silveira, M.F.; Sania, A.; Rosen, H.E.; Schmiegelow, C.; Adair, L.S.; et al. Estimates of burden and consequences of infants born small for gestational age in low and middle income countries with INTERGROWTH-21 standard: Analysis of CHERG datasets. *BMJ* **2017**, *358*, j3677. [CrossRef] [PubMed]
6. Shorer, D.T.; Wainstock, T.; Sheiner, E.; Landau, D.; Pariente, G. Long-term endocrine outcome of small for gestational age infants born to mothers with and without gestational diabetes mellitus. *Gynecol. Endocrinol.* **2019**, *35*, 1003–1009. [CrossRef]
7. Mousa, A.; Naqash, A.; Lim, S. Macronutrient and Micronutrient Intake during Pregnancy: An Overview of Recent Evidence. *Nutrients* **2019**, *11*, 443. [CrossRef]
8. Means, R.T. Iron Deficiency and Iron Deficiency Anemia: Implications and Impact in Pregnancy, Fetal Development, and Early Childhood Parameters. *Nutrients* **2020**, *12*, 447. [CrossRef]
9. Rasmussen, S.; Oian, P. First- and second-trimester hemoglobin levels. Relation to birth weight and gestational age. *Acta Obstet. Gynecol. Scand.* **1993**, *72*, 246–251. [CrossRef]
10. Steer, P.; Alam, M.A.; Wadsworth, J.; Welch, A. Relation between maternal haemoglobin concentration and birth weight in different ethnic groups. *BMJ* **1995**, *310*, 489–491. [CrossRef]
11. Dewey, K.G.; Oaks, B.M. U-shaped curve for risk associated with maternal hemoglobin, iron status, or iron supplementation. *Am. J. Clin. Nutr.* **2017**, *106*, 1694S–1702S. [CrossRef] [PubMed]
12. Stevens, G.A.; Finucane, M.M.; De-Regil, L.M.; Paciorek, C.J.; Flaxman, S.R.; Branca, F.; Peña-Rosas, J.P.; Bhutta, Z.A.; Ezzati, M. Global, regional, and national trends in haemoglobin concentration and prevalence of total and severe anaemia in children and pregnant and non-pregnant women for 1995-2011: A systematic analysis of population-representative data. *Lancet Glob. Health* **2013**, *1*, e16–e25. [CrossRef]
13. Goonewardene, M.; Shehata, M.; Hamad, A. Anaemia in pregnancy. *Best Pract. Res. Clin. Obstet. Gynaecol.* **2012**, *26*, 3–24. [CrossRef] [PubMed]
14. Haider, B.A.; Olofin, I.; Wang, M.; Spiegelman, D.; Ezzati, M.; Fawzi, W.W. Anaemia, prenatal iron use, and risk of adverse pregnancy outcomes: Systematic review and meta-analysis. *BMJ* **2013**, *346*, f3443. [CrossRef] [PubMed]
15. Rahman, M.M.; Abe, S.K.; Rahman, M.S.; Kanda, M.; Narita, S.; Bilano, V.; Ota, E.; Gilmour, S.; Shibuya, K. Maternal anemia and risk of adverse birth and health outcomes in low- and middle-income countries: Systematic review and meta-analysis. *Am. J. Clin. Nutr.* **2016**, *103*, 495–504. [CrossRef]
16. Hämäläinen, H.; Hakkarainen, K.; Heinonen, S. Anaemia in the first but not in the second or third trimester is a risk factor for low birth weight. *Clin. Nutr.* **2003**, *22*, 271–275. [CrossRef]
17. Ren, A.; Wang, J.; Ye, R.W.; Li, S.; Liu, J.M.; Li, Z. Low first-trimester hemoglobin and low birth weight, preterm birth and small for gestational age newborns. *Int. J. Gynaecol. Obstet.* **2007**, *98*, 124–128. [CrossRef]
18. Scanlon, K.S.; Yip, R.; Schieve, L.A.; Cogswell, M.E. High and low hemoglobin levels during pregnancy: Differential risks for preterm birth and small for gestational age. *Obstet. Gynecol.* **2000**, *96*, 741–748. [CrossRef]
19. Zhou, L.M.; Yang, W.W.; Hua, J.Z.; Deng, C.Q.; Tao, X.; Stoltzfus, R.J. Relation of hemoglobin measured at different times in pregnancy to preterm birth and low birth weight in Shanghai, China. *Am. J. Epidemiol.* **1998**, *148*, 998–1006. [CrossRef]
20. Gonzales, G.F.; Steenland, K.; Tapia, V. Maternal hemoglobin level and fetal outcome at low and high altitudes. *Am. J. Physiol. Regul. Integr. Comp. Physiol.* **2009**, *297*, R1477–R1485. [CrossRef]
21. Xiong, X.; Buekens, P.; Alexander, S.; Demianczuk, N.; Wollast, E. Anemia during pregnancy and birth outcome: A meta-analysis. *Am. J. Perinatol.* **2000**, *17*, 137–146. [CrossRef] [PubMed]
22. Chang, S.-C.; O'Brien, K.O.; Nathanson, M.S.; Mancini, J.; Witter, F.R. Hemoglobin concentrations influence birth outcomes in pregnant African-American adolescents. *J. Nutr.* **2003**, *133*, 2348–2355. [CrossRef] [PubMed]
23. Mohamed, M.A.; Ahmad, T.; Macri, C.; Aly, H. Racial disparities in maternal hemoglobin concentrations and pregnancy outcomes. *J. Perinat. Med.* **2012**, *40*, 141–149. [CrossRef] [PubMed]
24. Young, M.F.; Oaks, B.M.; Tandon, S.; Martorell, R.; Dewey, K.G.; Wendt, A.S. Maternal hemoglobin concentrations across pregnancy and maternal and child health: A systematic review and meta-analysis. *Ann. N. Y. Acad. Sci.* **2019**, *1450*, 47–68. [CrossRef] [PubMed]
25. Zhang, Q.; Ananth, C.V.; Li, Z.; Smulian, J.C. Maternal anaemia and preterm birth: A prospective cohort study. *Int. J. Epidemiol.* **2009**, *38*, 1380–1389. [CrossRef]
26. Ali, S.A.; Tikmani, S.S.; Saleem, S.; Patel, A.B.; Hibberd, P.L.; Goudar, S.S.; Dhaded, S.; Derman, R.J.; Moore, J.L.; McClure, E.M.; et al. Hemoglobin concentrations and adverse birth outcomes in South Asian pregnant women: Findings from a prospective Maternal and Neonatal Health Registry. *Reprod. Health* **2020**, *17*, 154. [CrossRef]
27. Li, S.; Mi, B.; Qu, P.; Liu, D.; Lei, F.; Wang, D.; Zeng, L.; Kang, Y.; Shen, Y.; Pei, L.; et al. Association of antenatal vitamin B complex supplementation with neonatal vitamin B status: Evidence from a cluster randomized controlled trial. *Eur. J. Nutr.* **2021**, *60*, 1031–1039. [CrossRef]
28. Perinatal medicine branch of Chinese Medical Association. Chinese clinical guidelines for the diagnosis and treatment of maternal anemia during pregnancy. *Zhonghua Wei Chan Yi Xue Za Zhi* **2014**, *7*, 451–454.

29. Wang, L.; Mei, Z.; Li, H.; Zhang, Y.; Liu, J.; Serdula, M.K. Modifying effects of maternal Hb concentration on infant birth weight in women receiving prenatal iron-containing supplements: A randomised controlled trial. *Br. J. Nutr.* **2016**, *115*, 644–649. [CrossRef]
30. Randall, D.A.; Patterson, J.A.; Gallimore, F.; Morris, J.M.; Simpson, J.M.; McGee, T.M.; Ford, J.B. Haemoglobin trajectories during pregnancy and associated outcomes using pooled maternity and hospitalization data from two tertiary hospitals. *Vox Sang.* **2019**, *114*, 842–852. [CrossRef]
31. WHO. *Haemoglobin Concentrations for the Diagnosis of Anaemia and Assessment of Severity.* WHO. 2011. Available online: https://apps.who.int/iris/handle/10665/85839 (accessed on 7 December 2021).
32. Pena-Rosas, J.P.; De-Regil, L.M.; Dowswell, T.; Viteri, F.E. Daily oral iron supplementation during pregnancy. *Cochrane Database Syst. Rev.* **2012**, *12*, CD004736. [PubMed]
33. Zhu, L.; Zhang, R.; Zhang, S.; Shi, W.; Yan, W.; Wang, X.; Lyu, Q.; Liu, L.; Zhou, Q.; Qiu, Q.; et al. Chinese neonatal birth weight curve for different gestational age. *Zhonghua Er Ke Za Zhi* **2015**, *53*, 97–103. [PubMed]
34. Li, S.; Liu, D.; Zhang, R.; Lei, F.; Liu, X.; Cheng, Y.; Li, C.; Xiao, M.; Guo, L.; Li, M.; et al. The association of maternal dietary folate intake and folic acid supplementation with small-for-gestational-age births: A cross-sectional study in Northwest China. *Br. J. Nutr.* **2019**, *122*, 459–467. [CrossRef] [PubMed]
35. Wang, Y.; Sun, M.; Xue, H.; Zhao, W.; Yang, X.; Zhu, X.; Zhao, L.; Yang, Y. Understanding the China Blue Paper on Obesity Prevention and Control and policy implications and recommendations for obesity prevention and control in China. *Zhonghua Yu Fang Yi Xue Za Zhi* **2019**, *53*, 875–884.
36. Hubbard, A.E.; Ahern, J.; Fleischer, N.L.; Van der Laan, M.; Lippman, S.A.; Jewell, N.; Bruckner, T.; Satariano, W.A. To GEE or not to GEE: Comparing population average and mixed models for estimating the associations between neighborhood risk factors and health. *Epidemiology* **2010**, *21*, 467–474. [CrossRef]
37. Roux, A.V.D. Neighborhoods and health: Where are we and were do we go from here? *Rev. Epidemiol. Sante Publique* **2007**, *55*, 13–21. [CrossRef]
38. Desquilbet, L.; Mariotti, F. Dose-response analyses using restricted cubic spline functions in public health research. *Stat. Med.* **2010**, *29*, 1037–1057. [CrossRef]
39. WHO. *Worldwide Prevalence of Anaemia 1993–2005: WHO Global Database on Anaemia*; WHO: Geneva, Switzerland, 2008; pp. 1–51.
40. Lin, L.; Wei, Y.; Zhu, W.; Wang, C.; Su, R.; Feng, H.; Yang, H. Prevalence, risk factors and associated adverse pregnancy outcomes of anaemia in Chinese pregnant women: A multicentre retrospective study. *BMC Pregnancy Childbirth* **2018**, *18*, 111. [CrossRef]
41. Yang, J.; Dang, S.; Cheng, Y.; Qiu, H.; Mi, B.; Jiang, Y.; Qu, P.; Zeng, L.; Wang, Q.; Li, Q.; et al. Dietary intakes and dietary patterns among pregnant women in Northwest China. *Public Health Nutr.* **2017**, *20*, 282–293. [CrossRef]
42. Jwa, S.C.; Fujiwara, T.; Yamanobe, Y.; Kozuka, K.; Sago, H. Changes in maternal hemoglobin during pregnancy and birth outcomes. *BMC Pregnancy Childbirth* **2015**, *15*, 80. [CrossRef]
43. Chen, J.H.; Guo, X.F.; Liu, S.; Long, J.H.; Zhang, G.Q.; Huang, M.C.; Qiu, X.Q. Impact and changes of maternal hemoglobin on birth weight in pregnant women of Zhuang Nationality, in Guangxi. *Zhonghua Liu Xing Bing Xue Za Zhi* **2017**, *38*, 154–157. [PubMed]
44. Steer, P.J. Maternal hemoglobin concentration and birth weight. *Am. J. Clin. Nutr.* **2000**, *71*, 1285S–1287S. [CrossRef] [PubMed]
45. Jung, J.; Rahman, M.M.; Rahman, M.S.; Swe, K.T.; Islam, M.R.; Rahman, M.O.; Akter, S. Effects of hemoglobin levels during pregnancy on adverse maternal and infant outcomes: A systematic review and meta-analysis. *Ann. N. Y. Acad. Sci.* **2019**, *1450*, 69–82. [CrossRef] [PubMed]
46. Grantz, K.L.; Kim, S.; Grobman, W.A.; Newman, R.; Owen, J.; Skupski, D.; Grewal, J.; Chien, E.K.; Wing, D.A.; Wapner, R.J.; et al. Fetal growth velocity: The NICHD fetal growth studies. *Am. J. Obstet. Gynecol.* **2018**, *219*, 285.e1–285.e36. [CrossRef]
47. Singla, P.N.; Tyagi, M.; Kumar, A.; Dash, D.; Shankar, R. Fetal growth in maternal anaemia. *J. Trop. Pediatr.* **1997**, *43*, 89–92. [CrossRef]
48. Zondervan, H.A.; Voorhorst, F.J.; Robertson, E.A.; Kurver, P.H.; Massen, C. Is maternal whole blood viscosity a factor in fetal growth? *Eur. J. Obstet. Gynecol. Reprod. Biol.* **1985**, *20*, 145–151. [CrossRef]
49. Fisher, A.L.; Nemeth, E. Iron homeostasis during pregnancy. *Am. J. Clin. Nutr.* **2017**, *106*, 1567S–1574S. [CrossRef]
50. Cogswell, M.E.; Parvanta, I.; Ickes, L.; Yip, R.; Brittenham, G.M. Iron supplementation during pregnancy, anemia, and birth weight: A randomized controlled trial. *Am. J. Clin. Nutr.* **2003**, *78*, 773–781. [CrossRef]
51. Li, N.; Liu, E.; Guo, J.; Pan, L.; Li, B.; Wang, P.; Liu, J.; Wang, Y.; Liu, G.; Baccarelli, A.A.; et al. Maternal prepregnancy body mass index and gestational weight gain on pregnancy outcomes. *PLoS ONE* **2013**, *8*, e82310. [CrossRef]

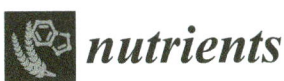

Article

Associations of B Vitamin-Related Dietary Pattern during Pregnancy with Birth Outcomes: A Population-Based Study in Northwest China

Shanshan Li [1,†], Danmeng Liu [2,†], Yijun Kang [2], Pengfei Qu [3], Baibing Mi [2], Zhonghai Zhu [2], Lixin Han [4,5], Yaling Zhao [2], Fangyao Chen [2], Leilei Pei [2], Lingxia Zeng [2], Duolao Wang [6], Hong Yan [2,7] and Shaonong Dang [2,*]

1. School of Public Health, Shandong First Medical University & Shandong Academy of Medical Sciences, Taian 271016, China; lishanshan@sdfmu.edu.cn
2. Department of Epidemiology and Health Statistics, Health Science Center, Xi'an Jiaotong University, Xi'an 710061, China; liudanmeng1214@stu.xjtu.edu.cn (D.L.); tjkyj@xjtu.edu.cn (Y.K.); xjtu.mi@xjtu.edu.cn (B.M.); zhonghai_zhu@xjtu.edu.cn (Z.Z.); zhaoyl666@xjtu.edu.cn (Y.Z.); chenfy@xjtu.edu.cn (F.C.); peileilei424@163.com (L.P.); tjzlx@xjtu.edu.cn (L.Z.); yanhonge@xjtu.edu.cn (H.Y.)
3. Translational Medicine Center, Northwest Women's and Children's Hospital, Xi'an 710061, China; xinxi3057@stu.xjtu.edu.cn
4. Key Laboratory of Trace Elements and Endemic Diseases of National Health Commission, Health Science Center, Xi'an Jiaotong University, Xi'an 710061, China; weijianweijikongchu@shaanxi.gov.cn
5. Disease Control and Prevention Division, Shaanxi Provincial Health Commission, Xi'an 710000, China
6. Department of Clinical Sciences, Liverpool School of Tropical Medicine, Liverpool L3 5QA, UK; duolao.wang@lstmed.ac.uk
7. Nutrition and Food Safety Engineering Research Center of Shaanxi Province, Xi'an 710061, China
* Correspondence: tjdshn@xjtu.edu.cn
† These authors contributed equally to this work.

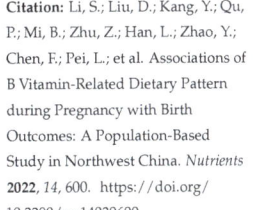

Citation: Li, S.; Liu, D.; Kang, Y.; Qu, P.; Mi, B.; Zhu, Z.; Han, L.; Zhao, Y.; Chen, F.; Pei, L.; et al. Associations of B Vitamin-Related Dietary Pattern during Pregnancy with Birth Outcomes: A Population-Based Study in Northwest China. *Nutrients* 2022, 14, 600. https://doi.org/10.3390/nu14030600

Academic Editor: Yunxian Yu

Received: 27 December 2021
Accepted: 27 January 2022
Published: 29 January 2022

Publisher's Note: MDPI stays neutral with regard to jurisdictional claims in published maps and institutional affiliations.

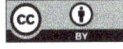

Copyright: © 2022 by the authors. Licensee MDPI, Basel, Switzerland. This article is an open access article distributed under the terms and conditions of the Creative Commons Attribution (CC BY) license (https://creativecommons.org/licenses/by/4.0/).

Abstract: This study aimed to derive a maternal dietary pattern to explain the variation in B vitamins during pregnancy and to investigate this pattern in relation to birth outcomes. A total of 7347 women who gave birth to live newborns less than one year were included. Their dietary pattern during pregnancy was derived using the reduced-rank regression method with six B vitamins as response variables. Associations between dietary pattern score and birth weight, gestational age at delivery, birth weight Z score, low birth weight, preterm, and small-for-gestational-age (SGA) were estimated using generalised linear mixed models. We identified a high B-vitamin dietary pattern characterised by high intakes of animal foods, vegetables, fungi and algae, legumes, and low intakes of oils and cereals. Women in the highest quartile of this pattern score had newborns with a 44.5 g (95% CI: 13.8, 75.2 g) higher birth weight, 0.101 (95% CI: 0.029, 0.172) higher birth weight Z score, and 27.2% (OR: 0.728; 95% CI: 0.582, 0.910) lower risk of SGA than those in the lowest quartile. Our study suggested that adherence to the high B-vitamin dietary pattern during pregnancy was associated with a higher birth weight and a lower risk of SGA.

Keywords: dietary pattern; B vitamins; pregnancy; birth weight; small-for-gestational-age; reduced rank regression

1. Introduction

Birth outcomes, which commonly refer to birth weight and gestational age, are not only closely related to the morbidity and mortality of infants and young children [1,2], but are also key predictors of chronic non-communicable diseases in adulthood [3–5]. As the economy grows by leaps and bounds, the health status of women and children in China has been greatly improved in the past few decades [6]. However, China has the largest population in the world, of more than 1.4 billion. According to the latest WHO data, China ranks among the top five countries worldwide in terms of the number of adverse birth outcomes such as preterm, low birth weight (LBW), and small-for-gestational-age (SGA) [7–9].

The aetiology of most types of adverse birth outcomes is complex. As a modifiable risk factor, maternal nutrition during pregnancy has been widely discussed for its potential to prevent adverse birth outcomes [10]. B vitamins are a class of water-soluble micronutrients that act as co-enzymes in numerous catabolic and anabolic enzymatic reactions [11]. To our knowledge, the associations of other B vitamins than folate (vitamin B9) with adverse birth outcomes remain unclear. Some epidemiologic studies have reported that maternal dietary intakes of B vitamins are inversely related to the risk of adverse birth outcomes [12–14]. Since B vitamins share similarities in food sources and biological functions, these studies failed to clarify the individual effect of specific B vitamins, nor did they capture the cumulative effect of multiple B vitamins [15].

Recent nutritional epidemiological studies have shifted the focus from single nutrients to dietary patterns, which describe the overall diet and better reflect the interactive or synergistic effects of different nutrients [16]. Of note, Hoffmann et al. proposed the reduced rank regression (RRR) method, by which dietary patterns are derived using a posteriori statistical analysis, but response variables (e.g., nutrients) are chosen using a priori knowledge that suggests these variables are hypothesized to be related to health outcomes [17]. The RRR method identifies the linear combination of food groups that account for as much variation as possible in a set of response variables. Compared to traditional methods (e.g., Health Eating Index and principal component analysis), the RRR method has the advantage of building biological pathways through which diet affects health outcomes [18].

Therefore, based on the cross-sectional data in northwest China, we aimed to identify a maternal dietary pattern that maximally explains the variation in B vitamins using the RRR method. Furthermore, we sought to assess the associations of this pattern with birth outcomes after controlling for covariates.

2. Materials and Methods

2.1. Study Design and Participants

The present study used data from a cross-sectional study conducted in Shaanxi Province of northwest China. The design and methodology of the cross-sectional study have been described previously in detail [19,20]. Briefly, 30,027 women who were pregnant during 2010–2013 and had pregnancy outcomes were selected using the stratified multistage random sampling method. First, twenty counties and ten districts were randomly selected from the Shaanxi Province according to the proportion of urban to rural population, population density and fertility rate. Second, six townships and three streets were randomly selected from the sampled counties and districts, separately. Third, six villages and communities were randomly selected from the sampled townships and streets, separately. Finally, thirty and sixty women were randomly selected from the sampled villages and communities, separately. All participants were interviewed from August to November 2013. Information on maternal general and pregnancy characteristics, and neonatal outcomes were collected by a standardised and structured questionnaire. Furthermore, 7750 women who gave birth to live newborns less than one year ago were interviewed to obtain information on dietary intakes during pregnancy. For this study, 403 women were excluded due to multiple births (n = 87) or implausible energy intake (<4500 or >20000 kJ/d) (n = 316) [21]. Consequently, a total of 7347 women were included in the final analysis, with a median of 3 months (10–90th percentiles: 0–7 months) after delivery. A flow chart of the selection of study participants is displayed in Figure S1.

2.2. Dietary Assessment

The dietary intakes during pregnancy were estimated retrospectively using a semi-quantitative food frequency questionnaire (FFQ). Since dietary intakes did not change to a great extent throughout pregnancy [22–24], and it was cumbersome to collect dietary data for different trimesters, we assessed the average dietary intakes over the whole pregnancy at one time. The FFQ applied in this study was established based on a validated FFQ designed for pregnant women during the third trimester in northwest China [25]. The validation study showed good correlations between nutrients estimated by the FFQ and six repeated 24 h recalls. Pearson's correlation coefficients ranged from 0.53 for cholesterol and carotene, to 0.70 for vitamin E and potassium [25]. The FFQ used in this study consisted of 107 items. For the five food items concerning edible oil and condiments, the weight consumed per month and the number of family members were recorded. For the other 102 food items, consumption frequencies were assessed on an eight-level scale (never or almost not, less than one time/month, one to three times/month, one time/week, two to four times/week, five to six times/week, one time/day, or more than two times/day), and portion sizes were estimated on a three-level scale (large, medium, or small) using the food photographs [26]. The daily intakes of total energy and nutrients were estimated by multiplying consumption frequency by the portion size of each food item and their corresponding nutrient content abstracted from the China Food Composition Table [27,28]. All nutrient intakes were adjusted for total energy intake with the use of the residual method [29].

2.3. Birth Outcomes

Neonatal outcomes, including sex, gestational age at birth, and birth weight were obtained from the Medical Certificate of Birth. Birth weight was measured to the nearest 10 g. Gestational age at birth was the number of weeks from the first day of the last menstrual period to the date of delivery. The sex- and gestational age-adjusted birth weight Z score was calculated based on the International Fetal and Newborn Growth Consortium for the 21st Century (INTERGROWTH-21st) standards [30]. LBW referred to a birth weight less than 2500 g [31]. Preterm was defined as gestational age at birth less than 37 weeks [32]. SGA referred to a birth weight Z score below the 10th percentile [33].

2.4. Covariates

The covariates selected based on previous studies can be categorised as maternal socio-demographic characteristics and health-related behaviours during pregnancy [34–36]. Socio-demographic characteristics comprised geographic area, residence, age at delivery, education, occupation, household wealth index, and parity. The principal component analysis was used to construct the household wealth index based on household income and expenditure, type of house, number of appliances, and number of vehicles [37]. Poor was defined as the first principal component below the 33.3rd percentile. Health-related behaviours included smoking, alcohol consumption, pregnancy complications, medication use, as well as folic acid, iron, calcium, and multivitamin supplementation. Only passive smoking was considered as a covariate because of pregnant women's low prevalence of active smoking in our study areas. Passive smoking was defined as a non-smoker being exposed to tobacco smoke for at least 15 min per day. Self-reported pregnancy complications consisted of anaemia, hypertension, diabetes, intrahepatic cholestasis, and so on.

2.5. Statistical Analysis

Maternal dietary pattern during pregnancy was obtained by the reduced rank regression (RRR) method using the PLS procedure in SAS [17]. Before conducting this analysis, 107 food items were categorised into 21 food groups according to their similarities in nutrient content and culinary usage (Table S1). The predictor variables were the daily intakes of 21 food groups in grams, while the response variables were the daily intakes of thiamin (vitamin B1), riboflavin (vitamin B2), niacin (vitamin B3), vitamin B6, folate, and vitamin B12 in grams. The number of RRR factors derived was equal to the number of response variables. Considering that the first RRR factor explained the highest proportion of the variation in response variables, only this factor was considered as the dietary pattern of interest [18,38]. Food groups with an absolute factor loading ≥ 0.2 were utilised to characterise the dietary pattern. The dietary pattern score of each participant was outputted by summing up the intakes of each food group and multiplying with the corresponding factor loadings and categorised into quartiles. Pearson's correlation coefficients and 95% CIs between the dietary pattern score and each response variable were calculated.

Binary and continuous variables were presented as n (%) and means ± SDs, respectively. Linear trends across the quartiles of dietary pattern score were estimated using Cochran-Armitage tests for maternal characteristics and univariate linear regression models for nutrient intakes. Given the significant within-group homogeneity for most birth outcomes at the county level, the generalised linear mixed model with a random intercept at the county level was employed to estimate the associations of maternal dietary pattern score with birth outcomes. The dietary pattern score was analysed both as a continuous variable (per 1-SD increase) and a categorised variable (the lowest quartile as the reference). To assess the robustness of these associations, a total of three models were constructed in sequence. Model 1 included no covariates. Model 2 included socio-demographic characteristics. Model 3 included all covariates in Model 2 plus health-related behaviours. The link functions of continuous and binary dependent variables were "identity" and "logit", separately. Linear trends for birth outcomes across the quartiles of dietary pattern score were assessed by putting the quartile number into models as an ordinal variable. Since multivitamins usually contain B vitamins, stratified analyses by folic acid and multivitamin supplementation were performed to test whether these supplements modified the associations of dietary pattern score with birth outcomes. Potential effect modifications were examined by including interaction terms in the fully adjusted models.

All statistical analyses were performed using SAS software (version 9.4; SAS Institute Inc., Cary, CA, USA). A two-sided $p < 0.05$ was considered statistically significant.

3. Results

3.1. Dietary Pattern

A total of six RRR factors were identified. The first RRR factor explained 42.27% of thiamin, 68.34% of riboflavin, 20.92% of niacin, 59.00% of vitamin B6, 56.16% of folate, 41.50% of vitamin B12, and 48.03% of the total variation of six B vitamins. The subsequent five RRR factors explained only 12.73%, 4.71%, 1.67%, 1.45%, and 1.01% of the total variation, separately. Therefore, only the first RRR factor was regarded as the dietary pattern of interest. Since the dietary pattern score was moderately to highly positively correlated with the intakes of six B vitamins (Table 1), this pattern was named the high B-vitamin dietary pattern.

Table 1. Associations between the dietary pattern score derived by reduced rank regression and B vitamins intakes.

	r (95% CI)	p
Thiamin	0.677 (0.664, 0.689)	<0.001
Riboflavin	0.866 (0.860, 0.872)	<0.001
Niacin	0.578 (0.562, 0.593)	<0.001
Vitamin B6	0.809 (0.801, 0.817)	<0.001
Folate	0.841 (0.834, 0.847)	<0.001
Vitamin B12	0.686 (0.674, 0.698)	<0.001

The factor loading values of the food groups in the high B-vitamin dietary pattern are shown in Figure 1. The dietary pattern was characterised by high intakes of organ meat; fungi and algae; green vegetables; other vegetables; meat and poultry; legumes; fish, shrimps, and crabs; and low intakes of oils and cereals. As displayed in Table S2, the mean intakes of the selected nutrient varied across quartiles of the high B-vitamin dietary pattern score. On the whole, with the increasing quartiles, women tended to have lower intakes of carbohydrates, the percentage of energy from carbohydrates, potassium, and sodium but higher intakes of protein, the percentage of energy from protein, and most vitamins and minerals.

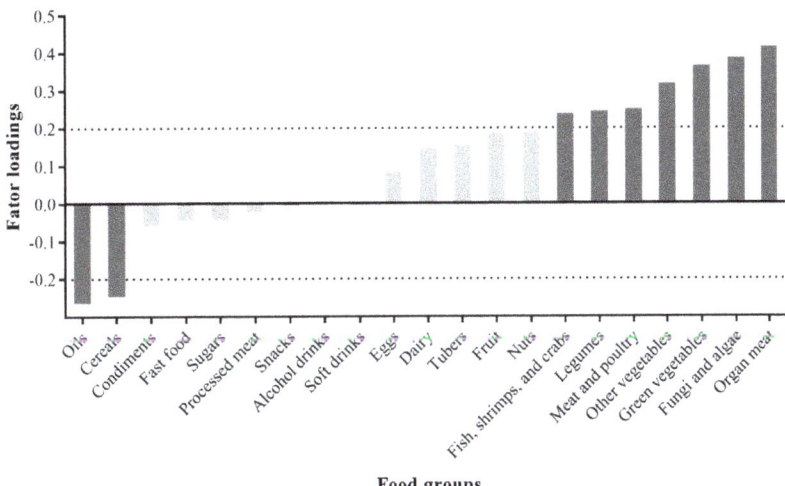

Figure 1. Factor loading of the food groups in the high B-vitamin dietary pattern score. Dark grey indicates absolute factor loading value ≥ 0.2.

3.2. Participants Characteristics

Maternal socio-demographic characteristics and health-related behaviours differed by quartiles of the high B-vitamin dietary pattern score (Table 2). Women in the highest quartile were more likely to be primiparous, give birth at the ages of 25–29 years, have more than junior school education, drink alcohol, and take iron, calcium, and folic acid supplements. By contrast, women in the highest quartile were less likely to be farmers, be poorer, be exposed to passive smoking, live in rural areas, have pregnancy complications, and use medication.

Table 2. Maternal characteristics according to quartiles of the high B-vitamin dietary pattern score.

Characteristics	Total	Quartile				p_{trend} [a]
		Q1	Q2	Q3	Q4	
N	7347	1837	1837	1837	1836	
Socio-demographic characteristics						
Geographic area (central Shaanxi)	3993 (54.35)	994 (54.11)	1002 (54.55)	956 (52.04)	1041 (56.70)	0.311
Residence (rural)	5612 (76.38)	1560 (84.92)	1530 (83.29)	1395 (75.94)	1127 (61.38)	<0.001
Age at delivery (25–29 years)	2721 (37.35)	650 (35.66)	664 (36.50)	667 (36.51)	740 (40.73)	0.003
Education (more than junior school)	2726 (37.23)	561 (30.62)	577 (31.46)	671 (36.67)	917 (50.19)	<0.001
Occupation (farmer)	5266 (72.21)	1406 (77.00)	1404 (76.93)	1332 (73.11)	1124 (61.76)	<0.001
Household wealth index (poor)	2474 (33.67)	684 (37.23)	686 (37.34)	592 (32.23)	512 (27.89)	<0.001
Parity (primiparous)	4570 (62.22)	1088 (59.23)	1080 (58.82)	1141 (62.15)	1261 (68.68)	<0.001
Health-related behaviours						
Passive smoking	1639 (22.37)	463 (25.23)	430 (23.50)	420 (22.93)	326 (17.81)	<0.001
Alcohol consumption	97 (1.32)	23 (1.25)	15 (0.82)	24 (1.31)	35 (1.91)	0.040
Pregnancy complications	1521 (20.71)	394 (21.46)	405 (22.07)	385 (20.96)	337 (18.37)	0.014
Medication use	1394 (19.02)	380 (20.71)	359 (19.61)	339 (18.49)	316 (17.26)	0.005
Folic acid supplementation	5430 (74.25)	1340 (73.18)	1333 (72.96)	1328 (72.57)	1429 (78.30)	0.001
Calcium supplementation	4796 (65.76)	1172 (64.18)	1194 (65.46)	1170 (63.93)	1260 (69.50)	0.004
Iron supplementation	727 (9.93)	156 (8.51)	171 (9.36)	196 (10.72)	204 (11.15)	0.003
Multivitamin supplementation	647 (8.85)	130 (7.10)	152 (8.33)	165 (9.03)	200 (10.93)	<0.001

Values are n (%). [a] Obtained from Cochran-Armitage trend tests.

3.3. Dietary Pattern and Birth Outcomes

Associations of the high B-vitamin dietary pattern score with birth outcomes are presented in Tables 3 and 4. After adjustment for socio-demographic characteristics and health-related behaviours, the 1-SD increase in the high B-vitamin dietary pattern score was associated with 16.4 g (95% CI: 5.4, 27.4 g) higher birth weight, 0.040 (95% CI: 0.014, 0.065) higher birth weight Z score, and 12.1% (OR: 0.879; 95% CI: 0.809, 0.955) lower risk of SGA. Compared with women in the lowest quartile, those in the highest quartile had newborns with a 44.5 g (95% CI: 13.8, 75.2 g; p_{trend} = 0.012) higher birth weight, 0.101 (95% CI: 0.029, 0.172; p_{trend} = 0.012) higher birth weight Z score, and 27.2% (OR: 0.728; 95% CI: 0.582, 0.910; p_{trend} = 0.026) lower risk of SGA.

Table 3. Associations between the high B-vitamin dietary pattern score and continuous birth outcomes [a].

	Continuous [b]	Quartile				p_{trend} [c]
		Q1	Q2	Q3	Q4	
Birth weight, g [d]						
Mean ± SD	3270.2 ± 448.1	3244.4 ± 452.0	3269.5 ± 451.5	3259.5 ± 451.0	3307.4 ± 435.6	
Model 1 [e]	18.1 (7.5, 28.7)	Ref	26.2 (−2.8, 55.3)	12.5 (−16.8, 41.8)	52.3 (22.5, 82.2)	0.002
Model 2 [f]	16.3 (5.5, 27.1)	Ref	25.3 (−3.9, 54.6)	8.3 (−21.2, 37.8)	45.4 (15.0, 75.7)	0.010
Model 3 [g]	16.4 (5.4, 27.4)	Ref	21.9 (−7.6, 51.5)	6.4 (−23.4, 36.1)	44.5 (13.8, 75.2)	0.012
Gestational age at birth, weeks						
Mean ± SD	39.54 ± 1.50	39.55 ± 1.32	39.55 ± 1.38	39.55 ± 1.60	39.53 ± 1.69	
Model 1 [e]	0.002 (−0.033, 0.038)	Ref	−0.020 (−0.116, 0.077)	−0.003 (−0.101, 0.094)	0.010 (−0.090, 0.109)	0.785
Model 2 [f]	0.002 (−0.034, 0.038)	Ref	−0.011 (−0.108, 0.086)	−0.002 (−0.100, 0.096)	0.012 (−0.089, 0.114)	0.777
Model 3 [g]	−0.001 (−0.037, 0.037)	Ref	−0.006 (−0.105, 0.092)	−0.004 (−0.104, 0.095)	0.008 (−0.095, 0.111)	0.870
Birth weight Z score						
Mean ± SD	−0.03 ± 1.04	−0.09 ± 1.05	−0.03 ± 1.04	−0.05 ± 1.07	0.07 ± 1.01	
Model 1 [e]	0.042 (0.017, 0.067)	Ref	0.073 (0.005, 0.140)	0.032 (−0.036, 0.100)	0.116 (0.047, 0.186)	0.002
Model 2 [f]	0.039 (0.014, 0.064)	Ref	0.069 (0.002, 0.137)	0.023 (−0.045, 0.091)	0.101 (0.030, 0.171)	0.010
Model 3 [g]	0.040 (0.014, 0.065)	Ref	0.059 (−0.009, 0.128)	0.019 (−0.050, 0.088)	0.101 (0.029, 0.172)	0.012

Ref, reference. [a] Two-level generalised linear mixed models were used to estimate mean differences and 95% CIs. [b] Per 1-SD increase in the high B-vitamin dietary pattern score. [c] Obtained using the median value of each dietary pattern quartile as a continuous variable in the regression models. [d] Precise to 10 g. [e] Unadjusted. [f] Adjusted for socio-demographic characteristics, including geographic area, residence, age at delivery, education, occupation, household wealth index and parity. [g] Adjusted for all variables in model 2 plus health-related behaviours, including passive smoking, alcohol consumption, pregnancy complications, medication use, as well as iron, calcium, folic acid, and multivitamin supplementation.

Table 4. Associations between the high B-vitamin dietary pattern score and dichotomous birth outcomes [a].

	Continuous [b]	Quartile				p_{trend} [c]
		Q1	Q2	Q3	Q4	
LBW						
n (%)	226 (3.10)	58 (3.20)	59 (3.24)	64 (3.51)	45 (2.47)	
Model 1 [d]	0.901 (0.782, 1.039)	Ref	1.018 (0.704, 1.473)	1.111 (0.773, 1.598)	0.771 (0.518, 1.149)	0.256
Model 2 [e]	0.909 (0.786, 1.052)	Ref	1.004 (0.693, 1.455)	1.129 (0.784, 1.626)	0.796 (0.529, 1.196)	0.375
Model 3 [f]	0.923 (0.797, 1.069)	Ref	1.009 (0.695, 1.465)	1.125 (0.780, 1.623)	0.833 (0.553, 1.255)	0.501
Preterm						
n (%)	227 (3.09)	60 (3.27)	64 (3.49)	57 (3.11)	46 (2.51)	
Model 1 [d]	0.940 (0.817, 1.081)	Ref	1.077 (0.751, 1.544)	0.925 (0.637, 1.344)	0.718 (0.481, 1.072)	0.077
Model 2 [e]	0.940 (0.815, 1.086)	Ref	1.065 (0.739, 1.534)	0.895 (0.613, 1.307)	0.699 (0.464, 1.053)	0.062
Model 3 [f]	0.944 (0.817, 1.092)	Ref	1.042 (0.721, 1.506)	0.885 (0.604, 1.295)	0.701 (0.463, 1.061)	0.070
SGA						
n (%)	843 (11.54)	244 (13.33)	205 (11.22)	234 (12.81)	160 (8.79)	
Model 1 [d]	0.852 (0.786, 0.924)	Ref	0.818 (0.669, 0.999)	0.977 (0.803, 1.189)	0.660 (0.532, 0.821)	0.001
Model 2 [e]	0.874 (0.805, 0.948)	Ref	0.811 (0.662, 0.992)	0.988 (0.810, 1.204)	0.705 (0.566, 0.879)	0.011
Model 3 [f]	0.879 (0.809, 0.955)	Ref	0.831 (0.678, 1.020)	1.016 (0.832, 1.241)	0.728 (0.582, 0.910)	0.026

LBW, low birth weight; Ref, reference; SGA, small-for-gestational-age. [a] Two-level generalised linear mixed models were used to estimate ORs and 95% CIs. [b] Per 1-SD increase in the high B-vitamin dietary pattern score. [c] Obtained using the median value of each dietary pattern quartile as a continuous variable in the regression models. [d] Unadjusted. [e] Adjusted for socio-demographic characteristics, including geographic area, residence, age at delivery, education, occupation, household wealth index and parity. [f] Adjusted for all variables in model 2 plus health-related behaviours, including passive smoking, alcohol consumption, pregnancy complications, medication use, as well as iron, calcium, folic acid, and multivitamin supplementation.

Stratified analyses according to folic acid and multivitamin supplementation are displayed in Figures S2–S4. A marginally significant interaction was observed between multivitamin supplementation and dietary pattern score on SGA risk ($P_{interaction}$ = 0.056). Among the women who did not use multivitamins, per 1-SD increase in the high B-vitamin dietary pattern score was related to 14.2% (OR: 0.858; 95% CI: 0.786, 0.937) lower risk of SGA. In contrast, the association was not significant among users ($p > 0.05$) (Figure S4).

4. Discussion

This population-based study conducted in northwest China identified a high B-vitamin dietary pattern, which was characterised by high intakes of animal foods, vegetables, fungi and algae, legumes, and low intakes of oils and cereals. A higher score for the dietary pattern corresponded to higher birth weight and Z score as well as a lower risk of SGA.

To our knowledge, only one other study examined the associations of maternal dietary patterns characterised by B vitamins with neonatal outcomes [39]. In a mother-child cohort in France, 1638 pregnant women before 24 weeks of gestation were recruited to report their diet in the year before pregnancy retrospectively. As compared with our study, the authors regarded one-carbon metabolism nutrients including riboflavin, vitamin B6, folate, vitamin B12, betaine, choline, and methionine as response variables. They also derived a dietary pattern rich in B vitamins, which was loaded positively with low-fat milk, meat, liver, fish, eggs, cereals, mixed vegetables, chicory, leek and cabbage, and broccoli but loaded negatively with snacks and confectionery and sugar-sweetened beverages [39]. The similarity between the dietary patterns in their study and those of ours was that food groups were diverse and balanced. The difference was that our pattern had low intakes of cereals, which may be attributed to the variation in response variables and composition of cereals. The cereals we classified included wheat and rice products, whereas the cereals in their study referred to breakfast cereals and cereal bar fruits. In general, as the bran and germ are removed, commercially available cereals contain small amounts of B vitamins (thiamin, riboflavin, niacin, and folate). Given the protective effects of folic acid on neural tube defects, many countries have created legislation to mandate the fortification of industrially milled cereals with folic acid [40]. However, such projects have not yet been implemented both in China and France. The authors indicated that, when controlling for potential confounders, adherence to the high B-vitamin dietary pattern before pregnancy was not related to birth weight, gestational age, and the risk of SGA [39]. However, in our study, adherence to this dietary pattern during pregnancy was positively associated with birth weight and inversely associated with the risk of SGA. These results may be partly explained by the wide gap in nutritional status between the two populations. The intakes of riboflavin, vitamin B6, folate, and vitamin B12 in our population were approximately 15–65% lower compared with theirs. The benefits of micronutrients were more likely to be observed in malnourished populations. In addition, the timing of interest in the two studies was different. In terms of intrauterine growth, the role of maternal nutrition during pregnancy was far more prominent than that of pre-pregnancy nutrition.

In the present study, it seemed that the high B-vitamins dietary pattern exerted protective effects against SGA only among pregnant women who did not take multivitamins. A plausible explanation for this finding was that multivitamins provided adequate B vitamins to meet the needs of fetal growth. Owing to the variation in the brands of multivitamins, the content of B vitamins in supplements cannot be directly compared with the dietary pattern. Based on a double-blind randomised controlled trial in rural Shaanxi Province, we previously reported that antenatal multiple micronutrients with a recommended allowance of B vitamins resulted in a 44 g increase in birth weight and a 0.19 week increase in gestational age in comparison with folic acid alone [41]. Overall, these studies suggested that prenatal nutrition intervention focusing on B vitamins is probably an effective approach to improve birth outcomes in northwest China.

This study found that neither the continuous nor binary variable of gestational age was relevant to the high B-vitamin dietary pattern. On the contrary, birth weight-related outcomes, including crude birth weight, gestational age- and sex-specific birth weight, and SGA, were all associated with the high B-vitamin dietary pattern. These results suggest that birth weight rather than length of gestation is susceptible to the dietary pattern. Birth weight is the most widely used anthropometric indicator for newborns, in which an increase indicates the promotion of growth and development [42]. In 2012, an estimated 874,000 babies were born SGA in China, with 15,100 attributable neonatal deaths [43]. Babies born SGA are also reported to have a higher risk of delayed neurodevelopment and of being underweight in early adolescence [44,45]. The finding that adherence to the high B-vitamin dietary pattern was associated with a moderate reduction in SGA risk provides one possibility for achieving Sustainable Development Goal 3 (ensuring healthy lives and promoting well-being at all ages). Well-designed longitudinal studies are warranted to validate our findings and to explore the long-term effects of maternal dietary patterns.

Mechanisms that relate antenatal B vitamins and birth weight are still unclear. Almost all B vitamins are involved in one-carbon metabolism and related pathways. Folate is the main carrier of one-carbon units, while riboflavin, vitamin B6, and vitamin B12 act as essential cofactors or precursors of key enzymes [46]. Importantly, one-carbon metabolism plays a role in cellular processes such as biosynthesis, amino acid homeostasis, epigenetic regulation, and redox defence [47]. A growing body of clinical trials have shown that prenatal B vitamins can reduce homocysteine concentrations or alter DNA methylation patterns among newborns [48–50], but whether these changes further interfere with birth weight remains to be understood.

It is noteworthy that although our dietary pattern was driven by the variability of B vitamins, the highest quartile was accompanied by the highest intakes of other nutrients, such as protein, vitamin A, vitamin C, calcium, and zinc. We cannot exclude the potential effects of these nutrients on birth weight. Rather than single out individual nutrients that could account for the benefits of the dietary pattern studied, it may be more realistic to explore the synergy of multiple nutrients or food groups.

The present study has some strengths. First, because of the stratified multistage random sampling method, our findings can be generalised to the whole Shaanxi Province. Second, in contrast with previous studies that investigated the role of individual B vitamins in neonatal outcomes, our study explored the beneficial effect of the B vitamins-related dietary pattern using the RRR method, which provides a better foundation for the development of dietary recommendations for pregnant women. Nevertheless, several limitations should be noted. First, temporality and causality cannot be demonstrated from this cross-sectional study. Second, residual confounding cannot be ruled out due to unmeasured or unknown socio-demographic or health-related factors. Third, women were asked to recall pregnancy characteristics within 0–12 months after delivery in our study. Although many studies have shown that pregnancy is a major event during which many features can be recalled well even after years [51,52], the accuracy of our data remains to be validated. Finally, given the convenience and low cost, we evaluated the average dietary intake throughout pregnancy, which was likely to underestimate the importance of maternal diets during a certain stage. Indeed, accumulating evidence indicates that fetal growth is most affected by micronutrient deficiencies at the very earliest embryonic stages [53,54]. Prospective cohort studies that collect maternal dietary intakes over multiple time points from the periconceptional period onwards are required.

5. Conclusions

In the cross-sectional study in northwest China, we derived a maternal dietary pattern that was rich in B vitamins using the RRR method and found that greater adherence to this dietary pattern during pregnancy was related to higher birth weight and a lower risk of SGA. Based on these findings, obstetricians should pay more attention to the B-vitamin status of pregnant women and advise women to increase the proportion of animal foods, vegetables, fungi and algae, and legumes in their diets to prevent adverse birth outcomes.

Supplementary Materials: The following supporting information can be downloaded at: https://www.mdpi.com/article/10.3390/nu14030600/s1, Table S1: Foods items within each food group; Table S2: Selected nutrient intakes according to quartiles of the high B-vitamin dietary pattern score; Figure S1: Flow chart of the selection of study participants; Figure S2: Associations of 1-SD increase in the high B-vitamin dietary pattern score with birth weight stratified by the use of B vitamins-containing supplements; Figure S3: Associations of 1-SD increase in the high B-vitamin dietary pattern score with birth weight Z score stratified by the use of B vitamins-containing supplements; Figure S4: Associations of 1-SD increase in the high B-vitamin dietary pattern score with SGA stratified by the use of B vitamins-containing supplements.

Author Contributions: L.Z., S.D. and H.Y. conceived and designed the cross-sectional study; Y.K., P.Q., B.M., Z.Z., L.P., L.Z. and S.D. conducted the study; S.L., D.L., L.H., Y.Z., F.C. and D.W. performed the statistical analysis; L.Z. and S.D. wrote the manuscript. All authors have read and agreed to the published version of the manuscript.

Funding: This research was funded by the National Key Research and Development Program of China (grant numbers: 2017YFC0907200 and 2017YFC0907201), the National Natural Science Foundation of China (grant numbers: 81230016 and 72174167), and the Project of birth defect control and prevention in Shaanxi (grant number: Sxwsjswzfcght2016-013).

Institutional Review Board Statement: The cross-sectional study was conducted following the Declaration of Helsinki, and approved by the ethics committee of the Xi'an Jiaotong University Health Science Center (No. 2012008).

Informed Consent Statement: Informed consent was obtained from all subjects involved in the study.

Acknowledgments: The authors are grateful to all participants and investigators in the present study.

Conflicts of Interest: The authors declare no conflict of interest. The funders had no role in the design of the study; in the collection, analyses, or interpretation of data; in the writing of the manuscript, or in the decision to publish the results.

References

1. Katz, J.; Lee, A.C.; Kozuki, N.; Lawn, J.E.; Cousens, S.; Blencowe, H.; Ezzati, M.; Bhutta, Z.A.; Marchant, T.; Willey, B.A.; et al. Mortality risk in preterm and small-for-gestational-age infants in low-income and middle-income countries: A pooled country analysis. *Lancet* **2013**, *382*, 417–425. [CrossRef]
2. Jin, J. JAMA patient page. Babies with low birth weight. *JAMA* **2015**, *313*, 432. [CrossRef]
3. Barker, D.J. Fetal origins of coronary heart disease. *BMJ* **1995**, *311*, 171–174. [CrossRef]
4. Barker, D.J.; Osmond, C. Infant mortality, childhood nutrition, and ischaemic heart disease in England and Wales. *Lancet* **1986**, *1*, 1077–1081. [CrossRef]
5. Osmond, C.; Barker, D.J.; Winter, P.D.; Fall, C.H.; Simmonds, S.J. Early growth and death from cardiovascular disease in women. *BMJ* **1993**, *307*, 1519–1524. [CrossRef]
6. Department of Maternal and Child Health. China Maternal and Child Health Development Report (2019). Available online: http://www.nhc.gov.cn/fys/s7901/201905/bbd8e2134a7e47958c5c9ef032e1dfa2.shtml (accessed on 23 December 2021).
7. Chawanpaiboon, S.; Vogel, J.P.; Moller, A.-B.; Lumbiganon, P.; Petzold, M.; Hogan, D.; Landoulsi, S.; Jampathong, N.; Kongwattanakul, K.; Laopaiboon, M.; et al. Global, regional, and national estimates of levels of preterm birth in 2014: A systematic review and modelling analysis. *Lancet Glob. Health* **2019**, *7*, e37–e46. [CrossRef]
8. Blencowe, H.; Krasevec, J.; de Onis, M.; Black, R.E.; An, X.; Stevens, G.A.; Borghi, E.; Hayashi, C.; Estevez, D.; Cegolon, L.; et al. National, regional, and worldwide estimates of low birthweight in 2015, with trends from 2000: A systematic analysis. *Lancet Glob. Health* **2019**, *7*, e849–e860. [CrossRef]
9. Lee, A.C.C.; Katz, J.; Blencowe, H.; Cousens, S.; Kozuki, N.; Vogel, J.P.; Adair, L.; Baqui, A.H.; Bhutta, Z.A.; Caulfield, L.E.; et al. National and regional estimates of term and preterm babies born small for gestational age in 138 low-income and middle-income countries in 2010. *Lancet Glob. Health* **2013**, *1*, e26–e36. [CrossRef]
10. Abu-Saad, K.; Fraser, D. Maternal nutrition and birth outcomes. *Epidemiol. Rev.* **2010**, *32*, 5–25. [CrossRef]
11. Lyon, P.; Strippoli, V.; Fang, B.; Cimmino, L. B Vitamins and one-carbon metabolism: Implications in human health and disease. *Nutrients* **2020**, *12*, 2867. [CrossRef]
12. Salcedo-Bellido, I.; Martínez-Galiano, J.M.; Olmedo-Requena, R.; Mozas-Moreno, J.; Bueno-Cavanillas, A.; Jimenez-Moleon, J.J.; Delgado-Rodríguez, M. Association between vitamin intake during pregnancy and risk of small for gestational age. *Nutrients* **2017**, *9*, 1277. [CrossRef]
13. Krapels, I.P.; van Rooij, I.A.; Ocké, M.C.; van Cleef, B.A.; Kuijpers-Jagtman, A.M.; Steegers-Theunissen, R.P. Maternal dietary B vitamin intake, other than folate, and the association with orofacial cleft in the offspring. *Eur. J. Nutr.* **2004**, *43*, 7–14. [CrossRef]

14. Verkleij-Hagoort, A.C.; de Vries, J.H.M.; Ursem, N.T.C.; de Jonge, R.; Hop, W.C.J.; Steegers-Theunissen, R.P.M. Dietary intake of B-vitamins in mothers born a child with a congenital heart defect. *Eur. J. Nutr.* **2006**, *45*, 478–486. [CrossRef]
15. Hu, F.B. Dietary pattern analysis: A new direction in nutritional epidemiology. *Curr. Opin. Lipidol.* **2002**, *13*, 3–9. [CrossRef]
16. Nakayama, A.T.; Lutz, L.J.; Hruby, A.; Karl, J.P.; McClung, J.P.; Gaffney-Stomberg, E. A dietary pattern rich in calcium, potassium, and protein is associated with tibia bone mineral content and strength in young adults entering initial military training. *Am. J. Clin. Nutr.* **2019**, *109*, 186–196. [CrossRef]
17. Hoffmann, K.; Schulze, M.B.; Schienkiewitz, A.; Nöthlings, U.; Boeing, H. Application of a new statistical method to derive dietary patterns in nutritional epidemiology. *Am. J. Epidemiol.* **2004**, *159*, 935–944. [CrossRef]
18. Hoffmann, K.; Zyriax, B.C.; Boeing, H.; Windler, E. A dietary pattern derived to explain biomarker variation is strongly associated with the risk of coronary artery disease. *Am. J. Clin. Nutr.* **2004**, *80*, 633–640. [CrossRef]
19. Li, S.; Liu, D.; Zhang, R.; Lei, F.; Liu, X.; Cheng, Y.; Li, C.; Xiao, M.; Guo, L.; Li, M.; et al. The association of maternal dietary folate intake and folic acid supplementation with small-for-gestational-age births: A cross-sectional study in Northwest China. *Br. J. Nutr.* **2019**, *122*, 459–467. [CrossRef]
20. Li, S.; Lei, F.; Zhang, R.; Liu, D.; Qu, P.; Cheng, Y.; Liu, X.; Chen, F.; Dang, S.; Yan, H. Socioeconomic disparity in the diet quality of pregnant women in Northwest China. *Asia Pac. J. Clin. Nutr.* **2019**, *28*, 330–340. [CrossRef]
21. Meltzer, H.M.; Brantsaeter, A.L.; Ydersbond, T.A.; Alexander, J.; Haugen, M. Methodological challenges when monitoring the diet of pregnant women in a large study: Experiences from the Norwegian Mother and Child Cohort Study (MoBa). *Matern. Child Nutr.* **2008**, *4*, 14–27. [CrossRef]
22. Rifas-Shiman, S.L.; Rich-Edwards, J.W.; Willett, W.C.; Kleinman, K.P.; Oken, E.; Gillman, M.W. Changes in dietary intake from the first to the second trimester of pregnancy. *Paediatr. Perinat. Epidemiol.* **2006**, *20*, 35–42. [CrossRef] [PubMed]
23. Cucó, G.; Fernández-Ballart, J.; Sala, J.; Viladrich, C.; Iranzo, R.; Vila, J.; Arija, V. Dietary patterns and associated lifestyles in preconception, pregnancy and postpartum. *Eur. J. Clin. Nutr.* **2006**, *60*, 364–371. [CrossRef] [PubMed]
24. Crozier, S.R.; Robinson, S.M.; Godfrey, K.M.; Cooper, C.; Inskip, H.M. Women's dietary patterns change little from before to during pregnancy. *J. Nutr.* **2009**, *139*, 1956–1963. [CrossRef] [PubMed]
25. Cheng, Y.; Yan, H.; Dibley, M.J.; Shen, Y.; Li, Q.; Zeng, L. Validity and reproducibility of a semi-quantitative food frequency questionnaire for use among pregnant women in rural China. *Asia Pac. J. Clin. Nutr.* **2008**, *17*, 166–177.
26. Cheng, Y.; Zhou, X.; Zhang, X.; Zeng, L.; Yan, H. *Food Frequency Questionnaire and Atlas*; Shaanxi Science and Technology Press: Xi'an, China, 2009.
27. Institute of Nutrition and Food Safety; China Center for Disease Control and Prevention. *China Food Composition Book 1*, 6th ed.; Peking University Medical Press: Beijing, China, 2018.
28. Institute of Nutrition and Food Safety; China Center for Disease Control and Prevention. *China Food Composition Book 2*, 6th ed.; Peking University Medical Press: Beijing, China, 2019.
29. Willett, W. *Nutritional Epidemiology*, 3rd ed.; Oxford University Press: New York, NY, USA, 2013.
30. Villar, J.; Cheikh Ismail, L.; Victora, C.G.; Ohuma, E.O.; Bertino, E.; Altman, D.G.; Lambert, A.; Papageorghiou, A.T.; Carvalho, M.; Jaffer, Y.A.; et al. International standards for newborn weight, length, and head circumference by gestational age and sex: The Newborn Cross-Sectional Study of the INTERGROWTH-21st Project. *Lancet* **2014**, *384*, 857–868. [CrossRef]
31. WHO. ICD-11 for Mortality and Morbidity Statistics. Available online: https://icd.who.int/browse11/l-m/en#/http://id.who.int/icd/entity/2041060050 (accessed on 23 December 2021).
32. WHO. Recommended definitions, terminology and format for statistical tables related to the perinatal period and use of a new certificate for cause of perinatal deaths. *Acta Obstet. Gynecol. Scand.* **1977**, *56*, 247–253.
33. de Onis, M.; Habicht, J.P. Anthropometric reference data for international use: Recommendations from a World Health Organization Expert Committee. *Am. J. Clin. Nutr.* **1996**, *64*, 650–658. [CrossRef]
34. Liu, X.; Lv, L.; Zhang, H.; Zhao, N.; Qiu, J.; He, X.; Zhou, M.; Xu, X.; Cui, H.; Liu, S.; et al. Folic acid supplementation, dietary folate intake and risk of preterm birth in China. *Eur. J. Nutr.* **2016**, *55*, 1411–1422. [CrossRef]
35. Timmermans, S.; Jaddoe, V.W.V.; Hofman, A.; Steegers-Theunissen, R.P.M.; Steegers, E.A.P. Periconception folic acid supplementation, fetal growth and the risks of low birth weight and preterm birth: The Generation R Study. *Br. J. Nutr.* **2009**, *102*, 777–785. [CrossRef]
36. Zheng, J.S.; Guan, Y.; Zhao, Y.; Zhao, W.; Tang, X.; Chen, H.; Xu, M.; Wu, L.; Zhu, S.; Liu, H.; et al. Pre-conceptional intake of folic acid supplements is inversely associated with risk of preterm birth and small-for-gestational-age birth: A prospective cohort study. *Br. J. Nutr.* **2016**, *115*, 509–516. [CrossRef]
37. Pei, L.; Kang, Y.; Zhao, Y.; Cheng, Y.; Yan, H. Changes in socioeconomic inequality of low birth weight and macrosomia in Shaanxi province of Northwest China, 2010-2013: A cross-sectional study. *Medicine* **2016**, *95*, e2471. [CrossRef] [PubMed]
38. Maddock, J.; Ambrosini, G.L.; Griffin, J.L.; West, J.A.; Wong, A.; Hardy, R.; Ray, S. A dietary pattern derived using B-vitamins and its relationship with vascular markers over the life course. *Clin. Nutr.* **2019**, *38*, 1464–1473. [CrossRef] [PubMed]
39. Lecorguillé, M.; Lioret, S.; de Lauzon-Guillain, B.; de Gavelle, E.; Forhan, A.; Mariotti, F.; Charles, M.A.; Heude, B. Association between dietary intake of one-carbon metabolism nutrients in the year before pregnancy and birth anthropometry. *Nutrients* **2020**, *12*, 838. [CrossRef] [PubMed]
40. Crider, K.S.; Bailey, L.B.; Berry, R.J. Folic acid food fortification-its history, effect, concerns, and future directions. *Nutrients* **2011**, *3*, 370–384. [CrossRef] [PubMed]

41. Zeng, L.; Dibley, M.J.; Cheng, Y.; Dang, S.; Chang, S.; Kong, L.; Yan, H. Impact of micronutrient supplementation during pregnancy on birth weight, duration of gestation, and perinatal mortality in rural western China: Double blind cluster randomised controlled trial. *BMJ* **2008**, *337*, a2001. [CrossRef] [PubMed]
42. Ba-Saddik, I.A.; Al-Asbahi, T.O. Anthropometric measurements of singleton live full-term newborns in Aden, Yemen. *Int. J. Pediatr. Adolesc. Med.* **2020**, *7*, 121–126. [CrossRef]
43. Estimates of burden and consequences of infants born small for gestational age in low and middle income countries with INTERGROWTH-21st standard: Analysis of CHERG datasets. *BMJ* **2017**, *358*, j4229. [CrossRef]
44. Zhu, Z.; Perumal, N.; Fawzi, W.W.; Cheng, Y.; Elhoumed, M.; Qi, Q.; Wang, L.; Dibley, M.J.; Zeng, L.; Sudfeld, C.R. Postnatal stature does not largely mediate the relation between adverse birth outcomes and cognitive development in mid-childhood and early adolescence in rural western China. *J. Nutr.* **2022**, *152*, 302–309. [CrossRef] [PubMed]
45. Elhoumed, M.; Andegiorgish, A.K.; Qi, Q.; Gebremedhin, M.A.; Wang, L.; Uwimana, G.; Cheng, Y.; Zhu, Z.; Zeng, L. Patterns and determinants of the double burden of malnutrition among adolescents: A 14-year follow-up of a birth cohort in rural China. *J. Pediatr.* **2021**. *Online ahead of print*. [CrossRef]
46. Anderson, O.S.; Sant, K.E.; Dolinoy, D.C. Nutrition and epigenetics: An interplay of dietary methyl donors, one-carbon metabolism and DNA methylation. *J. Nutr. Biochem.* **2012**, *23*, 853–859. [CrossRef]
47. Clare, C.E.; Brassington, A.H.; Kwong, W.Y.; Sinclair, K.D. One-carbon metabolism: Linking nutritional biochemistry to epigenetic programming of long-term development. *Annu. Rev. Anim. Biosci.* **2019**, *7*, 263–287. [CrossRef] [PubMed]
48. Li, S.; Mi, B.; Qu, P.; Liu, D.; Lei, F.; Wang, D.; Zeng, L.; Kang, Y.; Shen, Y.; Pei, L.; et al. Association of antenatal vitamin B complex supplementation with neonatal vitamin B12 status: Evidence from a cluster randomized controlled trial. *Eur. J. Nutr.* **2021**, *60*, 1031–1039. [CrossRef] [PubMed]
49. Caffrey, A.; Irwin, R.E.; McNulty, H.; Strain, J.J.; Lees-Murdock, D.J.; McNulty, B.A.; Ward, M.; Walsh, C.P.; Pentieva, K. Gene-specific DNA methylation in newborns in response to folic acid supplementation during the second and third trimesters of pregnancy: Epigenetic analysis from a randomized controlled trial. *Am. J. Clin. Nutr.* **2018**, *107*, 566–575. [CrossRef] [PubMed]
50. Duggan, C.; Srinivasan, K.; Thomas, T.; Samuel, T.; Rajendran, R.; Muthayya, S.; Finkelstein, J.L.; Lukose, A.; Fawzi, W.; Allen, L.H.; et al. Vitamin B-12 supplementation during pregnancy and early lactation increases maternal, breast milk, and infant measures of vitamin B-12 status. *J. Nutr.* **2014**, *144*, 758–764. [CrossRef] [PubMed]
51. Bunin, G.R.; Gyllstrom, M.E.; Brown, J.E.; Kahn, E.B.; Kushi, L.H. Recall of diet during a past pregnancy. *Am. J. Epidemiol.* **2001**, *154*, 1136–1142. [CrossRef]
52. Bosco, J.L.; Tseng, M.; Spector, L.G.; Olshan, A.F.; Bunin, G.R. Reproducibility of reported nutrient intake and supplement use during a past pregnancy: A report from the Children's Oncology Group. *Paediatr. Perinat. Epidemiol.* **2010**, *24*, 93–101. [CrossRef]
53. Nafee, T.M.; Farrell, W.E.; Carroll, W.D.; Fryer, A.A.; Ismail, K.M. Epigenetic control of fetal gene expression. *Bjog Int. J. Obstet. Gynaecol.* **2008**, *115*, 158–168. [CrossRef]
54. Waterland, R.A.; Jirtle, R.L. Early nutrition, epigenetic changes at transposons and imprinted genes, and enhanced susceptibility to adult chronic diseases. *Nutrition* **2004**, *20*, 63–68. [CrossRef]

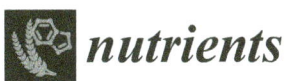

Article

Cord Blood Manganese Concentrations in Relation to Birth Outcomes and Childhood Physical Growth: A Prospective Birth Cohort Study

Yiming Dai [1,†], Jiming Zhang [1,†], Xiaojuan Qi [1,2], Zheng Wang [1], Minglan Zheng [1], Ping Liu [1], Shuai Jiang [1], Jianqiu Guo [1], Chunhua Wu [1] and Zhijun Zhou [1,*]

1 Key Laboratory of Public Health Safety of Ministry of Education, Key Laboratory of Health Technology Assessment of National Health Commission, School of Public Health, Fudan University, No.130 Dong'an Road, Shanghai 200032, China; 20111020031@fudan.edu.cn (Y.D.); zhangjiming@fudan.edu.cn (J.Z.); xjqi@cdc.zj.cn (X.Q.); 20211020149@fudan.edu.cn (Z.W.); mlzheng@cdc.zj.cn (M.Z.); 0557084@fudan.edu.cn (P.L.); jiangshuai12@fudan.edu.cn (S.J.); jqguo14@fudan.edu.cn (J.G.); chwu@fudan.edu.cn (C.W.)
2 Zhejiang Provincial Center for Disease Control and Prevention, No.3399 Binsheng Road, Hangzhou 310051, China
* Correspondence: zjzhou@fudan.edu.cn
† These authors contributed equally to this work.

Citation: Dai, Y.; Zhang, J.; Qi, X.; Wang, Z.; Zheng, M.; Liu, P.; Jiang, S.; Guo, J.; Wu, C.; Zhou, Z. Cord Blood Manganese Concentrations in Relation to Birth Outcomes and Childhood Physical Growth: A Prospective Birth Cohort Study. *Nutrients* **2021**, *13*, 4304. https://doi.org/10.3390/nu13124304

Academic Editor: Yunxian Yu

Received: 12 October 2021
Accepted: 26 November 2021
Published: 28 November 2021

Publisher's Note: MDPI stays neutral with regard to jurisdictional claims in published maps and institutional affiliations.

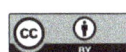

Copyright: © 2021 by the authors. Licensee MDPI, Basel, Switzerland. This article is an open access article distributed under the terms and conditions of the Creative Commons Attribution (CC BY) license (https://creativecommons.org/licenses/by/4.0/).

Abstract: Gestational exposure to manganese (Mn), an essential trace element, is associated with fetal and childhood physical growth. However, it is unclear which period of growth is more significantly affected by prenatal Mn exposure. The current study was conducted to assess the associations of umbilical cord-blood Mn levels with birth outcomes and childhood continuous physical development. The umbilical cord-blood Mn concentrations of 1179 mother–infant pairs in the Sheyang mini birth cohort were measured by graphite furnace atomic absorption spectrometry (GFAAS). The association of cord-blood Mn concentrations with birth outcomes, and the BMI z-score at 1, 2, 3, 6, 7 and 8 years old, were estimated separately using generalized linear models. The relationship between prenatal Mn exposure and BMI z-score trajectory was assessed with generalized estimating equation models. The median of cord-blood Mn concentration was 29.25 µg/L. Significantly positive associations were observed between Mn exposure and ponderal index (β, regression coefficient = 0.065, 95% CI, confidence interval: 0.021, 0.109; $p = 0.004$). Mn exposure was negatively associated with the BMI z-score of children aged 1, 2, and 3 years (β = −0.383 to −0.249, $p < 0.05$), while no significant relationships were found between Mn exposure and the BMI z-score of children at the age of 6, 7, and 8 years. Prenatal Mn exposure was related to the childhood BMI z-score trajectory (β = −0.218, 95% CI: −0.416, −0.021; $p = 0.030$). These results indicated that prenatal Mn exposure was positively related to the ponderal index (PI), and negatively related to physical growth in childhood, which seemed most significant at an early stage.

Keywords: manganese; cord blood; birth outcomes; childhood growth

1. Introduction

Manganese (Mn), an abundant heavy metal on Earth that occurs naturally [1], is widely used in industry, including the manufacturing of cosmetics, fertilizer, paints, fireworks, and the additive agents in gasoline and pesticides [2,3]. At the same time, Mn is an essential trace element and functions as a cofactor in critical biological processes that are involved in bone formation and the metabolism of carbohydrates, amino acids, and lipids [4,5]. However, excess Mn intake or exposure is associated with adverse neurological outcomes in children [6]. One review pointed out that Mn supplementation of infant formulas and excess Mn intake from drinking water should be avoided due to the potential hazards of excess Mn [7]. Animal studies have related both prenatal Mn deficiency and overexposure to decreased fetal size [8–10]. The primary route of typical Mn intake in humans is through diet and drinking water, but an additional amount of Mn can also enter the human body through the respiratory system and via skin contact from the environment [11]. Generally, 2 mg of Mn per day constitutes an adequate intake for pregnant women, with a tolerable upper intake level of 11 mg, according to the Food and Nutrition Board of the Institute of Medicine [12].

The fetus is particularly susceptible to environmental threats. Gestational exposure to environmental toxicants has been related not only to fetal growth and development but also to long-term health challenges [13–15]. Thus, assessing the relationship between prenatal pollutants exposure and the features of childhood growth is desirable, and identifying which period of growth is most sensitive to prenatal environmental pollutants exposure is essential for infants' and children's development. Mn can be transferred from the mother to the fetus via the placenta through active transport mechanisms [16]. Thus, the concentration of Mn in cord blood is able to clearly present the level of exposure to Mn of the fetus [17].

Since the required amount of Mn can be taken in through dietary sources, Mn deficiency is rare in humans. However, excess Mn exposure or Mn deficiency during pregnancy has been associated with fetal development. Several epidemiologic studies have revealed inconsistent relationships between Mn exposure during pregnancy and birth size [10,18,19]. For instance, a study in Wuhan in China has suggested that high levels of urinary Mn, even at levels that did not exceed the upper limit of reference (10 µg/L), are related to an increased risk of low birth weight [20]. However, data from Spain suggested that placental Mn was associated with slight increases in head circumference [21]. Nevertheless, limited evidence showed prenatal exposure to Mn was associated with continuous childhood anthropometric measures. Based on a longitudinal birth cohort in Jiangsu Province, China, this study aimed to assess the association of prenatal Mn exposure with birth size as well as childhood physical growth, and to explore which period of children's growth is most sensitive to prenatal Mn exposure.

2. Materials and Methods

2.1. Study Population

The Sheyang mini birth cohort study (SMBCS) is a prospective birth cohort study of fetal and childhood exposure to environmental chemicals and their impact on growth and neurodevelopment in children [22]. In total, 1303 pregnant women were recruited at a major maternity hospital between June 2009 and January 2010 in Sheyang County, Jiangsu Province, China [23–25]. Pregnant women who volunteered to participate in the study signed an informed consent form and agreed to donate cord blood samples. After the exclusion of 15 pregnant women with complications (14 with gestational diabetes mellitus and 1 with hyperthyroidism), 4 active smokers and 7 who consumed alcohol, 1 stillbirth, 9 congenital anomalies, 9 multiple births, 52 cases with incomplete information and 22 showing a lack of Mn concentrations in cord blood, eventually, 1179 mother–newborn pairs were eligible for analyzing birth outcomes. Subsequently, the present study focused on mother–child pairs that had at least one indicator of child anthropometry at ages 1, 2, 3, 6, 7 or 8 years (Figure S1). The recruited women provided written informed consents and each child's caregivers also signed for their child. The SMBCS protocol was approved by the Ethics Committee of the School of Public Health, Fudan University (IRB#2021−02−0875).

2.2. Umbilical-Cord Blood Mn Analysis

Umbilical cord blood samples were collected by professional midwives, using standard protocols [26]. Whole blood samples were collected in 5 mL sterile centrifuge tubes containing anticoagulant EDTA and were stored at -80 °C until analysis. Mn concentrations in umbilical-cord blood were measured using graphite furnace atomic absorption spectrometry (GFAAS, Perkin Elmer AA 800, Waltham, MA, USA), as described previously [27]. Briefly, samples were mixed with 1:9 (v/v) of 0.1% nitric acid (guaranteed reagent (GR)). The external quality-control program did not show any time trend in the accuracy of the Mn measurement. The recovery of cord blood Mn was 94.0% ~ 102.7% and relative standard deviation (RSD) was 1.0% ~ 5.2%. The limit of detection (LOD) was 0.062 µg/L.

2.3. Anthropometric Measurements

Anthropometric measurements of the newborns, including their weight, length and head circumference, were assessed by hospital staff [28]. Birth weight was measured using a digital scale and was rounded to the nearest 0.1 kg. Birth length was measured with extended legs and heels against the measuring board, using an infantometer, and rounded to the nearest 0.1 cm. Head circumference was measured to the closest 0.1 cm at the maximal occipital-frontal circumference, using a standard measuring tape. The ponderal index (PI), known to be a good indicator used to quantify asymmetric fetal growth restriction and to reflect adiposity in infants, was calculated using mass divided by the height, cubed ($PI = weight(g)/height(cm)^3 \times 100$) [29].

The children's weight and length were also measured when assessments were followed up at ages 1, 2, 3, 6, 7 and 8 years. In each visit, we measured the weight to the nearest 0.1 kg and height to the closest 0.1 cm. Body mass index (BMI) was calculated as the child's weight in kilograms divided by the square of their height in meters. We computed age- and sex-standardized z-scores using the World Health Organization (WHO)'s child growth standards. Therefore, the final measures of body sizes were z-scores for weight, height, head circumference, weight for height and BMI.

2.4. Covariates

Medical history, such as gestational age and gestational weight gain, was abstracted from medical records. A questionnaire was administered to each pregnant woman upon recruitment, to collect information on socio-demographic characteristics, living environment and lifestyles. The data on the child's health and behavior were collected with specifically designed questionnaires by trained study staff during the study's follow-up visits. Potential confounding variables were adjusted, including the known or suspected risk factors for the exposure or outcome a priori, based on the previous literature and a directed acyclic graph (DAG) (Figures S2 and S3). In the multivariable regression models, a set of potential confounders were included if they were related to Mn exposure and body size ($p < 0.10$) or changed the coefficients of Mn concentrations by more than 10% (Table S1). The following covariates for an analysis of birth outcomes were included: maternal age at delivery, pre-pregnancy BMI, gestational age, gestational weight gain, maternal education (<high school or ≥high school), family annual income (<30,000 RMB or ≥30,000 RMB), parity (0 or ≥1), passive smoking (yes or no), vitamin supplement during pregnancy (yes or no), child's sex and child's birth weight. The delivery mode was also adjusted in models for head circumference to correct head shape after spontaneous vaginal deliveries. The child's age in months and their time spent playing outdoors (<3 h or ≥3 h) were additionally included to investigate prenatal Mn exposure and childhood anthropometric parameters.

2.5. Statistical Analysis

Cord blood Mn concentrations were naturally logarithmically transformed to normalize their skewed distributions. Independent *t*-tests for continuous variables and Chi-square tests for categorical variables were used to assess potential differences in characteristics between initial mother–newborn pairs and included participants at each period. Missing values in the covariables were imputed by multiple imputations (less than 5%).

Generalized linear models were applied to evaluate the associations between Mn concentration and the anthropometric measurements of the children at each age stage. Separate models were fitted for Mn exposure and for each outcome. We further stratified the models according to the children's sex. Moreover, we assessed the linearity of each dose-response relationship between Mn exposure and each outcome, using generalized additive models (GAMs) with a three-degrees-of-freedom cubic spline function. Because no non-linear exposure-response relationship was observed, linear models were still used. Associations between prenatal Mn exposure and longitudinal BMI z-score were examined using multivariable generalized estimating equation models (GEE).

We performed GAM model analysis using SAS (version 9.4, SAS Institute Inc., Cary, NC, USA) and the other analyses in SPPS version 19.0. Statistical significance was considered as a two-sided p-value < 0.05.

2.6. Sensitivity Analysis

We performed several sensitivity analyses. Heavy metals could impact fetal and child growth; we further adjusted the lead and cadmium concentrations in cord blood to test the robustness of the results. We also restricted the participants, excluding low birth-weight infants and preterm births. Furthermore, we re-ran the multivariable generalized estimating equation models using the data of children who were followed up at all time points.

3. Results

3.1. General Characteristics

Table 1 presents mother–child pairs' characteristics from pregnancy until the child is 8 years of age. In total, 1072 (90.9%) pregnant women were younger than 35 years old at delivery. The gestational period of 1170 (99.2%) infants was over 37 weeks. Before conception, 149 (12.6%) women were underweight (BMI < 18.5 kg/m^2), 842 (71.4%) were normal weight (BMI between 18.5 and 23.9 kg/m^2), and 188 (16.0%) were overweight and obese (BMI $\geq$ 24 kg/m^2). A majority of women (63.9%) had less than a high-school education. In addition, approximately 52.5% of the newborns were boys. The status of socioeconomic information at childhood was similar to that during pregnancy; no significant difference was observed regarding the distributions of baseline characteristics among enrollments and in six follow-up visits.

Table 1. Maternal characteristics and sociodemographic characteristics in each subgroup. (N (%)).

Characteristics	Pregnancy (n = 1179)	1 Year Old (n = 567)	2 Years Old (n = 358)	3 Years Old (n = 409)	6 Years Old (n = 421)	7 Years Old (n = 388)	8 Years Old (n = 374)	p *
Maternal age (years)								
<35	1072 (90.9)	507 (89.4)	323 (90.2)	374 (91.4)	370 (87.9)	344 (88.7)	332 (88.8)	
$\geq$35	107 (9.1)	60 (10.6)	35 (9.8)	35 (8.6)	51 (12.1)	44 (11.3)	42 (11.2)	0.461
Gestational age (weeks)								
<37	9 (0.8)	3 (0.5)	2 (0.6)	2 (0.5)	4 (1.0)	3 (0.8)	2 (0.5)	
$\geq$37	1170 (99.2)	564 (99.5)	356 (99.4)	407 (99.5)	417 (99.0)	385 (99.2)	372 (99.5)	0.975
Pre-pregnancy BMI (kg/m^2)								
<18.5	149 (12.6)	74 (13.1)	52 (14.5)	53 (12.9)	43 (10.2)	41 (10.6)	42 (11.2)	
18.5–23.9	842 (71.4)	405 (71.4)	248 (69.3)	287 (70.2)	294 (69.8)	269 (69.3)	254 (67.9)	
$\geq$24	188 (16.0)	88 (15.5)	58 (16.2)	69 (16.9)	84 (20.0)	78 (20.1)	78 (20.9)	0.288
Maternal education								
<High school (9 years)	753 (63.9)	388 (68.4)	252 (70.4)	284 (69.4)	302 (71.7)	272 (70.1)	272 (72.7)	
$\geq$High school (9 years)	426 (36.1)	179 (31.6)	106 (29.6)	125 (30.6)	119 (28.3)	116 (29.9)	102 (27.3)	0.006
Neonatal sex								
Boys	619 (52.5)	296 (52.2)	194 (54.2)	202 (49.4)	227 (53.9)	216 (55.7)	203 (54.3)	
Girls	560 (47.5)	271 (47.8)	164 (45.8)	207 (50.6)	194 (46.1)	172 (44.3)	171 (45.7)	0.663
Parity								
0	613 (52.0)	293 (51.7)	196 (54.7)	224 (54.8)	225 (53.4)	212 (54.6)	192 (51.3)	
$\geq$1	566 (48.0)	274 (48.3)	162 (45.3)	185 (45.2)	196 (46.4)	176 (45.4)	182 (48.7)	0.848

* The differences in frequency distribution were established by chi-square tests. Abbreviation: BMI: body mass index.

3.2. Mn Concentrations in Cord Blood

Cord blood Mn levels were detectable in all samples. The median level of Mn in cord blood was 29.25 µg/L, ranging from 6.84 µg/L to 316.73 µg/L (Table S2). The geometric mean and geometric standard deviation of cord-blood Mn concentrations were 29.03 µg/L and 1.50 µg/L.

3.3. Cord-Blood Mn Concentration and Birth Outcomes

Associations between Mn exposure and size at birth were listed in Table 2. After controlling for potential confounders, each 1-unit increase in ln-transformed Mn concentrations in cord blood was associated with an increase of 0.065 (95% CI: 0.021, 0.109) in PI of newborns at birth ($p = 0.004$), about 2.51% of the mean PI (mean: 2.59). Prenatal exposure to Mn was associated with an increase in PI in the fourth quartiles of exposure compared to the lowest quartile ($\beta = 0.082$, 95% CI: 0.032, 0.132; $p = 0.001$). In addition, the infants among the highest quartile of prenatal Mn exposure had a higher birth weight compared to the lowest quartile ($\beta = 0.067$, 95% CI: 0.003, 0.131; $p = 0.041$).

Table 2. Regression coefficients (95% CI) for associations between Mn concentrations in cord blood and birth outcomes.

	Birth Weight (kg)		Birth Length (cm)		Head Circumference (cm)		Ponderal Index	
	β (95% CI)	p	β (95% CI)	p	β (95% CI)	p	β (95% CI)	p
All newborns [a]								
Ln (Mn)	0.044 (−0.012, 0.100)	0.124	−0.190 (−0.508, 0.128)	0.242	0.105 (−0.093, 0.303)	0.299	0.065 (0.021, 0.109)	0.004
Q1	Ref.		Ref.		Ref.		Ref.	
Q2	0.033 (−0.031, 0.096)	0.316	0.059 (−0.301, 0.420)	0.748	0.097 (−0.125, 0.320)	0.391	0.032 (−0.018, 0.081)	0.209
Q3	0.035 (−0.029, 0.098)	0.283	−0.031 (−0.391, 0.329)	0.865	0.012 (−0.211, 0.236)	0.914	0.042 (−0.008, 0.091)	0.101
Q4	0.067 (0.003, 0.131)	0.041	−0.160 (−0.522, 0.202)	0.385	0.193 (−0.031, 0.418)	0.091	0.082 (0.032, 0.132)	0.001
p-trend		0.051		0.331		0.172		0.002
Boys [b]								
Ln (Mn)	0.005 (−0.073, 0.083)	0.899	−0.378 (−0.804, 0.047)	0.082	0.104 (−0.183, 0.392)	0.477	0.052 (−0.005, 0.110)	0.073
Q1	Ref.		Ref.		Ref.		Ref.	
Q2	0.050 (−0.047, 0.146)	0.312	0.143 (−0.381, 0.667)	0.592	0.173 (−0.178, 0.524)	0.334	0.023 (−0.048, 0.093)	0.528
Q3	0.056 (−0.039, 0.151)	0.245	0.194 (0.323, 0.710)	0.462	0.090 (−0.258, 0.438)	0.611	0.002 (−0.068, 0.071)	0.962
Q4	0.054 (−0.039, 0.147)	0.256	−0.287 (−0.792, 0.219)	0.266	0.285 (−0.056, 0.626)	0.102	0.078 (0.010, 0.146)	0.024
p-trend		0.288		0.260		0.159		0.043
Girls [b]								
Ln (Mn)	0.090 (0.010, 0.170)	0.027	0.043 (−0.435, 0.521)	0.861	0.109 (−0.158, 0.376)	0.424	0.079 (0.011, 0.146)	0.022
Q1	Ref.		Ref.		Ref.		Ref.	
Q2	0.012 (−0.072, 0.095)	0.784	−0.035 (−0.531, 0.461)	0.889	0.027 (−0.248, 0.302)	0.848	0.035 (−0.035, 0.976)	0.323
Q3	0.011 (−0.073, 0.096)	0.792	−0.281 (−0.782, 0.221)	0.273	−0.038 (−0.317, 0.241)	0.788	0.081 (0.011, 0.152)	0.024
Q4	0.085 (−0.003, 0.172)	0.059	0.019 (−0.503, 0.542)	0.943	0.096 (−0.193, 0.385)	0.516	0.080 (0.006, 0.153)	0.034
p-trend		0.089		0.755		0.665		0.013

[a] Models were adjusted for maternal age at delivery, pre-pregnancy BMI, gestational age, gestational weight gain, maternal education, parity, family annual income, passive smoking, vitamin supplement during pregnancy, child's sex, delivery mode (just for head circumference).
[b] Models were adjusted for maternal age at delivery, pre-pregnancy BMI, gestational age, gestational weight gain, maternal education, parity, family annual income, passive smoking, vitamin supplement during pregnancy, delivery mode (just for head circumference).

In sex-stratified analyses, higher Mn exposure was in association with increases in PI among girls ($\beta = 0.079$, 95% CI: 0.011, 0.146; $p = 0.022$). In addition, among girls, prenatal Mn concentrations were positively related to birth weight ($\beta = 0.090$, 95% CI: 0.010, 0.170; $p = 0.027$). The dose-response relationships between prenatal Mn exposure and birth outcomes were shown in Figure 1. Generalized additive models suggested a linear relationship between cord blood Mn and PI among the total infants, and the same linear association between cord blood Mn and birth weight among girls.

3.4. Cord-Blood Mn Level and BMI of Children Aged 1, 2, 3, 6, 7, and 8 Years Old

As shown in Figure 2, prenatal Mn exposure was negatively associated with the BMI z-score of children at the ages of 1 year ($\beta = -0.383$, 95% CI: −0.668, −0.098; $p = 0.008$), 2 years ($\beta = -0.300$, 95% CI: −0.546, −0.055; $p = 0.017$), and 3 years ($\beta = -0.249$, 95% CI: −0.477, −0.020; $p = 0.033$). However, non-significantly inverse associations of prenatal Mn exposure with childhood BMI z-score at the ages of 6, 7 and 8 years were observed.

Regarding sex-specific difference (Table S3), Mn concentrations in cord blood were significantly inversely related to the BMI z-score in boys aged 1 year old ($\beta = -0.607$, 95% CI: −0.993, −0.220; $p = 0.002$) and 3 years old ($\beta = -0.358$, 95% CI: −0.710, −0.005; $p = 0.047$). A significant negative relationship between cord-blood Mn concentration and BMI z-score was observed in 2-year-old girls ($\beta = -0.434$, 95% CI: −0.805, −0.062; $p = 0.022$).

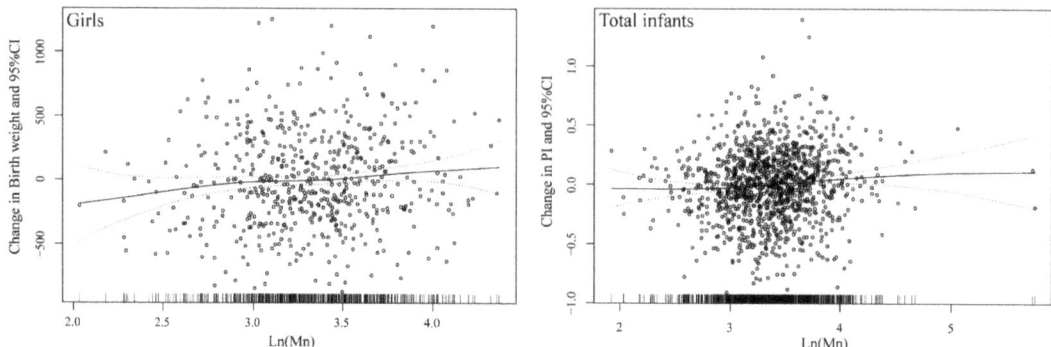

Figure 1. Generalized additive models for associations between prenatal Mn exposure and birth outcomes.

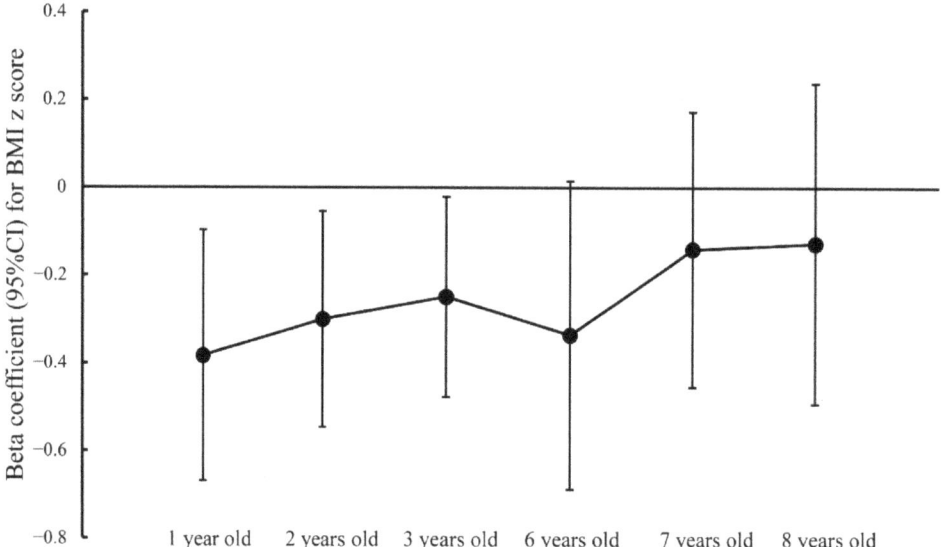

Figure 2. Generalized linear models for associations between prenatal Mn exposure and body mass index z score at different ages. (Abbreviation: BMI—body mass index).

In longitudinal analyses using GEE models (Figure 3, Table S4), prenatal Mn exposure was related to the childhood BMI z-score trajectory in children aged 1 to 8 years old ($\beta = -0.253$, 95% CI: -0.445, -0.060; $p = 0.010$). A significant trend was also observed from the first quartile to the fourth quartile ($p = 0.016$). Compared with the lowest Mn levels in cord blood, the BMI z-score was significantly decreased in the fourth quartile ($\beta = -0.234$, 95% CI: -0.460, -0.009; $p = 0.041$). These inverse associations between Mn exposure and childhood BMI trajectory were only observed in boys ($\beta = -0.388$, 95% CI: -0.678, -0.098; $p = 0.009$).

3.5. Sensitivity Analysis

Overall, effect estimates did not change in terms of complete analyses when adding other heavy metals, such as lead and cadmium (Table S5). Results were similar after excluding those children who were low-birth-weight infants and preterm births (Table S6). In addition, the data of children followed up at all time points made the coefficients become stronger (Table S7). Finally, the results remained robust after performing sensitivity analysis.

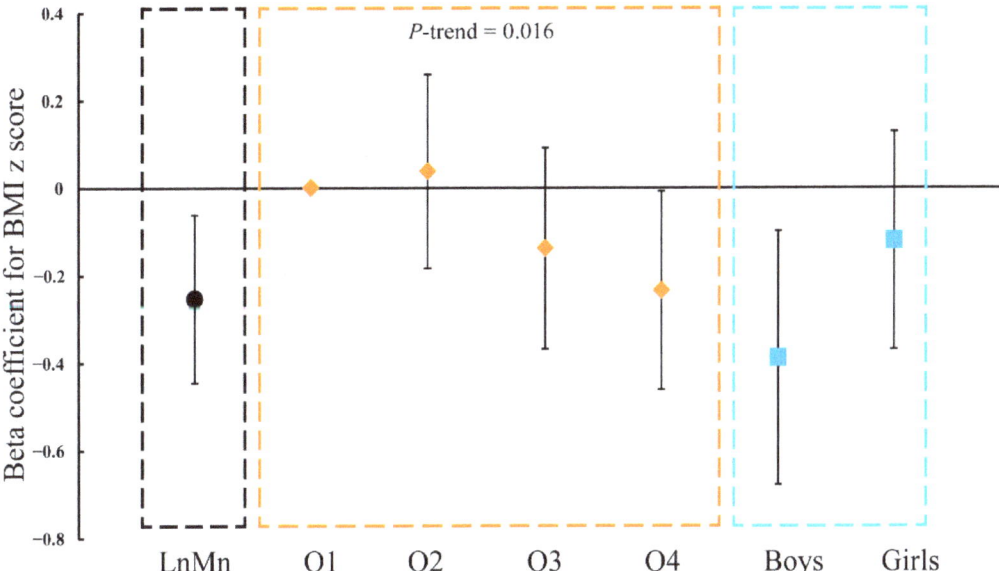

Figure 3. Generalized estimating equation models for associations of body mass. index z score with prenatal Mn exposure. (Abbreviation: BMI—body mass index).

4. Discussion

In this prospective birth cohort, we found significant associations of prenatal Mn exposure with birth size and physical development during childhood. Briefly, prenatal Mn exposure was associated with an increased PI among newborns. Higher Mn concentrations in cord blood were related to BMI during toddlerhood, but not in the school-age period. The association of Mn with the childhood BMI z-score trajectory feature was also observed.

The level of cord blood Mn in the present study (median = 29.25 µg/L, geometric mean = 29.03 µg/L, range: 6.84–316.73 µg/L) was within the range of levels seen in prior studies. Our measured level was comparable to the median value of Mn concentration, as measured in Germany (median = 28.8 µg/L) [30] and Canada (median = 31.8 µg/L) [31] but was much lower than the levels reported in the US, Mexico, and Beijing in China. (>40 µg/L, Table S8) [6,17,32]. The differences in cord-blood Mn concentrations across populations could be a result of environmental exposure levels and dietary intakes. Blood Mn has been advised as a biomarker of Mn exposure [33,34]. Cord-blood Mn represents fetal exposure during the third trimester because the half-life of Mn in the blood is 37 days [35]. However, further studies with sequential measures of Mn during pregnancy are needed to confirm our findings and explore whether the associations of Mn with birth outcomes and childhood physical development depend on the timing of Mn exposure.

Only a few epidemiologic research studies addressing cord-blood Mn and birth size with inconsistent results have been conducted [8,19,36,37]. Specifically, in a study of 1377 mother-infant pairs in Shanghai, China, the Mn concentrations in cord serum were significantly related to shorter birth length and higher PI [38]. In agreement with their findings, we observed positive associations between Mn in cord blood and the PI of infants. Similarly, our findings showed that cord-blood Mn concentrations were related to a reduction in birth length, but the association was not significant. At the same time, we found higher levels of cord-blood Mn were associated with increased birth weight compared with those showing the lowest Mn levels. Another Chinese study in northern China using data from 125 mother–infant pairs showed an inverse U-shaped relationship between cord-blood Mn levels (median = 77.20 µg/L) and birth weight [19]. In Spain, cord-blood Mn was not significantly associated with birth weight, probably due to the small sample size (n = 54) [8]. A study of 1519 mother–infant pairs in Canada found a negative association for cord-blood Mn with birth weight [36]. The level of exposure might be a reason for these inconsistent results of the associations between cord-blood Mn and birth weight. An animal study also suggested that prenatal exposure to Mn was related to reduced fetal body weight in mice [37]. Although some negative associations between cord-blood Mn and birth weight were found, the potential mechanisms might include oxidative stress caused by excess Mn exposure [39,40]. Mn is still an essential trace element that was shown to play a role in bone formation and fetal growth. The level of Mn concentrations in our study captured the ascending segment of the inverted U-shape dose-response relationship between Mn and birth weight. In addition, a study from Bangladesh suggested sex-specific positive and linear associations for Mn with birth weight [41]. Our sex-stratified results were similar. Potential mechanisms for the associations are unclear; prenatal sex-steroid hormones [42] and maternal iron deficiency [43] might play an important role.

As for postnatal growth, we found that prenatal Mn exposure was negatively associated with childhood BMI z-score, and the association was more significant when the toddlers were aged 1, 2, or 3 years old, but non-significant at the age of 6, 7, or 8 years. Human growth and development at different stages were influenced by several kinds of factors that include micronutrients (e.g., Mn, etc.) [44,45]. A cross-sectional study analyzing two cycles of NHANES revealed that the increase in the concentration of blood Mn was associated with an increased BMI in US children aged 6–12 years [46]. Another study of 470 preschool children on the southeast coast of China indicated that there was no significant association between children's blood Mn and BMI [15], in contrast to the present study. Mn exposure in utero or in childhood might have different effects on children's growth. According to the Development Origins of Health and Disease (DOHaD), prenatal exposure to environmental factors played a role in determining the development of human growth in childhood [47]. Associations between prenatal Mn and BMI in the development periods of children were found in the present study and were also found in the sensitivity analysis of data from the children followed up at all time points. However, which periods of childhood are mostly affected by prenatal Mn exposure was unclear. To the best of our knowledge, this is the first study that illuminated the associations between prenatal Mn exposure and BMI z-score at the ages of 1, 2, 3, 6, 7, or 8 years. We also found that prenatal Mn exposure was more sensitive in terms of BMI z-score in toddlerhood, and the associations became weaker in school-age childhood. Our further study is to explore longer-term effects, even physical development, in adolescence.

Benefiting from the continuous follow-up of our cohort, we could observe the physical growth of children from birth to the age of 8. Prenatal Mn exposure was associated with an increased PI at birth and decreased BMI z-score in childhood, especially toddlerhood. Catch-up, which is defined as accelerated rates of growth following a period of failure to reach the growth reference of normal preterm or term-born infants, seemed to explain the results [48]. As an essential element, moderate Mn intake in utero could ensure the normal growth of the fetus, prevent low birth weight, and avoid catch-up. Furthermore, Mn exposure was suspected to affect human health in a "U-shaped" dose-responsive manner [10,18]. Excess Mn exposure or Mn deficiency might have different mechanisms. The potential biological mechanisms caused by prenatal excess Mn exposure could be related to impairments in fetal development and childhood growth, but the processes were still unclear. The animal studies suggested that maternal excessive Mn exposure was related to reduced fetal weight, the restricted internal organ development of offspring, and impaired skeleton ossification [37,49,50]. Conversely, Mn deficiency also resulted in skeletal malformation and impaired growth in animals [4,51]. Moreover, high levels of Mn exposure were seen to cause oxidative stress in cells and impair the function and growth of cells [39]. Besides this, Mn deficiency was associated with impairments or dysfunctions in insulin production, lipoprotein metabolism, the oxidant defense system, and growth factor metabolism [52,53]. Therefore, more studies are needed to explore these unclear mechanisms.

Obviously, our study had several strengths and limitations. The repeated anthropometric data from a prospective cohort that had been followed for more than 8 years provided us with a good opportunity to explore the associations of cord-blood Mn with physical growth in utero and in toddlerhood, up to school-age childhood, although the research showed a lack of data for children at the ages of 4 and 5 years due to there being no follow-up. Reassuringly, participants who enrolled in the study could be representative of the full cohort and the presented results were still robust in the sensitivity analysis. On the other hand, potential confounders were obtained from face-to-face interviews, and recall bias was avoided. Although we adjusted the potential confounders as soon as possible, some other important determinants, such as some other microelements (e.g., Cu, Fe, Zn) [54], could not be controlled, which might bias the results. Therefore, future studies on the mixture effect of different microelements and other heavy metals on birth outcomes and childhood growth are needed.

5. Conclusions

In this prospective birth cohort study, we found that a high level of cord-blood Mn was associated with a significant increase in birth weight and ponderal index. Prenatal exposure to Mn was inversely related to childhood BMI z-score, especially in toddlerhood at the age of 1, 2, and 3 years. Further studies are warranted to confirm our findings and explore a longer-term effect in adolescence.

Supplementary Materials: The following are available online at https://www.mdpi.com/article/10.3390/nu13124304/s1, Figure S1: Recruitment and follow-up of pregnant women and their infants. Figure S2: Directed acyclic graph on covariates for assessment of prenatal manganese exposure for birth outcomes. Figure S3. Directed acyclic graph on covariates for assessment of prenatal manganese exposure for childhood BMI. Table S1. Associations between potential covariates and prenatal Mn exposure and birth outcomes. Table S2. Manganese concentrations (g/L) in umbilical cord blood. Table S3. Regression coefficients (95% CI) for associations of BMI-z score with umbilical cord blood manganese concentrations. Table S4. Generalized estimating equation models for associations of body mass index z score with Mn exposure. Table S5. Sensitivity analysis of generalized estimating equation models for associations of body mass index z-score with Mn exposure (Adding Ln (Pb), Ln (Cd) as covariates). Table S6. Sensitivity analysis of Generalized estimating equation models for associations of body mass index z score with Mn exposure (excluding low birth weight infants and preterm births). Table S7. Generalized estimating equation models for associations of body mass index z-score with Mn exposure (including children followed up at all time points, $N = 83$). Table S8. Comparison of manganese concentrations in cord blood in the previous literature.

Author Contributions: Conceptualization, Y.D. and Z.Z.; methodology, X.Q., Z.Z. and C.W.; software, Y.D.; formal analysis, Y.D.; investigation, Y.D., J.Z., Z.W., M.Z., P.L., S.J., J.G.; resources, Z.Z.; data curation, J.Z.; writing—original draft preparation, Y.D.; writing—review and editing, Y.D., C.W. and Z.Z.; visualization, Y.D.; project administration, J.Z.; funding acquisition, Z.Z. All authors have read and agreed to the published version of the manuscript.

Funding: The study was partly financially supported by the Three-year Public Health Action Plan of Shanghai (GWV−10.1-XK11) and National Natural Science Foundation of China (82073501).

Institutional Review Board Statement: The study had been performed in accordance with the 1964 Helsinki declaration and its later amendments or comparable ethical standards. The study protocol was approved by the Ethics Committee of the School of Public Health, Fudan University.

Informed Consent Statement: Informed consent was obtained from all subjects involved in the study.

Data Availability Statement: The data presented in this study are available on request from the corresponding author. The data are not publicly available due to privacy.

Acknowledgments: We are very grateful to all subjects in Sheyang Mini Birth Cohort Study and the staffs in Sheyang County People's Hospital. We also thank doctors worked in Sheyang Maternal and Child Health Care Centre for their support for follow-up.

Conflicts of Interest: The authors declare no conflict of interest.

References

1. Nadaska, G.; Lesny, J.; Michalik, I. Environmental aspect of manganese chemistry. *Hung. Electron. J. Sci. HEJ.* **2012**, 1–16. Available online: http://heja.szif.hu/ENV/ENV-100702-A/env100702a.pdf (accessed on 11 October 2021).
2. Boudissa, S.M.; Lambert, J.; Müller, C.; Kennedy, G.; Gareau, L.; Zayed, J. Manganese concentrations in the soil and air in the vicinity of a closed manganese alloy production plant. *Sci. Total Environ.* **2006**, *361*, 67–72. [CrossRef] [PubMed]
3. Aelion, C.M.; Davis, H.T.; McDermott, S.; Lawson, A.B. Metal concentrations in rural topsoil in South Carolina: Potential for human health impact. *Sci. Total Environ.* **2008**, *402*, 149–156. [CrossRef] [PubMed]
4. Aschner, J.L.; Aschner, M. Nutritional aspects of manganese homeostasis. *Mol. Asp. Med.* **2005**, *26*, 353–362. [CrossRef] [PubMed]
5. Harischandra, D.S.; Ghaisas, S.; Zenitsky, G.; Jin, H.; Kanthasamy, A.; Anantharam, V.; Kanthasamy, A.G. Manganese-Induced Neurotoxicity: New Insights into the Triad of Protein Misfolding, Mitochondrial Impairment, and Neuroinflammation. *Front. Neurosci.* **2019**, *13*, 654. [CrossRef] [PubMed]
6. Claus Henn, B.; Bellinger, D.C.; Hopkins, M.R.; Coull, B.A.; Ettinger, A.S.; Jim, R.; Hatley, E.; Christiani, D.C.; Wright, R.O. Maternal and Cord Blood Manganese Concentrations and Early Childhood Neurodevelopment among Residents near a Mining-Impacted Superfund Site. *Environ. Health Perspect.* **2017**, *125*, 67020. [CrossRef] [PubMed]
7. Mitchell, E.J.; Frisbie, S.H.; Roudeau, S.; Carmona, A.; Ortega, R. How much manganese is safe for infants? A review of the scientific basis of intake guidelines and regulations relevant to the manganese content of infant formulas. *J. Trace Elem. Med. Biol.* **2021**, *65*, 126710. [CrossRef] [PubMed]
8. Bermúdez, L.; García-Vicent, C.; López, J.; Torró, M.I.; Lurbe, E. Assessment of ten trace elements in umbilical cord blood and maternal blood: Association with birth weight. *J. Transl. Med.* **2015**, *13*, 291. [CrossRef] [PubMed]
9. Mora, A.M.; van Wendel De Joode, B.; Mergler, D.; Córdoba, L.; Cano, C.; Quesada, R.; Smith, D.R.; Menezes-Filho, J.A.; Eskenazi, B. Maternal blood and hair manganese concentrations, fetal growth, and length of gestation in the ISA cohort in Costa Rica. *Environ. Res.* **2015**, *136*, 47–56. [CrossRef]
10. Eum, J.; Cheong, H.; Ha, E.; Ha, M.; Kim, Y.; Hong, Y.; Park, H.; Chang, N. Maternal blood manganese level and birth weight: A MOCEH birth cohort study. *Environ. Health* **2014**, *13*, 31. [CrossRef]
11. Yoon, M.; Nong, A.; Clewell, H.J.; Taylor, M.D.; Dorman, D.C.; Andersen, M.E. Evaluating Placental Transfer and Tissue Concentrations of Manganese in the Pregnant Rat and Fetuses after Inhalation Exposures with a PBPK Model. *Toxicol. Sci.* **2009**, *112*, 44–58. [CrossRef]
12. Oulhote, Y.; Mergler, D.; Bouchard, M.F. Sex- and age-differences in blood manganese levels in the U.S. general population: National health and nutrition examination survey 2011–2012. *Environ. Health* **2014**, *13*, 87. [CrossRef] [PubMed]
13. Andiarena, A.; Irizar, A.; Molinuevo, A.; Urbieta, N.; Babarro, I.; Subiza-Pérez, M.; Santa-Marina, L.; Ibarluzea, J.; Lertxundi, A. Prenatal Manganese Exposure and Long-Term Neuropsychological Development at 4 Years of Age in a Population-Based Birth Cohort. *Int. J. Environ. Res. Public Health* **2020**, *17*, 1665. [CrossRef] [PubMed]
14. Li, Y.; Cha, C.; Lv, X.; Liu, J.; He, J.; Pang, Q.; Meng, L.; Kuang, H.; Fan, R. Association between 10 urinary heavy metal exposure and attention deficit hyperactivity disorder for children. *Environ. Sci. Pollut. Res.* **2020**, *27*, 31233–31242. [CrossRef] [PubMed]
15. Zeng, X.; Xu, X.; Qin, Q.; Ye, K.; Wu, W.; Huo, X. Heavy metal exposure has adverse effects on the growth and development of preschool children. *Environ. Geochem. Health* **2019**, *41*, 309–321. [CrossRef]
16. Krachler, M.; Rossipal, E.; Micetic-Turk, D. Trace element transfer from the mother to the newborn—Investigations on triplets of colostrum, maternal and umbilical cord sera. *Eur. J. Clin. Nutr.* **1999**, *53*, 486–494. [CrossRef] [PubMed]
17. Li, A.; Zhuang, T.; Shi, J.; Liang, Y.; Song, M. Heavy metals in maternal and cord blood in Beijing and their efficiency of placental transfer. *J. Environ. Sci.* **2019**, *80*, 99–106. [CrossRef]
18. Chen, L.; Ding, G.; Gao, Y.; Wang, P.; Shi, R.; Huang, H.; Tian, Y. Manganese concentrations in maternal–infant blood and birth weight. *Environ. Sci. Pollut. Res.* **2014**, *21*, 6170–6175. [CrossRef]
19. Guan, H.; Wang, M.; Li, X.; Piao, F.; Li, Q.; Xu, L.; Kitamura, F.; Yokoyama, K. Manganese concentrations in maternal and umbilical cord blood: Related to birth size and environmental factors. *Eur. J. Public Health* **2014**, *24*, 150–157. [CrossRef]
20. Hu, J.; Wu, C.; Zheng, T.; Zhang, B.; Xia, W.; Peng, Y.; Liu, W.; Jiang, M.; Liu, S.; Buka, S.L.; et al. Critical Windows for Associations between Manganese Exposure during Pregnancy and Size at Birth: A Longitudinal Cohort Study in Wuhan, China. *Environ. Health Perspect.* **2018**, *126*, 127006. [CrossRef]
21. Freire, C.; Amaya, E.; Gil, F.; Murcia, M.; LLop, S.; Casas, M.; Vrijheid, M.; Lertxundi, A.; Irizar, A.; Fernández-Tardón, G.; et al. Placental metal concentrations and birth outcomes: The Environment and Childhood (INMA) project. *Int. J. Hyg. Environ. Health* **2019**, *222*, 468–478. [CrossRef] [PubMed]

22. Qi, X.; Zheng, M.; Wu, C.; Wang, G.; Feng, C.; Zhou, Z. Urinary pyrethroid metabolites among pregnant women in an agricultural area of the Province of Jiangsu, China. *Int. J. Hyg. Environ. Health* **2012**, *215*, 487–495. [CrossRef] [PubMed]
23. Guo, J.; Wu, C.; Zhang, J.; Qi, X.; Lv, S.; Jiang, S.; Zhou, T.; Lu, D.; Feng, C.; Chang, X.; et al. Prenatal exposure to mixture of heavy metals, pesticides and phenols and IQ in children at 7 years of age: The SMBCS study. *Environ. Int.* **2020**, *139*, 105692. [CrossRef] [PubMed]
24. Zhang, J.; Guo, J.; Wu, C.; Qi, X.; Jiang, S.; Zhou, T.; Xiao, H.; Li, W.; Lu, D.; Feng, C.; et al. Early-life carbamate exposure and intelligence quotient of seven-year-old children. *Environ. Int.* **2020**, *145*, 106105. [CrossRef] [PubMed]
25. Liu, P.; Wu, C.; Chang, X.; Qi, X.; Zheng, M.; Zhou, Z. Adverse Associations of both Prenatal and Postnatal Exposure to Organophosphorous Pesticides with Infant Neurodevelopment in an Agricultural Area of Jiangsu Province, China. *Environ. Health Perspect.* **2016**, *124*, 1637–1643. [CrossRef] [PubMed]
26. Guo, J.; Wu, C.; Qi, X.; Jiang, S.; Liu, Q.; Zhang, J.; Cao, Y.; Chang, X.; Zhou, Z. Adverse associations between maternal and neonatal cadmium exposure and birth outcomes. *Sci. Total Environ.* **2017**, *575*, 581–587. [CrossRef] [PubMed]
27. Zhou, T.; Guo, J.; Zhang, J.; Xiao, H.; Qi, X.; Wu, C.; Chang, X.; Zhang, Y.; Liu, Q.; Zhou, Z. Sex-Specific Differences in Cognitive Abilities Associated with Childhood Cadmium and Manganese Exposures in School-Age Children: A Prospective Cohort Study. *Biol. Trace Elem. Res.* **2020**, *193*, 89–99. [CrossRef]
28. Guo, J.; Wu, C.; Lv, S.; Lu, D.; Feng, C.; Qi, X.; Liang, W.; Chang, X.; Xu, H.; Wang, G.; et al. Associations of prenatal exposure to five chlorophenols with adverse birth outcomes. *Environ. Pollut.* **2016**, *214*, 478–484. [CrossRef] [PubMed]
29. Landmann, E.; Reiss, I.; Misselwitz, B.; Gortner, L. Ponderal index for discrimination between symmetric and asymmetric growth restriction: Percentiles for neonates from 30 weeks to 43 weeks of gestation. *J. Matern. Fetal Neonatal Med.* **2006**, *19*, 157–160. [CrossRef] [PubMed]
30. Kopp, R.S.; Kumbartski, M.; Harth, V.; Brüning, T.; Käfferlein, H.U. Partition of metals in the maternal/fetal unit and lead-associated decreases of fetal iron and manganese: An observational biomonitoring approach. *Arch. Toxicol.* **2012**, *86*, 1571–1581. [CrossRef] [PubMed]
31. Arbuckle, T.E.; Liang, C.L.; Morisset, A.S.; Fisher, M.; Weiler, H.; Cirtiu, C.M.; Legrand, M.; Davis, K.; Ettinger, A.S.; Fraser, W.D. Maternal and fetal exposure to cadmium, lead, manganese and mercury: The MIREC study. *Chemosphere* **2016**, *163*, 270–282. [CrossRef] [PubMed]
32. Kupsco, A.; Sanchez-Guerra, M.; Amarasiriwardena, C.; Brennan, K.J.M.; Estrada-Gutierrez, G.; Svensson, K.; Schnaas, L.; Pantic, I.; Téllez-Rojo, M.M.; Baccarelli, A.A.; et al. Prenatal manganese and cord blood mitochondrial DNA copy number: Effect modification by maternal anemic status. *Environ. Int.* **2019**, *126*, 484–493. [CrossRef]
33. Laohaudomchok, W.; Lin, X.; Herrick, R.F.; Fang, S.C.; Cavallari, J.M.; Christiani, D.C.; Weisskopf, M.G. Toenail, blood, and urine as biomarkers of manganese exposure. *J. Occup. Environ. Med.* **2011**, *53*, 506–510. [CrossRef] [PubMed]
34. O'Neal, S.L.; Zheng, W. Manganese Toxicity upon Overexposure: A Decade in Review. *Curr. Environ. Health. Rep.* **2015**, *2*, 315–328. [CrossRef] [PubMed]
35. Milne, D.B.; Sims, R.L.; Ralston, N.V. Manganese content of the cellular components of blood. *Clin. Chem.* **1990**, *36*, 450–452. [CrossRef] [PubMed]
36. Ashley-Martin, J.; Dodds, L.; Arbuckle, T.E.; Ettinger, A.S.; Shapiro, G.D.; Fisher, M.; Monnier, P.; Morisset, A.; Fraser, W.D.; Bouchard, M.F. Maternal and cord blood manganese (Mn) levels and birth weight: The MIREC birth cohort study. *Int. J. Hyg. Environ. Health* **2018**, *221*, 876–882. [CrossRef]
37. Colomina, T.; Domingo, J.; Llobet, J.; Corbella, J. Effect of day of exposure on the developmental toxicity of manganese in mice. *Vet. Hum. Hum. Toxicol.* **1996**, *38*, 7–9.
38. Yu, X.; Cao, L.; Yu, X. Elevated cord serum manganese level is associated with a neonatal high ponderal index. *Environ. Res.* **2013**, *121*, 79–83. [CrossRef] [PubMed]
39. Erikson, K.M.; Dorman, D.C.; Fitsanakis, V.; Lash, L.H.; Aschner, M. Alterations of oxidative stress biomarkers due to in utero and neonatal exposures of airborne manganese. *Biol. Trace Elem. Res.* **2006**, *111*, 199–215. [CrossRef]
40. Duhig, K.; Chappell, L.C.; Shennan, A.H. Oxidative stress in pregnancy and reproduction. *Obstet. Med.* **2016**, *9*, 113–116. [CrossRef] [PubMed]
41. Rahman, M.L.; Oken, E.; Hivert, M.; Rifas-Shiman, S.; Lin, P.D.; Colicino, E.; Wright, R.O.; Amarasiriwardena, C.; Claus Henn, B.G.; Gold, D.R.; et al. Early pregnancy exposure to metal mixture and birth outcomes—A prospective study in Project Viva. *Environ. Int.* **2021**, *156*, 106714. [CrossRef]
42. Rivera-Núñez, Z.; Ashrap, P.; Barrett, E.S.; Watkins, D.J.; Cathey, A.L.; Vélez-Vega, C.M.; Rosario, Z.; Cordero, J.F.; Alshawabkeh, A.; Meeker, J.D. Association of biomarkers of exposure to metals and metalloids with maternal hormones in pregnant women from Puerto Rico. *Environ. Int.* **2021**, *147*, 106310. [CrossRef]
43. Kupsco, A.; Estrada-Gutierrez, G.; Cantoral, A.; Schnaas, L.; Pantic, I.; Amarasiriwardena, C.; Svensson, K.; Bellinger, D.C.; Tellez-Rojo, M.M.; Baccarelli, A.A.; et al. Modification of the effects of prenatal manganese exposure on child neurodevelopment by maternal anemia and iron deficiency. *Pediatr. Res.* **2020**, *88*, 325–333. [CrossRef]
44. Balasundaram, P.; Avulakunta, I.D. *Human Growth and Development*; StatPearls Publishing: Treasure Island, FL, USA, 2021.
45. Castillo-Durán, C.; Cassorla, F. Trace minerals in human growth and development. *J. Pediatr. Endocrinol. Metab.* **1999**, *12*, 589–601. [CrossRef]

46. Fan, Y.; Zhang, C.; Bu, J. Relationship between Selected Serum Metallic Elements and Obesity in Children and Adolescent in the U.S. *Nutrients* **2017**, *9*, 104. [CrossRef]
47. Kajee, N.; Sobngwi, E.; Macnab, A.; Daar, A.S. The Developmental Origins of Health and Disease and Sustainable Development Goals: Mapping the way forward. *J. Dev. Orig. Health Dis.* **2018**, *9*, 5–9. [CrossRef]
48. Toftlund, L.H.; Halken, S.; Agertoft, L.; Zachariassen, G. Catch-Up Growth, Rapid Weight Growth, and Continuous Growth from Birth to 6 Years of Age in Very-Preterm-Born Children. *Neonatology* **2018**, *114*, 285–293. [CrossRef]
49. Treinen, K.A.; Gray, T.J.; Blazak, W.F. Developmental toxicity of mangafodipir trisodium and manganese chloride in Sprague-Dawley rats. *Teratology* **1995**, *52*, 109–115. [CrossRef] [PubMed]
50. Sánchez, D.J.; Domingo, J.; Llobet, J.M.; Keen, C.L. Maternal and developmental toxicity of manganese in the mouse. *Toxicol. Lett.* **1993**, *69*, 45–52. [CrossRef]
51. Hansen, S.L.; Spears, J.W.; Lloyd, K.E.; Whisnant, C.S. Feeding a Low Manganese Diet to Heifers During Gestation Impairs Fetal Growth and Development. *J. Dairy Sci.* **2006**, *89*, 4305–4311. [CrossRef]
52. Tarale, P.; Daiwile, A.; Sivanesan, S.D.; Stöger, R.; Bafana, A.; Naoghare, P.; Parmar, D.; Chakrabarti, T.; Krishnamurthi, K. Manganese exposure: Linking down-regulation of miRNA−7 and miRNA−433 with α-synuclein overexpression and risk of idiopathic Parkinson's disease. *Toxicol. Vitr.* **2017**, *46*, 94–101. [CrossRef] [PubMed]
53. Keen, C.; Ensunsa, J.L.; Watson, M.H.; Baly, D.; Donovan, S.; Monaco, M.; Clegg, M. Nutritional aspects of manganese from experimental studies. *Neurotoxicology* **1999**, *20*, 213–223. [PubMed]
54. Lewandowska, M.; Lubiński, J. Serum Microelements in Early Pregnancy and their Risk of Large-for-Gestational Age Birth Weight. *Nutrients* **2020**, *12*, 866. [CrossRef] [PubMed]

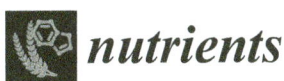

Article

The Association of Gene Variants in the Vitamin D Metabolic Pathway and Its Interaction with Vitamin D on Gestational Diabetes Mellitus: A Prospective Cohort Study

Minjia Mo [1,2,†], Bule Shao [1,3,†], Xing Xin [1,2], Wenliang Luo [1,2], Shuting Si [1,2], Wen Jiang [4], Shuojia Wang [1,2], Yu Shen [1,2], Jinhua Wu [4] and Yunxian Yu [1,2,*]

1. Department of Public Health, and Department of Anesthesiology, Second Affiliated Hospital of Zhejiang University School of Medicine, Hangzhou 310058, China; minjiamo@zju.edu.cn (M.M.); shaobl@163.com (B.S.); 21818488@zju.edu.cn (X.X.); 21918155@zju.edu.cn (W.L.); 21818499@zju.edu.cn (S.S.); wangsj2015@163.com (S.W.); shenyu_yoner@126.com (Y.S.)
2. Department of Epidemiology & Health Statistics, School of Public Health, School of Medicine, Zhejiang University, Hangzhou 310027, China
3. Department of Gastroenterology, Sir Run Run Shaw Hospital, School of Medicine, Zhejiang University, Hangzhou 310058, China
4. Zhoushan Maternal and Child Care Hospital, Zhoushan 316004, China; 21618436@zju.edu.cn (W.J.); 2012302170059@whu.edu.cn (J.W.)
* Correspondence: yunxianyu@zju.edu.cn; Tel.: +86-5718-8208-191
† These authors contributed equally to this work.

Abstract: The present prospective study included 2156 women and investigated the effect of gene variants in the vitamin D (VitD) metabolic and glucose pathways and their interaction with VitD levels during pregnancy on gestational diabetes mellitus (GDM). Plasma 25(OH)D concentrations were measured at the first and second trimesters. GDM subtype 1 was defined as those with isolated elevated fasting plasma glucose; GDM subtype 2 were those with isolated elevated postprandial glucose at 1 h and/or 2 h; and GDM subtype 3 were those with both elevated fasting plasma glucose and postprandial glucose. Six Gc isoforms were categorized based on two *GC* gene variants rs4588 and rs7041, including 1s/1s, 1s/2, 1s/1f, 2/2, 1f/2 and 1f/1f. *VDR*-rs10783219 and *MTNR1B*-rs10830962 were associated with increased risks of GDM and GDM subtype 2; interactions between each other as well as with *CDKAL1*-rs7754840 were observed ($P_{interaction} < 0.05$). Compared with the 1f/1f isoform, the risk of GDM subtype 2 among women with 1f/2, 2/2, 1s/1f, 1s/2 and 1s/1s isoforms and with prepregnancy body mass index ≥ 24 kg/m^2 increased by 5.11, 10.01, 10, 14.23, 19.45 times, respectively. Gene variants in VitD pathway interacts with VitD deficiency at the first trimester on the risk of GDM and GDM subtype 2.

Keywords: gestational diabetes mellitus; subtypes; gene polymorphism; vitamin D

1. Introduction

Gestational diabetes mellitus (GDM) is a growing public health problem [1,2] and associated with adverse perinatal and neonatal outcomes, including increased risks of gestational hypertension [3], preterm birth [4] and cardiovascular diseases [5]. Although a few risk factors of GDM have been identified, the etiology has not fully been elucidated [6].

Some research has focused on the genetic susceptibility of GDM. Moen et al. [7] found that *MAP3K1*-rs116745876, *PRKCE*-rs11682804 and *NUAK1*-rs11112715 were associated with higher fasting glucose levels at the first trimester and higher 2 h post-oral glucose levels at the second trimester in pregnant women. Other two single nucleotide polymorphisms (SNPs) *CDKAL1*-rs7754840 and *MTNR1B*-rs10830962 identified from a genome-wide association study of GDM were found to be highly correlated with GDM, and another one, *IGF2BP2*-rs1470579, was relatively weakly correlated [8]. On the other hand, genetic variants in the vitamin D (VitD) metabolic pathway were also found to be involved in the pathogenesis of insulin resistance and GDM [9–11]. The main circulating metabolite is 25(OH)D, a biomarker of VitD status. VitD metabolism is highly regulated, and variation in the expression or activity of key proteins may modify its level or effects. Key metabolic enzymes include: 25-hydroxylase (*CYP3A4*), which converts VitD to 25(OH)D; 1-hydroxylase (*CYP27B1*), which activates 25(OH)D to 1,25(OH)$_2$D; 24-hydroxylase (*CYP24A1*), which inactivates 25(OH)D and 1,25(OH)$_2$D; and megalin (*LRP2*), which reabsorbs 25(OH)D through endocytosis in the renal tubules. Other key components include vitamin D-binding protein (*GC*), which transports circulating metabolites, and the VitD receptor (*VDR*), which binds 1,25(OH)$_2$D to activate gene transcription and regulates VitD metabolism [12]. Compared to pregnant women with the CC genotype at *VDR*-rs1544410, the risk of GDM in pregnant women with the CT genotype was approximately doubled; compared to AA genotype at *VDR*-rs731236, the risk of GDM in pregnant women with the GA genotype was 1.42 times higher [13]. In addition, two SNPs, rs4588 and rs7041 on the *GC* gene, can form three allelic combinations (Gc1f, Gc1s and Gc2) and six different Gc isoforms, namely, 1s/1s, 1s/2, 1s/1f, 2/2, 1f/2 and 1f/1f [14,15]. According to the free hormone hypothesis, only free 25(OH)D and free 1,25(OH)$_2$D can directly exert biological functions [16,17], the proportion of which in blood were mostly influenced by the binding affinity of different Gc isoforms [18]. The polymorphism of VitD metabolic pathway genes, especially on the *GC* genes, may be good candidates to better understand how VitD levels are involved in the pathogenesis of GDM.

Most previous studies have regarded GDM as a homogenous disease, and little attention has been paid to GDM subtypes on the basis of the different time-point glucose levels of the oral glucose tolerance test (OGTT) [8,13]. Studies in non-pregnant women found that both isolated impaired fasting glucose (IFG) and isolated impaired glucose tolerance (IGT) patients were insulin resistance (IR) factors, but the target organs or tissues of IR were different [19–22]. Individuals with isolated IFG primarily manifest hepatic IR and relatively normal muscle IR. Otherwise, individuals with isolated IGT have normal to subtle hepatic IR and moderate to severe muscle IR. Thus, individuals with both IFG and IGT have both hepatic and muscle IR [19]. The different pathophysiological mechanisms of fasting and post-glycemic abnormalities result from distinct insulin sensitivity characteristics of the liver and muscle, respectively [20,21]. In addition, our previous population-based study found that VitD was associated with the occurrence of GDM with abnormal fasting glucose, especially among overweight/obese pregnant women, but not the occurrence of abnormal post-load glucose [23]. However, previous studies principally treated GDM as a dichotomous outcome when investigating the effects of gene variants on the VitD metabolic and glucose pathways on GDM, ignoring the different pathophysiological mechanisms of fasting and post-load glycemic abnormality [24].

Thus, the aim of this study was to explore the effect of gene variants in the VitD and glucose metabolic-pathway-related genes, and their interactions with 25(OH)D concentrations on the development of GDM and GDM subtypes.

2. Materials and Methods

2.1. Study Design and Participants

This prospective cohort study was based on the data of Zhoushan Pregnant Women Cohort (ZPWC) from August 2011 to May 2018, which is an ongoing prospective cohort conducted in Zhoushan Maternal and Child Health Care Hospital, Zhejiang. Pregnant women were invited to participate in the cohort at their first prenatal visit. A more detailed description of the inclusion and exclusion criteria has previously been described in detail [23]. Briefly, pregnant women aged between 18 and 45 years without serious physical, mental health disease, threatened abortion or fetal malformation, and who received OGTT were included in the study. Informed consent was obtained from all participants before the investigation.

2.2. Collection of Data and Blood Sample

A structured questionnaire was administrated face-to-face by an interviewer to collect information on socio-demographic, lifestyle, and health behavior at the first trimester (T1: 8th–14th gestational week), second trimester (T2: 24th–28th gestational week), third trimester (T3: 32nd–36th gestational week) and 42nd day postpartum. OGTT was conducted during T2 according to a conventional pregnant care program. A 5 mL fasting venous blood sample was drawn at each visit and centrifuged under 4 °C; then, the plasma and white blood cells were divided and stored under −80 °C until use. The results of the OGTT were extracted from the electronic medical records system.

2.3. Measurement of 25(OH)D Concentrations

Liquid chromatography–tandem mass spectrometry (API 3200MD (Applied Biosystems/MDS Sciex, Framingham, MA, USA)) was used to measure plasma $25(OH)D_2$ and $25(OH)D_3$ concentrations. The plasma 25(OH)D concentrations were reported in ng/mL, and the lowest sensitivity of the measurement was 2 ng/mL for $25(OH)D_2$ and 5 ng/mL for $25(OH)D_3$. The intra-assay coefficient variance values were 1.47–7.24% and 2.50–7.59% for $25(OH)D_2$ and $25(OH)D_3$, respectively. The inter-assay coefficients variances were 4.48–6.74% and 4.44–6.76% for $25(OH)D_2$ and $25(OH)D_3$, respectively [23]. The 25(OH)D concentrations were the sum of $25(OH)D_2$ and $25(OH)D_3$. The laboratory located in Hangzhou, Zhejiang Province, is CAP-accredited and annually participates in CAP Proficiency Tests and China NCCL Trueness Verification Plan of 25(OH)D Assays, for which satisfactory results in these PT or EQA tests have been obtained in consecutive years.

2.4. Covariates Assessment

Plasma 25(OH)D < 20 ng/mL (50 nmol/L) was defined as VitD deficiency according to Endocrine Society clinical practice guidelines [25], and 25(OH)D concentrations ≥20 ng/mL as VitD non-deficiency. Body mass index (BMI) = weight (kg)/height^2 (m^2). Prepregnancy BMI was divided into four categories based on the Working Group on Obesity in China [26]: underweight, BMI < 18.5 kg/m^2; normal, BMI 18.5–23.9 kg/m^2; overweight, BMI 24.0–27.9 kg/m^2; obesity, BMI ≥ 28 kg/m^2. VitD supplementation was categorized as "Yes", "No" and "Unknown". According to the sunshine intensity and duration in different months [27], the seasons of blood sampling were divided as follows: spring (March to May), summer (June to August), fall (September to November) and winter (December to February).

2.5. GDM and Its Subtypes Classification

GDM screening has become a routine examination among pregnant women in China. OGTT was conducted between the 24th and 28th weeks of gestation. After an overnight fast (at least 8 h), 75 g glucose resolved in 300 mL water was given and drunk within 5 min the next morning. Venous blood samples were taken at 0 h, 1 h and 2 h during OGTT for measuring plasma glucose levels. Plasma glucose levels were immediately measured by the hexokinase method with commercially available kits (Beckman AU5800, Beckman Coulter Inc., Brea, CA, USA). Using criteria proposed by the International Association of the Diabetes and Pregnancy Study Group [28], GDM was diagnosed if any one of the following criteria were met: fasting plasma glucose (FBG) at 0 h ≥5.1 mmol/L, postprandial glucose at 1 h (PG1H) ≥10 mmol/L, or postprandial glucose at 2 h (PG2H) ≥8.5 mmol/L. In addition, according to different types of insulin resistance represented by the blood glucose level at the three time-point glucose levels examined by OGTT [22–24], GDM was further categorized into the following three subtypes: GDM subtype 1, with isolated FBG ≥ 5.1 mmol/L; GDM subtype 2, with isolated PG1H ≥ 10 mmol/L and/or PG2H ≥ 8.5 mmol/L; and GDM subtype 3, with both elevated FBG (≥5.1 mmol/L) and post-load plasma glucose (PG1H ≥ 10 mmol/L and/or PG2H ≥ 8.5 mmol/L).

2.6. SNP Selection and Genotyping

GDM-related SNP selection: to verify the previous findings by Kwak et al. [8] in Korean pregnant women and Moen et al. [7] among pregnant women in Norway, 3 SNPs (*CDKAL1*-rs7754840, *MTNR1B*-rs10830962 and *IGF2BP2*-rs1470579) related to GDM [8] and 3 SNPs (*MAP3K1*-rs116745876, *PRKCE*-rs11682804 and *NUAK1*-rs11112715) related to blood glucose during pregnancy were selected [7]. According to the minor allele frequency ≥ 10 of each SNP in the Chinese population from the 1000 Genomes Project database, 4 GDM-related SNPs, *CDKAL1*-rs7754840, *MTNR1B*-rs10830962, *IGF2BP2*-rs1470579 and *PRKCE*-rs11682804, were finally included.

VitD-related SNP selection: the selection conditions of the VitD-related SNP in the study were as follows (satisfy any one) [15]: (1) a positive association between SNP and 25(OH)D concentration reported in the literature, and the minimum allele frequency (Minor allele frequency, MAF) $\geq 10\%$; (2) SNPs displayed in the functional region in the NCBI database: exon region, intron splicing point, 5′end and 3′end regulatory regions, and MAF $\geq 10\%$; (3) HapMap Chinese database, including gene regions, SNPs within 1500 bp at the 5′end and 3′end, using HaploView to select SNPs, and the conditions are: MAF $\geq 10\%$; $R^2 \geq 0.8$ [15]. In addition, *VDR* is closely related to insulin secretion [29,30], and *VDR*-rs11568820 is a functional SNP of the *VDR* gene. Previous studies found that rs10783219 and rs11568820 on *VDR* have high LD ($r^2 = 0.98$). Therefore, the rs10783219 was selected as the surrogate SNP of rs11568820 [15]. Finally, a total of 13 SNPs related to 25(OH)D concentration in the VitD metabolic pathway were selected (*CYP24A1*: rs2209314, *CYP3A4*: rs2242480, *GC*: rs1155563, rs16846876, rs17467825, rs2282679, rs2298849, rs2298850, rs3755967, rs4588, rs7041, *LRP2*: rs10210408 and *VDR*: rs10783219).

Gc isoforms: based on two SNPs, rs4588 and rs7041, on the *GC* gene, the Gc isoform was categorized into six different isoforms, including 1s/1s, 1s/2, 1s/1f, 2/2, 1f/2 and 1f/1f, of which the proportions of free 25(OH)D were successively reduced. The 1f/1f isoform with the highest proportion of free 25(OH)D was used as the reference group.

The conventional phenol–chloroform extraction method was used to extract DNA from the peripheral blood leukocytes, which was then stored in TE-buffer at -80 °C. For SNP analysis, DNA was then diluted to 10 ng/μL using a Nanodrop® ND-1000 Spectrophotometer (Thermo Fisher Scientific Inc., Wilmington, NC, USA). A Sequenom MassARRAY iPLEX Gold platform (Sequenom, San Diego, CA, USA) was used for SNP genotyping. In total, 17 SNPs were available for further analysis. The call rate of these SNPs was over 98%, which conformed to the Hardy–Weinberg equilibrium.

2.7. Statistical Analysis

t-tests and Wilcoxon signed-rank tests were used to compare the characteristics between GDM and non-GDM groups for continuous variables. Variance analysis was used to compare the characteristics between different GDM subtypes for continuous variables, and chi-squared tests were used for categorical variables between groups. Multiple linear regression models were used to analyze the association of SNPs in VitD and glucose metabolic-pathway-related genes, and their interactions with 25(OH)D concentrations at T1 and T2 with the blood glucose levels of each OGTT timepoint in a co-dominant genetic model. Multiple logistic regression models were used to analyze the relationship of SNPs, Gc isoforms and their interaction with 25(OH)D concentration at T1 and T2 with GDM as well as its subtypes in a co-dominant genetic model. Furthermore, stratification analysis by prepregnancy BMI was carried out to investigate the association between Gc isoforms and the risk of GDM and its subtypes [23]. To investigate the interaction between *VDR*-rs10783219, *CDKAL1*-rs7754840 and *MTNR1B*-rs10830962 on the risk of GDM and its subtypes, stratification analysis was carried out. In addition, to investigate the joint association of VitD status at T1 or/and T2 with Gc isoforms on the risk of GDM and its subtypes, we classified Gc isoforms into three groups—1f/1f and 1f/2; 2/2 and 1s/1f; and 1s/2 and 1s/1s—and crossover analysis was carried out. The hierarchical analysis was used to investigate the interaction between each SNP and 25(OH)D concentration on the risk of GDM, and the *p*-value of the interaction term was calculated. To investigate whether there was a dose–effect relationship between Gc isoforms and subtypes of GDM, a trend test was applied in the multiple logistic regression model and Gc isoforms were treated as continuous variables for different isoforms (1s/1s, 1s/2, 1s/1f, 2/2, 1f/2 and 1f/1f), of which the proportion of free 25(OH)D was successively reduced. The above multi-factor models were all adjusted for possible confounding, including maternal age, prepregnancy BMI, OGTT season, etc. All test results were considered statistically significant at a value of $p < 0.05$. All analyses were performed using SAS (version 9.2, SAS Institute).

Sample size calculation: in the present study, the risks of GDM subtype 2 of GG genotype in *MTNR1B*-rs10830962 were 1.85 times greater than compared with the CC genotype. The prevalence of GDM in this study was 23.8%; among them, 58.5% were GDM subtype 2. We hypothesized that $\alpha = 0.05$, power = 80%, $OR_{gene} = 1.85$, and the genotype frequency for SNP was 18%. Through QUANTO software, it was determined that the minimum case number for the GDM subtype 2 was 118, and the minimum case number for GDM was 202, which is lower than the number of GDM cases in this study ($n = 513$). Therefore, the sample size was large enough for the analysis of different GDM subtypes.

3. Results

3.1. Subject Characteristics

A total of 2156 pregnant women were included in this study, and the characteristics of the participants are shown in Table 1. Of these, 513 (23.8%) women were diagnosed with GDM. The mean age and prepregnancy BMI of participants were 28.8 years old and 20.7 kg/m², respectively. Compared with non-GDM women, women with GDM had higher prepregnancy BMI, lower 25(OH)D concentrations at T2 and lower educational levels. As shown in Supplementary Table S1, compared with participants with GDM subtype 1, those with GDM subtype 2 and 3 were older and had higher VitD levels at T1 and T2.

Table 1. Baseline characteristics of pregnant women.

Variables	Total	non-GDM	GDM	*p*
	$n = 2156$	$n = 1643$	$n = 513$	
Age, years	28.8 (3.7)	28.5 (3.5)	29.6 (4.0)	<0.0001
Prepregnancy BMI (kg/m²)	20.7 (2.8)	20.6 (2.7)	21.3 (3.0)	<0.0001
25(OH)D at T1 (ng/mL) *	18.9 (8.7)	18.7 (8.7)	19.5 (8.6)	0.0884
25(OH)D$_3$	18.1 (8.6)	17.9 (8.6)	18.7 (8.6)	0.0530
25(OH)D$_2$ ¶	0.6 (0.5)	0.6 (0.5)	0.5 (0.4)	0.9761 ⁋
25(OH)D at T2 (ng/mL) †	25.6 (11.5)	26.0 (11.7)	24.1 (10.7)	0.0149
25(OH)D$_3$	24.6 (11.5)	24.9 (11.7)	23.3 (10.8)	0.0310
25(OH)D$_2$ ¶	0.7 (0.7)	0.6 (0.7)	0.7 (0.6)	0.6255 ⁋
VitD deficiency at T1 *	1281 (62.3%)	983 (62.8%)	298 (60.7%)	0.3979
VitD deficiency at T2 †	499 (36.4%)	374 (34.8%)	125 (42.2%)	0.0180
GDM rate	513 (23.8%)	—	—	—
OGTT season				0.0920
Summer/fall	1045 (48.5%)	813 (49.5%)	232 (45.2%)	
Winter/spring	1111 (51.5%)	830 (50.5%)	281 (54.8%)	
Educational level				0.0179
≤High school	589 (27.3%)	428 (26.0%)	161 (31.4%)	
>High school	1567 (72.7%)	1215 (74.0%)	352 (68.6%)	
Income per capita, RMB				0.3659
<30,000	191 (8.9%)	143 (8.7%)	48 (9.4%)	
≥30,000	1647 (76.4%)	1269 (77.2%)	378 (73.7%)	
Not sure	180 (8.3%)	132 (8.0%)	48 (9.4%)	
Unknown	138 (6.4%)	99 (6.0%)	39 (7.6%)	
Planned pregnancy				0.0411
No	709 (32.9%)	563 (34.3%)	146 (28.5%)	
Yes	1313 (60.9%)	983 (59.8%)	330 (64.3%)	
Unknown	134 (6.2%)	97 (5.9%)	37 (7.2%)	

Table 1. Cont.

Variables	Total n = 2156	non-GDM n = 1643	GDM n = 513	p
Marital status				0.5033
Not married	47 (2.2%)	35 (2.1%)	12 (2.3%)	
Married	1976 (91.7%)	1512 (92.0%)	464 (90.4%)	
Unknown	133 (6.2%)	96 (5.8%)	37 (7.2%)	
VitD supplement				0.4623
0/week	765 (35.5%)	593 (36.1%)	172 (33.5%)	
>0/week	1233 (57.2%)	934 (56.8%)	299 (58.3%)	
Unknown	158 (7.3%)	116 (7.1%)	42 (8.2%)	
Primiparity				0.1854
No	491 (22.8%)	359 (21.9%)	132 (25.7%)	
Yes	1498 (69.5%)	1156 (70.4%)	342 (66.7%)	
Unknown	167 (7.7%)	128 (7.8%)	39 (7.6%)	
Physical exercise				0.0775
0/week	1717 (79.6%)	1326 (80.7%)	391 (76.2%)	
>0/week	292 (13.5%)	213 (13.0%)	79 (15.4%)	
Unknown	147 (6.8%)	104 (6.3%)	43 (8.4%)	

Abbreviations: GDM, gestational diabetes mellitus; VitD, vitamin D; T1, first trimester; T2, second trimester; OGTT, oral glucose tolerance test. * n = 2056, † n = 1372, ¶ Presented as the median (interquartile range), P compared by Wilcoxon signed-rank test.

3.2. Associations of SNPs and Its Interaction with VitD on GDM and GDM Subtypes

Compared with the wild-type genotype, the PG1H and/or PG2H levels of mutant genotypes were lower for *LRP2*-rs10210408, and higher for *VDR*-rs10783219, *CDKAL1*-rs7754840 and *MTNR1B*-rs10830962. Interactions between 25(OH)D concentrations at T1 and the CT genotype in *CYP3A4*-rs2242480, GA genotype in *GC*-rs2298849 and CC genotype in *CDKAL1*-rs7754840 on PG1H level, and the CT genotype in *CYP24A1*-rs2209314, TT genotype in *GC*-rs16846876 and GA genotype in *GC*-rs2298849 on PG2H level were observed (Supplementary Table S2, all $P_{interaction}$ < 0.05). The risks of GDM and GDM subtype 2 of TA genotype in *VDR*-rs10783219 were 1.26 and 1.33 times greater compared with the AA genotype (Table 2). Compared with the CC genotype, GG genotypes in *MTNR1B*-rs10830962 were at higher risk of GDM (Table 2, OR = 2.08, 95% CI: 1.46–2.97), GDM subtype 1 (Table 2, OR = 3.26, 95% CI: 1.62–6.59) and subtype 2 (Table 2, OR = 1.85, 95% CI: 1.22–2.81). Compared with the wild-type genotypes, interactions between 25(OH)D concentrations at T1 and the CT genotype in *CYP3A4*-rs2242480, and the TT genotype in *LRP2*-rs10210408 on the risk of GDM and GDM subtype 2 were found (Table 2). However, interactions between SNPs and 25(OH)D concentrations at T2 on FBG, PG1H and PG2H levels of OGTT as well as GDM and its subtypes were not observed.

As shown in Table 3, significant interactions between *CDKAL1*-rs7754840 and *VDR*-rs10783219 on the risk of GDM and GDM subtype 2 ($P_{interaction}$: 0.0121 and 0.0432) as well as interactions between *CDKAL1*-rs7754840 and *MTNR1B*-rs10830962 on the risk of GDM and GDM subtype 1 ($P_{interaction}$: 0.0082 and 0.0071) were found.

3.3. Associations of Gc Isoforms and VitD with GDM and GDM Subtypes

Compared to women with Gc isoforms of 1f/1f, those with Gc isoforms of 2/2 and 1s/2 had higher levels of PG1H and PG2H among women with prepregnancy BMI ≥ 24 kg/m^2 (Supplementary Table S3). In addition, after adjusting for potential confounders, dose–effect relationships of Gc isoforms with GDM and GDM subtype 2 (P_{trend}: 0.0046 and 0.0011, Supplementary Table S4) were observed among women with prepregnancy BMI ≥ 24 kg/m^2. Compared to women with Gc isoforms of 1f/1f and 1f/2 and VitD non-deficiency at T1 and T2, those with Gc isoforms of 1s/2 and 1s/1s had increased risk of GDM and GDM subtype 2 (OR = 2.21, 95% CI: 1.14–4.30; OR = 2.79, 95% CI: 1.20–6.49, Table 4). However, combined effect of 25(OH)D concentrations at T1 or T2 with Gc isoforms on the risk of GDM and GDM subtypes were not observed (Table 4).

Table 2. Relationship of SNPs in VitD and glucose metabolic pathway and its interaction with 25(OH)D concentrations at T1 and T2 with GDM and GDM subtypes *.

SNPs	Genotypes	n	GDM † Case (%)	GDM † OR (95% CI)	GDM Subtype 1 ‡ Case (%)	GDM Subtype 1 ‡ OR (95% CI)	GDM Subtype 2 ‡ Case (%)	GDM Subtype 2 ‡ OR (95% CI)	GDM Subtype 3 ‡ Case (%)	GDM Subtype 3 ‡ OR (95% CI)
			VitD-related SNPs							
CYP24A1 rs2209314	TT	770	193 (25.1)	Ref	62 (8.1)	Ref	106 (13.8)	Ref	25 (3.2)	Ref
	CT	1039	244 (23.5)	0.93 (0.75–1.17)	62 (6.0)	0.71 (0.49–1.04)	151 (14.5)	1.07 (0.81–1.42)	31 (3.0)	0.92 (0.53–1.61)
	CC	335	75 (22.4)	0.86 (0.63–1.17)	20 (6.0)	0.72 (0.42–1.23)	42 (12.5)	0.89 (0.60–1.33)	13 (3.9)	1.10 (0.54–2.27)
CYP3A4 rs2242480	CC	1229	292 (23.8)	Ref	85 (6.9)	Ref	170 (13.8)	Ref	37 (3.0)	Ref
	CT	790	191 (24.2)	1.04 (0.84–1.29) ‖	54 (6.8)	1.13 (0.78–1.63)	109 (13.8)	0.97 (0.74–1.26)	28 (3.5)	1.32 (0.78–2.23)
	TT	125	28 (22.4)	0.96 (0.61–1.51)	5 (4.0)	0.59 (0.23–1.53)	19 (15.2)	1.08 (0.63–1.82)	4 (3.2)	1.30 (0.43–3.92)
GC rs1155563	TT	761	169 (22.2)	Ref	47 (6.2)	Ref	95 (12.5)	Ref	27 (3.5)	Ref
	TC	1019	248 (24.3)	1.15 (0.91–1.44)	72 (7.1)	1.16 (0.78–1.72)	146 (14.3)	1.20 (0.90–1.60)	30 (2.9)	0.90 (0.52–1.57)
	CC	362	94 (26.0)	1.19 (0.88–1.60)	25 (6.9)	1.13 (0.67–1.89)	57 (15.7)	1.29 (0.89–1.86)	12 (3.3)	0.89 (0.43–1.84) ‖
rs16846876	AA	1017	229 (22.5)	Ref	63 (6.2)	Ref	126 (12.4)	Ref	40 (3.9)	Ref
	AT	899	220 (24.5)	1.09 (0.87–1.35)	62 (6.9)	1.10 (0.76–1.60)	137 (15.2)	1.25 (0.95–1.63)	21 (2.3)	0.54 (0.31–0.94)
	TT	231	61 (26.4)	1.17 (0.84–1.64)	19 (8.2)	1.31 (0.75–2.29)	34 (14.7)	1.25 (0.82–1.90)	8 (3.5)	0.78 (0.34–1.75)
rs17467825	AA	1008	228 (22.6)	Ref	61 (6.1)	Ref	132 (13.1)	Ref	35 (3.5)	Ref
	GA	909	224 (24.6)	1.10 (0.89–1.36)	66 (7.3)	1.15 (0.79–1.66)	132 (14.5)	1.15 (0.88–1.50)	26 (2.9)	0.79 (0.46–1.35)
	GG	234	59 (25.2)	1.08 (0.77–1.51)	16 (6.8)	1.05 (0.58–1.89)	35 (15.0)	1.18 (0.78–1.80)	8 (3.4)	0.81 (0.36–1.85)
rs2282679	TT	1009	227 (22.5)	Ref	61 (6.0)	Ref	130 (12.9)	Ref	36 (3.6)	Ref
	GT	899	224 (24.9)	1.13 (0.91–1.40)	67 (7.5)	1.18 (0.81–1.71)	132 (14.7)	1.20 (0.92–1.57)	25 (2.8)	0.75 (0.44–1.29)
	GG	241	60 (24.9)	1.07 (0.76–1.50)	16 (6.6)	1.00 (0.55–1.81)	36 (14.9)	1.20 (0.80–1.82)	8 (3.3)	0.77 (0.34–1.74)
rs2298849	AA	894	216 (24.2)	Ref	66 (7.4)	Ref	120 (13.4)	Ref	30 (3.4)	Ref
	GA	960	231 (24.1)	1.03 (0.83–1.28)	58 (6.0)	0.82 (0.56–1.20)	145 (15.1)	1.16 (0.88–1.52)	28 (2.9)	0.93 (0.54–1.61)
	GG	299	65 (21.7)	0.87 (0.63–1.19)	20 (6.7)	0.89 (0.52–1.51)	34 (11.4)	0.80 (0.53–1.21)	11 (3.7)	1.08 (0.52–2.26)
rs2298850	GG	982	221 (22.5)	Ref	60 (6.1)	Ref	127 (12.9)	Ref	34 (3.5)	Ref
	CG	911	227 (24.9)	1.13 (0.91–1.40)	67 (7.4)	1.17 (0.81–1.70)	134 (14.7)	1.19 (0.91–1.55)	26 (2.9)	0.80 (0.47–1.38)
	CC	240	59 (24.6)	1.06 (0.75–1.48)	16 (6.7)	0.99 (0.55–1.80)	35 (14.6)	1.17 (0.77–1.78)	8 (3.3)	0.81 (0.36–1.83)
rs3755967	CC	1005	226 (22.5)	Ref	61 (6.1)	Ref	130 (12.9)	Ref	35 (3.5)	Ref
	CT	907	226 (24.9)	1.14 (0.91–1.41)	67 (7.4)	1.17 (0.81–1.70)	133 (14.7)	1.20 (0.91–1.57)	26 (2.9)	0.80 (0.47–1.37)
	TT	241	60 (24.9)	1.07 (0.76–1.50)	16 (6.6)	1.00 (0.55–1.80)	36 (14.9)	1.20 (0.79–1.81)	8 (3.3)	0.79 (0.35–1.79)
rs4588	GG	994	226 (22.7)	Ref	61 (6.1)	Ref	129 (13.0)	Ref	36 (3.6)	Ref
	GT	909	226 (24.9)	1.11 (0.89–1.38)	67 (7.4)	1.15 (0.80–1.67)	134 (14.7)	1.18 (0.90–1.55)	25 (2.8)	0.73 (0.42–1.25)
	TT	241	59 (24.5)	1.02 (0.73–1.44)	16 (6.6)	0.97 (0.54–1.75)	35 (14.5)	1.14 (0.75–1.73)	8 (3.3)	0.75 (0.33–1.70)
rs7041	AA	1162	271 (23.3)	Ref	79 (6.8)	Ref	153 (13.2)	Ref	39 (3.4)	Ref
	CA	826	201 (24.3)	1.08 (0.87–1.34)	57 (6.9)	1.07 (0.74–1.54)	119 (14.4)	1.13 (0.86–1.47)	25 (3.0)	0.93 (0.55–1.59)
	CC	162	41 (25.3)	1.22 (0.82–1.79)	8 (4.9)	0.89 (0.42–1.93)	28 (17.3)	1.38 (0.87–2.18)	5 (3.1)	1.25 (0.46–3.35)
LRP2 rs10210408	CC	703	181 (25.7)	Ref	45 (6.4)	Ref	110 (15.6)	Ref	26 (3.7)	Ref
	TC	1065	229 (21.5)	0.78 (0.62–0.99)	67 (6.3)	0.92 (0.61–1.37)	132 (12.4)	0.73 (0.55–0.97)	30 (2.8)	0.77 (0.44–1.34)
	TT	385	102 (26.5)	1.07 (0.80–1.43) ‖	32 (8.3)	1.32 (0.81–2.16)	57 (14.8)	0.97 (0.68–1.39) ‖	13 (3.4)	1.09 (0.54–2.21)
VDR rs10783219	AA	809	173 (21.4)	Ref	51 (6.3)	Ref	100 (12.4)	Ref	22 (2.7)	Ref
	TA	1010	254 (25.1)	1.26 (1.00–1.58) §	67 (6.6)	1.08 (0.73–1.60)	154 (15.2)	1.33 (1.01–1.76) §	33 (3.3)	1.32 (0.74–2.33)
	TT	332	86 (25.9)	1.32 (0.98–1.80)	26 (7.8)	1.35 (0.81–2.25)	46 (13.9)	1.24 (0.84–1.82)	14 (4.2)	1.66 (0.81–3.41)
rs10783219	AA	809	173 (21.4)	Ref	51 (6.3)	Ref	100 (12.4)	Ref	22 (2.7)	Ref
	TA/TT	1342	340 (25.3)	1.28 (1.03–1.58) §	93 (6.9)	1.15 (0.80–1.65)	200 (14.9)	1.31 (1.01–1.71) §	47 (3.5)	1.40 (0.82–2.40)
			GDM-related SNPs							
CDKAL1 rs7754840	GG	635	128 (20.2)	Ref	24 (3.8)	Ref	85 (13.4)	Ref	19 (3.0)	Ref
	GC	820	164 (20.0)	0.99 (0.76–1.29)	31 (3.8)	1.11 (0.63–1.95)	111 (13.5)	1.01 (0.74–1.38)	22 (2.7)	0.89 (0.46–1.70)
	CC	264	63 (23.9)	1.35 (0.95–1.92)	12 (4.5)	1.40 (0.67–2.91)	39 (14.8)	1.25 (0.82–1.91)	12 (4.5)	1.82 (0.84–3.95)
rs7754840	GG/GC	1455	292 (20.1)	Ref	55 (3.8)	Ref	196 (13.5)	Ref	41 (2.8)	Ref
	CC	264	63 (23.9)	1.43 (1.03–1.97) §	12 (4.5)	1.32 (0.68–2.56)	39 (14.8)	1.24 (0.85–1.83)	12 (4.5)	1.94 (0.97–3.88)
IGF2BP2 rs1470579	AA	966	203 (21.0)	Ref	39 (4.0)	Ref	136 (14.1)	Ref	28 (2.9)	Ref
	CA	664	133 (20.0)	0.95 (0.73–1.22)	25 (3.8)	0.94 (0.55–1.59)	85 (12.8)	0.89 (0.66–1.20)	23 (3.5)	1.25 (0.70–2.24)
	CC	89	18 (20.2)	0.96 (0.55–1.66)	3 (3.4)	0.87 (0.26–2.96)	13 (14.6)	1.02 (0.54–1.92)	2 (2.2)	0.83 (0.19–3.76)
MTNR1B rs10830962	CC	572	91 (15.9)	Ref	17 (3.0)	Ref	62 (10.8)	Ref	12 (2.1)	Ref
	GC	850	186 (21.9)	1.52 (1.14–2.03) §	30 (3.5)	1.45 (0.77–2.72)	122 (14.4)	1.43 (1.02–2.00) §	34 (4.0)	2.38 (1.18–4.81) §
	GG	297	78 (26.3)	2.08 (1.46–2.97) §	20 (6.7)	3.26 (1.62–6.59) §	51 (17.2)	1.85 (1.22–2.81) §	7 (2.4)	1.83 (0.68–4.88)
PRKCE rs11682804	GG	839	158 (18.8)	Ref	30 (3.6)	Ref	106 (12.6)	Ref	22 (2.6)	Ref
	AG	745	166 (22.3)	1.21 (0.94–1.56)	29 (3.9)	1.17 (0.69–2.01)	112 (15.0)	1.23 (0.91–1.66)	25 (3.4)	1.26 (0.69–2.31)
	AA	138	31 (22.5)	1.22 (0.78–1.90)	8 (5.8)	1.60 (0.69–3.71)	17 (12.3)	0.95 (0.54–1.69)	6 (4.3)	1.91 (0.73–4.98)

Abbreviations: GDM, gestational diabetes mellitus; VitD, vitamin D; subtype 1, elevated fasting glucose and normal post-load glucose; subtype 2, normal fasting glucose and elevated post-load glucose; subtype 3, elevated fasting and post-load glucose. * Adjusted for maternal age, prepregnancy BMI, parity, educational level, income, physical exercise and OGTT season. † Binomial logistic regression model; ‡ multinomial logistic regression model. § $p < 0.05$; ‖ p-value of the interaction term SNPs * 25(OH)D concentration at the first trimester < 0.05.

Table 3. Interactions between CDKAL1, MTNR1B and VDR on risk of GDM and GDM subtypes *.

SNPs	Risk Allele of GDM	n	GDM [†]		GDM Subtype 1 [‡]		GDM Subtype 2 [‡]		GDM Subtype 3 [‡]	
			Case (%)	OR (95% CI)	Case (%)	OR (95% CI)	Case (%)	OR (95% CI)	Case (%)	OR (95% CI)
CDKAL1-rs7754840	VDR-rs10783219									
GG	T	633	128 (20.2)	0.81 (0.60–1.09)	24 (3.8)	0.80 (0.43–1.50)	85 (13.4)	0.76 (0.53–1.08)	19 (3.0)	1.05 (0.52–2.10)
GC	T	819	164 (20.0)	1.35 (1.05–1.75) [§]	31 (3.8)	1.55 (0.91–2.63)	111 (13.6)	1.34 (1.00–1.81) [§]	22 (2.7)	1.14 (0.61–2.13)
CC	T	264	63 (23.8)	1.36 (0.89–2.08)	12 (4.6)	1.36 (0.52–3.59)	39 (14.8)	1.16 (0.69–1.95)	12 (4.6)	2.82 (0.99–8.04)
GC/CC	T	1083	227 (21.0)	1.37 (1.10–1.70) [§]	43 (4.0)	1.51 (0.95–2.38)	150 (13.9)	1.31 (1.02–1.70) [§]	34 (3.1)	1.49 (0.90–2.44)
			$P_{interaction}$ = 0.0121		$P_{interaction}$ = 0.2036		$P_{interaction}$ = 0.0432		$P_{interaction}$ = 0.1768	
MTNR1B-rs10830962	VDR-rs10783219									
CC	T	572	91 (15.9)	1.26 (0.91–1.76)	17 (3.0)	1.35 (0.64–2.87)	62 (10.8)	1.27 (0.85–1.88)	12 (2.1)	1.31 (0.54–3.18)
GC	T	848	186 (21.9)	0.90 (0.71–1.16)	30 (3.5)	0.72 (0.40–1.27)	122 (14.4)	0.89 (0.67–1.19)	34 (4.0)	1.15 (0.69–1.94)
GG	T	296	78 (26.4)	1.88 (1.20–2.94) [§]	20 (6.8)	2.99 (1.34–6.68) [§]	51 (17.2)	1.59 (0.94–2.69)	7 (2.4)	1.70 (0.50–5.76)
			$P_{interaction}$ = 0.5882		$P_{interaction}$ = 0.2611		$P_{interaction}$ = 0.9631		$P_{interaction}$ = 0.8731	
MTNR1B-rs10830962	CDKAL1-rs7754840									
CC	C	572	91 (15.9)	0.89 (0.63–1.24)	17 (3.0)	0.77 (0.37–1.61)	62 (10.8)	0.97 (0.65–1.45)	12 (2.1)	0.74 (0.31–1.74)
GC	C	848	186 (21.9)	1.08 (0.84–1.38)	30 (3.5)	0.86 (0.48–1.53)	122 (14.4)	1.08 (0.81–1.44)	34 (4.0)	1.32 (0.78–2.24)
GG	C	297	78 (26.3)	1.89 (1.23–2.91) [§]	20 (6.7)	3.06 (1.41–6.66) [§]	51 (17.2)	1.48 (0.90–2.46)	7 (2.4)	3.66 (0.94–14.26)
			$P_{interaction}$ = 0.0082		$P_{interaction}$ = 0.0071		$P_{interaction}$ = 0.1849		$P_{interaction}$ = 0.0653	

Abbreviations: GDM, gestational diabetes mellitus; subtype 1, elevated fasting glucose and normal post-load glucose; subtype 2, normal fasting glucose and elevated post-load glucose; subtype 3, elevated fasting and post-load glucose. * Adjusted for maternal age, prepregnancy BMI, parity, educational level, income, physical exercise and OGTT season. [†] Binomial logistic regression model; [‡] multinomial logistic regression model. [§] $p < 0.05$.

Table 4. The relationship of VitD status at T1 and T2, Gc isoforms with GDM and GDM subtypes *.

VitD Deficiency T1	VitD Deficiency T2	Gc Isoforms	n	GDM [a]		GDM Subtype 1 [b]		GDM Subtype 2 [b]		GDM Subtype 3 [b]	
				Case (%)	OR (95% CI)	Case (%)	OR (95% CI)	Case (%)	OR (95% CI)	Case (%)	OR (95% CI)
No	No	1f/1f and 1f/2	148	24 (16.2)	Ref	7 (4.7)	Ref	12 (8.1)	Ref	5 (3.4)	Ref
		2/2 and 1s/1f	116	17 (14.7)	0.98 (0.49–1.95)	4 (3.5)	0.73 (0.20–2.60)	9 (7.8)	1.12 (0.44–2.82)	4 (3.5)	1.13 (0.28–4.56)
		1s/2 and 1s/1s	85	23 (27.1)	2.21 (1.14–4.30) [▸]	3 (3.5)	1.02 (0.25–4.14)	15 (17.7)	2.79 (1.20–6.49) [▸]	5 (5.9)	2.55 (0.66–9.92)
No	Yes	1f/1f and 1f/2	31	11 (35.5)	2.91 (1.19–7.14) [▸]	6 (19.4)	4.31 (1.23–15.05) [▸]	2 (6.5)	1.31 (0.26–6.58)	3 (9.7)	3.83 (0.74–19.89)
		2/2 and 1s/1f	27	7 (25.9)	2.16 (0.80–5.84)	3 (11.1)	2.19 (0.50–9.71)	3 (11.1)	2.37 (0.59–9.56)	1 (3.7)	1.69 (0.17–17.04)
		1s/2 and 1s/1s	26	5 (19.2)	1.36 (0.46–4.05)	5 (19.2)	3.39 (0.95–12.09)	0 (0.0)	—	0 (0.0)	—
Yes	No	1f/1f and 1f/2	195	43 (22.05)	1.94 (1.09–3.45) [▸]	12 (6.2)	1.89 (0.71–5.08)	27 (13.9)	2.27 (1.07–4.82) [▸]	4 (2.1)	1.24 (0.30–5.14)
		2/2 and 1s/1f	163	33 (20.3)	1.67 (0.92–3.06)	10 (6.1)	1.83 (0.66–5.08)	21 (12.9)	1.95 (0.89–4.25)	2 (1.2)	0.60 (0.11–3.37)
		1s/2 and 1s/1s	100	21 (21.0)	1.87 (0.95–3.67)	4 (4.0)	1.28 (0.36–4.65)	17 (17.0)	2.56 (1.11–5.87) [▸]	0 (0.0)	—
Yes	Yes	1f/1f and 1f/2	165	35 (21.2)	1.71 (0.94–3.11)	22 (13.3)	3.04 (1.21–7.61) [▸]	8 (4.9)	0.80 (0.30–2.11)	5 (3.0)	1.57 (0.41–6.07)
		2/2 and 1s/1f	113	31 (27.4)	2.27 (1.22–4.22) [▸]	16 (14.2)	3.59 (1.38–9.33) [▸]	12 (10.6)	1.81 (0.75–4.36)	3 (2.7)	1.40 (0.31–6.38)
		1s/2 and 1s/1s	95	22 (23.2)	1.84 (0.94–3.60)	9 (9.5)	2.29 (0.79–6.58)	8 (8.4)	1.37 (0.51–3.64)	5 (5.3)	2.59 (0.67–10.02)

Abbreviations: GDM, gestational diabetes mellitus; VitD, vitamin D; T1, first trimester; T2, second trimester; subtype 1, elevated fasting glucose and normal post-load glucose; subtype 2, normal fasting glucose and elevated post-load glucose; subtype 3, elevated fasting and post-load glucose. * Adjusted for maternal age, prepregnancy BMI, parity, educational level, income, physical exercise and OGTT season. [a] Binomial logistic regression model; [b] multinomial logistic regression model. [▸] $p < 0.05$.

4. Discussion

The current study demonstrated significant associations of variant genotype of SNPs at VDR-rs10783219 and MTNR1B-rs10830962 with the risk of GDM and GDM subtype 2. Furthermore, CDKAL1-rs7754840 interacts with VDR-rs10783219 and MTNR1B-rs10830962 on GDM subtypes. In addition, among women with prepregnancy BMI ≥ 24 kg/m^2, a dose–effect relationship between Gc isoforms and GDM subtype 2 was observed.

The LRP2 gene plays an important role in the preservation of vitamin D metabolites and delivery of the precursor to the kidney for the generation of 1α,25(OH)$_2$D$_3$ [15,31], polymorphisms of which were associated with increased risks of severe VitD deficiency and related bone disease [32]. Our study initially found that variation at *LRP2*-rs10210408 was related to higher postprandial glucose levels among pregnant women. In addition, interactions between *LRP2*-rs10210408 and VitD level at T1 on the risk of GDM and GDM subtype 2 were found, which indicated that variations of the A allele to T at *LRP2*-rs10210408 might influence glucose metabolism through VitD during pregnancy.

VDR-rs11568820 is a functional SNP and its variant may improve the islet activity of the calcium-sensing receptor, which further inhibits insulin secretion [33]. Only one study has reported that the variant at *VDR*-rs11568820 impairs the secretion of pancreatic islets and increases the risk of type 2 diabetes in the adult cohort and PG2H in children [30]. In the present study, we identified that the homozygous variant at *VDR*-rs10783219 in pregnant women was associated with higher PG1H ($\beta = 0.24$, $p = 0.0212$), and higher risks of GDM (TA/TT vs. AA: OR = 1.28) and GDM subtype 2 (TA/TT vs. AA: OR = 1.31). According to the high-linkage relationship between *VDR*-rs10783219 and *VDR*-rs11568820 in this population [15], we could speculate that it might be the highly interlinked *VDR*-rs11568820 that exhibits the biological functions. *VDR*-rs11568820 not only plays an important role in the development of type 2 diabetes, but also of GDM. Significant associations between *CDKAL1*-rs7754840 and PG2H, as well as GDM, were also observed in our study, which was consistent with the genome-wide association study reported by Kwak et al. [8]. Variants at *CDKAL1*-rs7754840 may affect the conversion process from proinsulin to insulin [34]. This study further confirmed that variants at *CDKAL1*-rs7754840 increased the risk of GDM in Chinese populations. Furthermore, we also found that for each additional G risk allele at *MTNR1B*-rs10830962, the risk of GDM increased by 52% and 108%, and GDM subtype 2 by 43% and 85%, respectively, which was consistent with previous studies [8,35]. The *MTNR1B* gene encodes melatonin receptor 2 (MTNR2), which could significantly inhibit the expression of $3'5'$-cyclic adenosine monophosphate in cells, and subsequently reduces insulin secretion [36,37]. Therefore, variants of the C allele to G at *MTNR1B*-rs10830962 are likely to inhibit the release of insulin in islet cells and increase the risk of GDM.

Meanwhile, we also identified a significant interaction between *VDR*-rs10783219 and *CDKAL1*-rs7754840 as well as *MTNR1B*-rs10830962 on GDM. Variants at *VDR*-rs10783219 increased the risk of GDM and GDM subtype 2 among women with a variant at *CDKAL1*-rs7754840, suggesting that the protective effect of VitD on GDM was more obvious in patients with abnormal islet cell functions. In addition, the T allele at *VDR*-rs10783219 and the C allele at *CDKAL1*-rs7754840 separately increased the risk of GDM subtype 1 among women with the GG genotype at *MTNR1B*-rs10830962 (OR = 2.99, 95%CI: 1.34–6.68; OR = 3.06, 95%CI: 1.41–6.66) ($P_{interaction} = 0.2611$; $P_{interaction} = 0.0071$). Given that the *MTNR1B* gene could reduce the secretion of insulin, the conversion obstacles of proinsulin to insulin mediated by the *CDKAL1* gene might be strengthened with reduced insulin secretion. The above interaction between SNPs found in this study provides a new perspective for the study of the pathogenesis of GDM, but the specific biological mechanism still needs to be verified by further studies.

Traditionally, 25(OH)D was thought to be taken up by cells of the kidney binding to vitamin D-binding protein through megalin/cubilin-mediated endocytosis. However, studies [38,39] have found that although the levels of both 25(OH)D and 1,25(OH)$_2$D in blood and urine were low in megalin knockout and vitamin D-binding protein knockout mice, vitamin D-binding protein knockout mice did not show symptoms of VitD deficiency, unlike megalin knockout mice. In addition, vitamin D-binding protein knockout mice would rapidly manifest symptoms of VitD deficiency when fed with a VitD-deficient diet. In 2019, the first case of the human homozygous deletion of a *GC* gene reported by Henderson et al. [17] confirmed that this mechanism found in animals also applies to humans. The above research indicates that free 25(OH)D or 1,25(OH)$_2$D is the main form to exert the biological VitD effects. Furthermore, the proportion of free 25(OH)D of individuals with different Gc isoforms is different: individuals with the 1f/1f isoform have the highest free 25(OH)D concentrations, and individuals with 1s/1s have the lowest, followed by 1f/2,

2/2, 1s/1f and 1s/2 [16]. This study initially reported that the associations of Gc isoforms with GDM and GDM subtypes during pregnancy were different in pregnant women with different prepregnancy BMI. Significant associations were only observed among women who were overweight or obese before pregnancy. The distribution of Gc isoforms was significantly different between blacks and whites along with the distribution of fat with the same BMI [40]. More than 90% of blacks were of Gc1f type, whereas the majority of whites are of Gc1s type; Asians were in between [41]. The accumulation of abdominal fat is a risk factor for insulin resistance and metabolic syndrome [42]. Given the strong association between BMI and insulin resistance [43], we speculated that overweight and obese pregnant women might have underlying insulin resistance before pregnancy, and the difference in insulin resistance among pregnant women with different Gc isoforms may be caused by the difference in body fat distribution. In this study, it was found that compared with the 1f/1f isoform, pregnant women with 1s/2 and 1s/1s isoforms had higher risk of GDM subtype 2, indicating higher visceral and liver fat content, and thus, higher muscle insulin resistance. However, the specific pathophysiological mechanism needs to be confirmed by further studies.

Our previous study [23] found that serum 25(OH)D only affected FBG and GDM subtypes with abnormal fasting glucose. However, this study found that free 25(OH)D (represented by Gc isoforms) mainly influences postprandial glucose levels and GDM subtype 2. The difference between serum 25(OH)D and free 25(OH)D on glucose and GDM risk indicates that the proportion of free 25(OH)D is mainly related to muscle insulin resistance or insulin secretion, and serum 25(OH)D in circulation is not mainly mediated by free 25(OH)D, which may be related to fasting gluconeogenesis levels in the liver, and plays its role in lowering glucose levels through megalin/cubilin-mediated endocytosis through the kidney or parathyroid cells [44]. However, combined effects of 25(OH)D concentrations at T1 or T2 with Gc isoforms on the risk of GDM and GDM subtypes were not observed.

Strengths of the current study included the prospective cohort design and the relatively large sample size, which may guarantee the authenticity of the research results and higher statistical test efficiency. Furthermore, we initially divided GDM into different subtypes based on the different mechanisms of insulin resistance. The risks of GDM and GDM subtypes in pregnant women with different Gc isoforms have been investigated for the first time, and the effect of prepregnancy BMI and longitudinal changes in VitD during pregnancy on the association between Gc isoforms and GDM as well as its subtypes was considered. However, there were several potential limitations in this study. Insulin levels, which could more accurately distinguish different types of insulin resistance in GDM, were not detected simultaneously during the OGTT examination in this study. In addition, the average prepregnancy BMI of the population in this study was low, and about 12% of the pregnant women were overweight (10.3%) or obese (2.1%). Furthermore, in this study, we investigated whether there was a VitD supplementation of participants during pregnancy, but did not consider the supplementation dose because the clinically recommended supplementation dose of VitD for pregnant women is between 400 and 600 IU. However, the type of VitD supplementation was unknown, which restricted the study to further explore how the SNP affected the response to VitD supplementation on serum 25(OH)D concentrations and its impact on GDM. Therefore, the results of this study may be limited when extrapolating to obese or severely obese pregnant women.

5. Conclusions

In conclusion, our results showed that variants of SNPs at *VDR*-rs10783219 and *MTNR1B*-rs10830962 significantly increased the risk of GDM and GDM subtypes with normal fasting glucose and elevated post-load glucose, and interactions were investigated between each other as well as with *CDKAL1*-rs7754840. With lower Gc isoforms, the proportions of free 25(OH)D were related to an increased risk of GDM with abnormal postprandial blood glucose in prepregnancy overweight and obese women. The present study explored whether gene variants in the VitD metabolic and glucose pathway would affect the risk of GDM from a genetic point of view. In addition, the 25(OH)D concentration is very unstable and can easily be affected by exposure factors such as supplementation and sunlight exposure. Identifying the effect of gene variants in the VitD and glucose metabolic-pathway-related genes on the development of GDM and GDM subtypes could more objectively evaluate the relationship between VitD and GDM and provide standards for subsequent clinical applications.

Supplementary Materials: The following are available online at https://www.mdpi.com/article/10.3390/nu13124220/s1, Supplementary Table S1. Baseline characteristics of pregnant women with different GDM subtypes, Supplementary Table S2. Association of SNPs and its interaction with VitD level at T1 and T2 on three time-point plasma glucose levels of OGTT, Supplementary Table S3. Association of Gc isoforms and different time-point plasma glucose levels of OGTT, Supplementary Table S4. Association of Gc isoforms with GDM and GDM subtypes among women with different prepregnancy BMI values.

Author Contributions: Conceptualization, Y.Y.; Methodology, B.S.; Validation, M.M.; Resources, X.X. and W.L.; Formal Analysis, J.W.; Investigation, W.J.; Writing—Review and Editing, B.S. and M.M.; Visualization, S.S., S.W. and Y.S. All authors have read and agreed to the published version of the manuscript.

Funding: This study was funded by Chinese National Natural Science Foundation (81973055), the national key research and development program of China (2016YFC1305301) and the Fundamental Research Funds for the Central Universities.

Institutional Review Board Statement: The study was conducted according to the guidelines of the Declaration of Helsinki, and approved by the institutional review board of Zhejiang University School of Medicine on 2 March 2016 ((2016) Lun Shen Yan (Shen 017)).

Informed Consent Statement: Informed consent was obtained from all subjects involved in the study.

Data Availability Statement: The data presented in this study are available on request from the corresponding author. The data are not publicly available because they contain information that could compromise the privacy of research participants.

Acknowledgments: We thank all the participants who took part in this study. We acknowledge the support of Zhoushan Maternal and Child Care Hospital and fellows there who conducted and managed the cohort.

Conflicts of Interest: The authors declare that they have no conflict of interest.

References

1. American Diabetes Association. Diagnosis and classification of diabetes mellitus. *Diabetes Care* **2014**, *37* (Suppl. 1), S81–S90. [CrossRef]
2. Federation, I. *International Diabetes Federation*; IDF Diabetes Atlas: Brussels, Belgium, 2019.
3. Bryson, C.L.; Ioannou, G.N.; Rulyak, S.J.; Critchlow, C. Association between gestational diabetes and pregnancy-induced hypertension. *Am. J. Epidemiol.* **2003**, *158*, 1148–1153. [CrossRef]
4. Hedderson, M.M.; Ferrara, A.; Sacks, D.A. Gestational diabetes mellitus and lesser degrees of pregnancy hyperglycemia: Association with increased risk of spontaneous preterm birth. *Obstet. Gynecol.* **2003**, *102*, 850–856. [CrossRef] [PubMed]
5. Yu, Y.; Arah, O.A.; Liew, Z.; Cnattingius, S.; Olsen, J.; Sørensen, H.T.; Qin, G.; Li, J. Maternal diabetes during pregnancy and early onset of cardiovascular disease in offspring: Population based cohort study with 40 years of follow-up. *BMJ* **2019**, *367*, l6398. [CrossRef] [PubMed]
6. Casagrande, S.S.; Linder, B.; Cowie, C.C. Prevalence of gestational diabetes and subsequent Type 2 diabetes among U.S. women. *Diabetes Res. Clin. Pract.* **2018**, *141*, 200–208. [CrossRef]
7. Moen, G.H.; LeBlanc, M.; Sommer, C.; Prasad, R.B.; Lekva, T.; Normann, K.R.; Qvigstad, E.; Groop, L.; Birkeland, K.I.; Evans, D.M.; et al. Genetic determinants of glucose levels in pregnancy: Genetic risk scores analysis and GWAS in the Norwegian STORK cohort. *Eur. J. Endocrinol.* **2018**, *179*, 363–372. [CrossRef] [PubMed]
8. Kwak, S.H.; Kim, S.H.; Cho, Y.M.; Go, M.J.; Cho, Y.S.; Choi, S.H.; Moon, M.K.; Jung, H.S.; Shin, H.D.; Kang, H.M.; et al. A genome-wide association study of gestational diabetes mellitus in Korean women. *Diabetes* **2012**, *61*, 531–541. [CrossRef]
9. Shi, A.; Wen, J.; Liu, G.; Liu, H.; Fu, Z.; Zhou, J.; Zhu, Y.; Liu, Y.; Guo, X.; Xu, J. Genetic variants in vitamin D signaling pathways and risk of gestational diabetes mellitus. *Oncotarget* **2016**, *7*, 67788–67795. [CrossRef]

10. Wang, Y.; Wang, O.; Li, W.; Ma, L.; Ping, F.; Chen, L.; Nie, M. Variants in Vitamin D Binding Protein Gene Are Associated with Gestational Diabetes Mellitus. *Medicine* **2015**, *94*, e1693. [CrossRef]
11. Apaydin, M.; Beysel, S.; Eyerci, N.; Pinarli, F.A.; Ulubay, M.; Kizilgul, M.; Ozdemir, O.; Caliskan, M.; Cakal, E. The VDR gene FokI polymorphism is associated with gestational diabetes mellitus in Turkish women. *BMC Med. Genet.* **2019**, *20*, 82. [CrossRef]
12. Barry, E.L.; Rees, J.R.; Peacock, J.L.; Mott, L.A.; Amos, C.I.; Bostick, R.M.; Figueiredo, J.C.; Ahnen, D.J.; Bresalier, R.S.; Burke, C.A.; et al. Genetic variants in CYP2R1, CYP24A1, and VDR modify the efficacy of vitamin D3 supplementation for increasing serum 25-hydroxyvitamin D levels in a randomized controlled trial. *J. Clin. Endocrinol. Metab.* **2014**, *99*, E2133–E2137. [CrossRef] [PubMed]
13. Zhu, B.; Huang, K.; Yan, S.; Hao, J.; Zhu, P.; Chen, Y.; Ye, A.; Tao, F. VDR Variants rather than Early Pregnancy Vitamin D Concentrations Are Associated with the Risk of Gestational Diabetes: The Ma'anshan Birth Cohort (MABC) Study. *J. Diabetes Res.* **2019**, *2019*, 8313901. [CrossRef] [PubMed]
14. Arnaud, J.; Constans, J. Affinity differences for vitamin D metabolites associated with the genetic isoforms of the human serum carrier protein (DBP). *Hum. Genet.* **1993**, *92*, 183–188. [CrossRef] [PubMed]
15. Shao, B.; Jiang, S.; Muyiduli, X.; Wang, S.; Mo, M.; Li, M.; Wang, Z.; Yu, Y. Vitamin D pathway gene polymorphisms influenced vitamin D level among pregnant women. *Clin. Nutr.* **2018**, *37*, 2230–2237. [CrossRef]
16. Mendel, C.M. The free hormone hypothesis: A physiologically based mathematical model. *Endocr. Rev.* **1989**, *10*, 232–274. [CrossRef]
17. Henderson, C.M.; Fink, S.L.; Bassyouni, H.; Argiropoulos, B.; Brown, L.; Laha, T.J.; Jackson, K.J.; Lewkonia, R.; Ferreira, P.; Hoofnagle, A.N.; et al. Vitamin D-Binding Protein Deficiency and Homozygous Deletion of the GC Gene. *N. Engl. J. Med.* **2019**, *380*, 1150–1157. [CrossRef]
18. Schwartz, J.B.; Gallagher, J.C.; Jorde, R.; Berg, V.; Walsh, J.; Eastell, R.; Evans, A.L.; Bowles, S.; Naylor, K.E.; Jones, K.; et al. Determination of Free 25(OH)D Concentrations and Their Relationships to Total 25(OH)D in Multiple Clinical Populations. *J. Clin. Endocrinol. Metab.* **2018**, *103*, 3278–3288. [CrossRef]
19. Nathan, D.M.; Davidson, M.B.; DeFronzo, R.A.; Heine, R.J.; Henry, R.R.; Pratley, R.; Zinman, B. Impaired fasting glucose and impaired glucose tolerance: Implications for care. *Diabetes Care* **2007**, *30*, 753–759. [CrossRef]
20. Ahlqvist, E.; Storm, P.; Karajamaki, A.; Martinell, M.; Dorkhan, M.; Carlsson, A.; Vikman, P.; Prasad, R.; Aly, D.M.; Almgren, P.; et al. Novel subgroups of adult-onset diabetes and their association with outcomes: A data-driven cluster analysis of six variables. *Lancet Diabetes Endocrinol.* **2018**, *6*, 361–369. [CrossRef]
21. Faerch, K.; Witte, D.R.; Tabak, A.G.; Perreault, L.; Herder, C.; Brunner, E.J.; Kivimäki, M.; Vistisen, D. Trajectories of cardiometabolic risk factors before diagnosis of three subtypes of type 2 diabetes: A post-hoc analysis of the longitudinal Whitehall II cohort study. *Lancet Diabetes Endocrinol.* **2013**, *1*, 43–51. [CrossRef]
22. Faerch, K.; Johansen, N.B.; Witte, D.R.; Lauritzen, T.; Jorgensen, M.E.; Vistisen, D. Relationship Between Insulin Resistance and beta-Cell Dysfunction in Subphenotypes of Prediabetes and Type 2 Diabetes. *J. Clin. Endocrinol. Metab.* **2015**, *100*, 707–716. [CrossRef] [PubMed]
23. Shao, B.L.; Mo, M.J.; Xin, X.; Jiang, W.; Wu, J.; Huang, M.; Wang, S.; Muyiduli, X.; Si, S.; Shen, Y.; et al. The interaction between prepregnancy BMI and gestational vitamin D deficiency on the risk of gestational diabetes mellitus subtypes with elevated fasting blood glucose. *Clin. Nutr.* **2020**, *39*, 2265–2273. [CrossRef] [PubMed]
24. Ferrannini, E.; Bjorkman, O.; Reichard, G.A.; Pilo, A.; Olsson, M.; Wahren, J.; DeFronzo, R.A. The disposal of an oral glucose load in healthy subjects. A quantitative study. *Diabetes* **1985**, *34*, 580–588. [CrossRef] [PubMed]
25. Holick, M.F.; Binkley, N.C.; Bischoff-Ferrari, H.A.; Gordon, C.M.; Hanley, D.A.; Heaney, R.P.; Murad, M.H.; Weaver, C.M. Evaluation, treatment, and prevention of vitamin D deficiency: An Endocrine Society clinical practice guideline. *J. Clin. Endocrinol. Metab.* **2011**, *96*, 1911–1930. [CrossRef] [PubMed]
26. Zhou, B.F.; Cooperative Meta-Analysis Group of the Working Group on Obesity in China. Predictive values of body mass index and waist circumference for risk factors of certain related diseases in Chinese adults–study on optimal cut-off points of body mass index and waist circumference in Chinese adults. *Biomed. Environ. Sci.* **2002**, *15*, 83–96.
27. Thorne, H.C.; Jones, K.H.; Peters, S.P.; Archer, S.N.; Dijk, D.-J. Daily and seasonal variation in the spectral composition of light exposure in humans. *Chronobiol. Int.* **2009**, *26*, 854–866. [CrossRef]
28. International Association of Diabetes; Pregnancy Study Groups Consensus Panel. International association of diabetes and pregnancy study groups recommendations on the diagnosis and classification of hyperglycemia in pregnancy. *Diabetes Care* **2010**, *33*, 676–682. [CrossRef] [PubMed]
29. Goltzman, D. Vitamin D Action: Lessons learned from genetic mouse models. *Ann. N. Y. Acad. Sci.* **2010**, *1192*, 145–152. [CrossRef]
30. Sentinelli, F.; Bertoccini, L.; Barchetta, I.; Capoccia, D.; Incani, M.; Pani, M.; Loche, S.; Angelico, F.; Arca, M.; Morini, S.; et al. The vitamin D receptor (VDR) gene rs11568820 variant is associated with type 2 diabetes and impaired insulin secretion in Italian adult subjects, and associates with increased cardio-metabolic risk in children. *Nutr. Metab. Cardiovasc. Dis.* **2016**, *26*, 407–413. [CrossRef] [PubMed]
31. Nykjaer, A.; Dragun, D.; Walther, D.; Vorum, H.; Jacobsen, C.; Herz, J.; Melsen, F.; Christensen, E.I.; Willnow, T.E. An endocytic pathway essential for renal uptake and activation of the steroid 25-(OH) vitamin D3. *Cell* **1999**, *96*, 507–515. [CrossRef]

32. Wang, C.; Hu, Y.M.; He, J.W.; Gu, J.M.; Zhang, H.; Hu, W.W.; Yue, H.; Gao, G.; Xiao, W.J.; Yu, J.B.; et al. Association between Low Density Lipoprotein Receptor-Related Protein 2 Gene Polymorphisms and Bone Mineral Density Variation in Chinese Population. *PLoS ONE* **2011**, *6*, e28874. [CrossRef] [PubMed]
33. Arai, H.; Miyamoto, K.I.; Yoshida, M.; Yamamoto, H.; Taketani, Y.; Morita, K.; Kubota, M.; Yoshida, S.; Ikeda, M.; Watabe, F.; et al. The polymorphism in the caudal-related homeodomain protein Cdx-2 binding element in the human vitamin D receptor gene. *J. Bone Miner. Res.* **2001**, *16*, 1256–1264. [CrossRef] [PubMed]
34. Palmer, C.J.; Bruckner, R.J.; Paulo, J.A.; Kazak, L.; Long, J.Z.; Mina, A.I.; Deng, Z.; LeClair, K.B.; Hall, J.A.; Hong, S.; et al. Cdkal1, a type 2 diabetes susceptibility gene, regulates mitochondrial function in adipose tissue. *Mol. Metab.* **2017**, *6*, 1212–1225. [CrossRef] [PubMed]
35. Xie, K.; Chen, T.; Zhang, Y.; Wen, J.; Cui, X.; You, L.; Zhu, L.; Xu, B.; Ji, C.; Guo, X. Association of rs10830962 polymorphism with gestational diabetes mellitus risk in a Chinese population. *Sci. Rep.* **2019**, *9*, 5357. [CrossRef] [PubMed]
36. Kemp, D.M.; Ubeda, M.; Habener, J.F. Identification and functional characterization of melatonin Mel 1a receptors in pancreatic beta cells: Potential role in incretin-mediated cell function by sensitization of cAMP signaling. *Mol. Cell. Endocrinol.* **2002**, *191*, 157–166. [CrossRef]
37. Peschke, E. Melatonin, endocrine pancreas and diabetes. *J. Pineal Res.* **2008**, *44*, 26–40. [CrossRef]
38. Safadi, F.F.; Thornton, P.; Magiera, H.; Hollis, B.W.; Gentile, M.; Haddad, J.G.; Liebhaber, S.A.; Cooke, N.E. Osteopathy and resistance to vitamin D toxicity in mice null for vitamin D binding protein. *J. Clin. Investig.* **1999**, *103*, 239–251. [CrossRef]
39. Zella, L.A.; Shevde, N.K.; Hollis, B.W.; Cooke, N.E.; Pike, J.W. Vitamin D-binding protein influences total circulating levels of 1,25-dihydroxyvitamin D3 but does not directly modulate the bioactive levels of the hormone in vivo. *Endocrinology* **2008**, *149*, 3656–3667. [CrossRef]
40. Chung, S.T.; Courville, A.B.; Onuzuruike, A.U.; La Cruz, M.G.-D.; Mabundo, L.S.; DuBose, C.W.; Kasturi, K.; Cai, H.; Gharib, A.M.; Walter, P.J.; et al. Gluconeogenesis and risk for fasting hyperglycemia in Black and White women. *JCI Insight* **2018**, *3*, e121495. [CrossRef]
41. Powe, C.E.; Evans, M.K.; Wenger, J.; Zonderman, A.B.; Berg, A.H.; Nalls, M.; Tamez, H.; Zhang, D.; Bhan, I.; Karumanchi, S.A.; et al. Vitamin D-binding protein and vitamin D status of black Americans and white Americans. *N. Engl. J. Med.* **2013**, *369*, 1991–2000. [CrossRef]
42. Wagenknecht, L.E.; Langefeld, C.D.; Scherzinger, A.L.; Norris, J.M.; Haffner, S.M.; Saad, M.F.; Bergman, R.N. Insulin sensitivity, insulin secretion, and abdominal fat: The Insulin Resistance Atherosclerosis Study (IRAS) Family Study. *Diabetes* **2003**, *52*, 2490–2496. [CrossRef] [PubMed]
43. Baptiste-Roberts, K.; Barone, B.B.; Gary, T.L.; Golden, S.H.; Wilson, L.M.; Bass, E.; Nicholson, W.K. Risk factors for type 2 diabetes among women with gestational diabetes: A systematic review. *Am. J. Med.* **2009**, *122*, 207–214.e204. [CrossRef] [PubMed]
44. Knutson, A.; Hellman, P.; Akerstrom, G.; Westin, G. Characterization of the human Megalin/LRP-2 promoter in vitro and in primary parathyroid cells. *DNA Cell Biol.* **1998**, *17*, 551–560. [CrossRef] [PubMed]

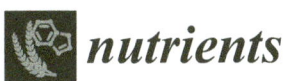

Systematic Review

Vitamin D Levels in Early and Middle Pregnancy and Preeclampsia, a Systematic Review and Meta-Analysis

Kai-Lun Hu [1,2,†], Chun-Xi Zhang [1,†], Panpan Chen [1], Dan Zhang [1,2,*] and Sarah Hunt [3]

1. Key Laboratory of Reproductive Genetics (Ministry of Education), Department of Reproductive Endocrinology, Women's Hospital, Zhejiang University School of Medicine, Hangzhou 310006, China; hukailun@bjmu.edu.cn (K.-L.H.); zhangcxi@zju.edu.cn (C.-X.Z.); 12018523@zju.edu.cn (P.C.)
2. Key Laboratory of Women's Reproductive Health of Zhejiang Province, Zhejiang University, Hangzhou 310006, China
3. Department of Obstetrics and Gynaecology, Monash University, Clayton, VIC 3168, Australia; sarah_prema@hotmail.com
* Correspondence: zhangdan@zju.edu.cn; Tel./Fax: +86-0571-89991008
† These authors contributed equally to this work.

Abstract: Vitamin D (VitD) shows a beneficial role in placentation, the immune system, and angiogenesis, and thus, VitD status may link to the risk of preeclampsia. A meta-analysis was conducted to investigate the association between VitD status in early and middle pregnancy and the risk of preeclampsia. A total of 22 studies with 25,530 participants were included for analysis. Women with VitD insufficiency or deficiency had a higher preeclampsia rate compared to women with replete VitD levels (OR 1.58, 95% CI 1.39–1.79). Women with VitD deficiency had a higher preeclampsia rate compared to women with replete or insufficient VitD levels (OR 1.35, 95% CI 1.10–1.66). Women with insufficient VitD levels had a higher preeclampsia rate compared to women with replete VitD levels (OR 1.44, 95% CI 1.24–1.66). Women with deficient VitD levels had a higher preeclampsia rate compared to women with replete VitD levels (OR 1.50, 95% CI 1.05–2.14). Sensitivity analysis showed the results were stable after excluding any one of the included studies. In conclusion, our systematic review suggested that VitD insufficiency or deficiency was associated with an increased risk of preeclampsia.

Keywords: vitamin D; preeclampsia; pregnancy; systematic review; meta-analysis

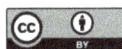

1. Introduction

Preeclampsia is a multisystem disease during pregnancy, characterized by the new-onset of gestational hypertension and proteinuria. It occurs in around 3–8% of all pregnancies and is associated with increased maternal and fetal morbidity and mortality [1,2]. Maternal preeclampsia is also associated with a higher incidence of cardiovascular and kidney disease in the later life of the child [3–5]. Currently, delivery is the only curative therapy for preeclampsia, and pharmacological management is symptomatic treatment only. Therapies aimed at preventing preeclampsia therefore are a priority for ongoing investigation.

VitD deficiency is common during pregnancy, with a prevalence ranging from 8–70% depending on skin pigmentation and sunlight exposure [6–9]. Accumulating evidence suggests that VitD deficiency may be implicated in recurrent pregnancy loss, adverse obstetrical and neonatal outcomes [10,11]. More recently, attention has been paid to the potential association between VitD levels in pregnancy and the risk of preeclampsia. It has been postulated that increased VitD levels may improve the invasion of the human extravillous trophoblast, which is required for normal placentation [12]. Additionally, accumulating evidence suggested that VitD has a beneficial effect on endothelial repair and angiogenesis [13–15] and that VitD deficiency is associated with the pathogenesis of cardiovascular diseases and arterial hypertension [16,17]. Therefore, it is likely that VitD has a role in improving endothelial repair and angiogenesis and controlling blood pressure in preeclampsia [18]. Furthermore, the immunomodulatory properties of VitD may also reduce the risk of preeclampsia development [13,19,20]. Indeed, previous observational studies have demonstrated significant association between VitD deficiency and increased preeclampsia risk [21–23], whereas others suggest no association between maternal VitD deficiency and preeclampsia rate [11,24–26]. Overall, the epidemiological evidence from observational data is conflicting and most studies are limited by small sample sizes. Additionally, there is a lack of consensus regarding definition of VitD deficiency and the potential threshold level associated with preeclampsia risk. Although there have been several systematic review and meta-analysis papers related to the association of VitD with preeclampsia [27–30], some important studies were not included in these meta-analyses. Additionally, most studies included in these systematic reviews were case-control studies that investigated women in late pregnancy. Even when the association between VitD deficiency in late pregnancy and obstetric complications is detected, the prevention of these diseases by the modification of VitD status is too late.

In this systematic review, we aimed to determine the association between VitD levels in early or middle pregnancy ($\leq$24 weeks) and the risk of pre-eclampsia.

2. Methods

2.1. Eligibility Criteria

The protocol of this systematic review was prospectively registered in PROSPERO (reference: CRD42021271154). We reported this systematic review according to the guideline of The Preferred Reporting Items for Systematic reviews and Meta-Analyses (PRISMA) statement 2020 [31]. We included all studies that investigated the association of VitD levels with the rate of preeclampsia. Because the detection of the association between VitD deficiency in early or middle pregnancy (rather than late pregnancy) and later obstetric complications may allow the prevention of these diseases by screening and modification of VitD status in early or middle pregnancy [24], we excluded studies if they investigated pregnant women over 24 gestational weeks. Reviews, case report studies, and study protocols were also excluded.

2.2. Search Strategy

Two authors (KLH and CXZ) independently searched the database of PubMed, EMBASE, Cochrane library, and Web of Science from January 1990 to July 2021. The search terms included "preeclampsia", "vitamin D", and "hypertensive disorder of pregnancy". The detailed search terms could be seen in Table S1.

2.3. Selection Process

Two authors (KLH and CXZ) independently reviewed the titles and abstracts based on the predefined eligibility criteria. The full manuscripts were obtained when the titles and abstracts were considered to be related. Any disagreement between the two authors was resolved by a third review author. References from all included studies were checked to identify relevant articles not captured by the electronic searches.

2.4. Risk of Bias Assessment

Two reviewers (KLH and CXZ) independently assessed the quality of the included studies. Cohort and case-control studies were assessed according to The Newcastle-Ottawa Quality Assessment Scales [32]. Cross-sectional studies were assessed using the Agency for Healthcare Research and Quality (AHRQ).

2.5. Data Collection Process

Two reviewers (KLH and CXZ) independently extracted the data from included studies. If a study with multiple publications was found, the main report was used as the reference with additional details supplemented from other papers.

VitD levels were stratified into three groups according to Endocrine Society recommendations [9]: the replete level (>30 ng/mL or >75 nmol/L), the insufficient level (20–30 ng/mL or 50–75 nmol/L), and the deficient level (<20 ng/mL or <50 nmol/L). A few studies used 15 ng/mL (37.5 nmol/L) as the cutoff, and thus <15 ng/mL was considered as the deficient level in these studies. The primary outcome was preeclampsia, defined by the new-onset of gestational hypertension and proteinuria.

2.6. Synthesis Methods

The Stata 15.0 (StataCorp, College Station, TX, USA) was as used to perform the meta-analysis using either the inverse-variance weighted model (fixed-effect) or the DerSimonian and Laird model (random-effect). Both were displayed in the forest plot, and the fixed-effect model was applied if no significant heterogeneity was identified ($I^2 < 50\%$), whereas a random-effect model was used a significant heterogeneity was detected ($I^2 > 50\%$),. The combined data was shown in a pooled odds ratio (OR) with a 95% confidence interval (CI). Publication bias was assessed by funnel plot asymmetry as well as Egger's test. Sensitivity analysis was conducted by omitting each individual study in turn to explore the effect of a single study on the overall meta-analysis. Subgroup analysis was conducted according to the gestational weeks of pregnancy (early $\leq$ 14 weeks, middle 15–24 weeks, early and middle not specified) and study design (case-control, cohort, cross-sectional). Statistical significance was set at α equals to 0.05.

3. Results

3.1. Characteristics of the Included Studies

Diagramatic representation of the review process is outlined in Figure S1. A total of 22 studies with a sample size of 25,530 were included for analysis [11,21,22,24–26,33–48]. The characteristics of the included studies are shown in Table 1. Study quality assessment were shown in Table S2 (case-control studies), Table S3 (cohort studies), and Table S4 (cross-sectional studies).

The included studies varied in publication date from 2007 to 2020. Eleven were case-control studies; eight were cohort studies and three were cross-sectional studies (Table 1). Sample sizes varied from 142 women to 5109 women. Six studies focused on women in early pregnancy and three studies included women in middle pregnancy (Table 1). While most studies defined insufficiency and deficiency at 30 ng/mL and 20 ng/mL, respectively, four studies used 15 ng/mL as the diagnostic cutoff [11,25,34,35] (Table S5). Nearly all studies used multivariable analysis; however, the number and type of potential confounders controlled for in the final analyses was not uniform between studies (Table S5).

Table 1. Characteristics of included studies.

Studies	Study Type	Eligibility for Pregnant Women	Method of Measurement	Gestational Weeks of Sampling	Sample Size	Location
[11]	Nested case-control	Women with multiple gestations, fetal anomalies, or maternal medical complications were excluded.	LCMS	15-21	266	Birmingham, America /52.3° N
[33]	Nested case-control	Women with multiple gestations, major congenital fetal anomalies, pregestational hypertension, kidney disease, diabetes mellitus, known thrombophilias, PCMD were excluded.	LCMS	15-20	241	Boston, America /52.58° N
[26]	Cohort	Women with abnormal liver function, chronic disease and tumor; severe infections, trauma or in perioperative, before 13 weeks of gestation, and women who take corticosteroids, drug abuse (including alcohol) were excluded.	ECLIA	16-20	1953	Guangzhou, China /23.1° N
[34]	Nested case-control	Women with adverse pregnancy outcomes were excluded	CLIA	10-14	5109	New South Wales, Australia /33.9°
[25]	Nested case-control	Women with GDM or give birth to SGA infants	LCMS	≤14	170	Boston, America /52.58° N
[22]	Nested case-control	Women who had aneuploidy screening at 20 weeks or less gestation and who subsequently delivered live born infants.	LCMS	≤20	2327	Pennsylvania, America /40.3°
[35]	Nested case-control	Nulliparous women aged 14-44 years, carrying singleton infants.	ELISA	≤22	265	Pennsylvania, America /40.3°
[36]	Nested case-control	Women with multiple gestations, calcium imbalance, hypertension, renal insufficiency, bone disease, lithium therapy, bowel malabsorption, or kidney stone disease were excluded.	RIA	≤15	402	six centers: one in Belgium and five in France
[21]	Nested case-control	Women with preexisting hypertension, missing essential outcome information (no gestational age at enrollment), or multiple gestations were excluded.	CLIA	≤20	2048	Quebec, Canada /46.5° N
[37]	Cross-sectional	Women with increased risks for intrauterine fetal growth restriction, hereditary thrombophilias, or acquired thrombophilias were excluded.	ECLIA	11-14	466	Almeria, Spain /36.8°
[38]	Cross-sectional	NA	CLIA	≤24	1382	Bern, Switzerland /46.5°
[39]	Cross-sectional	Women with PCMD, metabolic bone disease, liver, kidney, or gastrointestinal diseases and the use of vitamin D supplements.	ELISA	≤12	1000	Saudi Arabia /24.3°
[40]	Cohort	Nulliparous women with a low-risk singleton pregnancy. Pregnancies at increased risk of pre-eclampsia, SGA, or spontaneous preterm birth or medical history, known major fetal anomaly or abnormal karyotype were excluded.	LCMS	<16	1754	Cork, Ireland /51.9° N

Table 1. Cont.

Studies	Study Type	Eligibility for Pregnant Women	Method of Measurement	Gestational Weeks of Sampling	Sample Size	Location
[24]	Nested case-control	Maternal age between 18 and 39 years and not a current smoker or a user of other nicotine products. Women with PCMD, multiple pregnancies, vitamin D taken (>2000 IU per day), fetal anomalies, or ART use were excluded.	CLIA	16–18	157	United States
[41]	Cohort	Women who regularly took 200 mg/d for vitamin C and/or 50 IU/d for vitamin E, or warfarin, or with fetal abnormalities, or with PCMD, or with repeated spontaneous abortion were excluded.	CLIA	12–18	697	Canada and Mexico
[42]	Cohort	Healthy, nulliparous women aged 18 years or older without PCMD or infertility treatment. Patients with predictors for hypovitaminosis D or a prior pregnancy that had progressed beyond the first trimester and resulted in a fetal loss were excluded.	ELISA	8–12	235	United States
[43]	Cohort	Women aged ≥ 18 years with either clinical or biochemical risk factors for pre-eclampsia	RIA	10–20	221	Canada/49° N
[44]	Cohort	Nulliparous women with a singleton pregnancy.	ELISA	<17	2074	Amsterdam, the Netherlands
[45]	Cohort	Gestational age < 24 weeks, resident in Rotterdam at the date of delivery, expected delivery date lies between June 2002 and July 2004	LCMS	<24	3323	Rotterdam, the Netherlands
[46]	Cohort	Healthy pregnant women. Gravidae with serious nonobstetric problems are not eligible.	LCMS	<20	1141	Camden, United States
[47]	Nested case-control	Suspected PE over 20 weeks of gestation between January 2010 and March 2013. Women who were diagnosed with PE before their presentation at the emergency department were not included.	CLIA	9–12	142	Oviedo, Spain
[48]	Nested case-control	After identifying women who developed preeclampsia, the control group was drawn by random selection and comprised 10 women delivered in each month of the year	CLIA	Mean (SD): 12 (3)	157	Malmo, Sweden /55°37′ N

Abbreviations: Premature rupture of membranes, PROM; preeclampsia, PE; gestational diabetes mellitus, GDM; small-for-gestational-age, SGA; diabetes mellitus, DM; preexisting chronic medical disease, PCMD; liquid chromatography–tandem mass spectrometry, LCMS; enzyme-linked immunosorbent assay, ELISA; electrochemiluminescence immunoassay, ECLIA; radioimmunoassay, RIA; chemiluminescent immunoassay, CLIA; assisted reproductive techniques, ART.

3.2. Replete Levels of VitD (≥30 ng/mL) versus Insufficient or Deficient Levels of VitD (<30 ng/mL)

A total of 17,719 pregnant women (n = 12,908 with replete levels of VitD and n = 4811 with insufficient or deficient levels of VitD) from 14 studies were included. Women with VitD < 30 ng/mL showed an increased preeclampsia rate compared to women with VitD ≥ 30 ng/mL (OR 1.58, 95% CI 1.39–1.79, I^2 = 34%, fixed-effect) (Figure 1). No publication bias was detected (Figure S2a, Egger's test: p = 0.069). Sensitivity analysis demonstrated the results were stable after excluding any one of the included studies (Figure S3a). There was a trend toward an increased risk of preeclampsia in women with VitD < 30 ng/mL in both early pregnancy and middle pregnancy, but they were not statistically significant (early pregnany: OR 1.29, 95% CI 0.93–1.79, I^2 = 0%, fixed-effect; middle pregnancy: OR 1.41, 95% CI 0.97–2.06, I^2 = 18%, fixed-effect) (Figure 1a). The pooled data from studies with a case-control design showed a significantly higher risk of preeclampsia in women with VitD < 30 ng/mL, but it was not seen in pooled data from cohort studies or cross-sectional studies (case-control: OR 1.80, 95% CI 1.56–2.09, I^2 = 0%, fixed-effect; cohort: OR 1.09, 95% CI 0.85–1.40, I2 = 0%, fixed-effect; cross-sectional: OR 0.76, 95% CI 0.18–3.19, I^2 = 0%, fixed-effect) (Figure 1b).

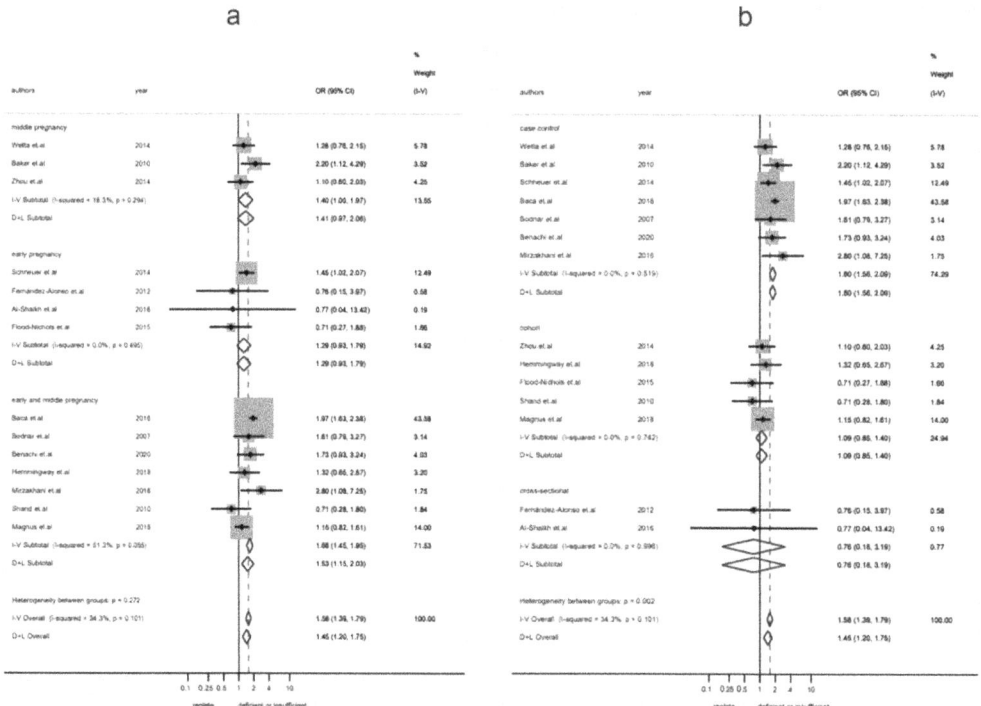

Figure 1. Studies evaluating replete vitamin D levels versus insufficient or deficient vitamin D levels. (**a**): Studies were stratified by gestational weeks (early, middle, and early and middle not specified); (**b**): studies were stratified by the study design.

3.3. Replete or Insufficient Levels of VitD (≥20 ng/mL) versus Deficient Levels of VitD (<20 ng/mL or < 15 ng/mL)

A total of 23,217 pregnant women (n = 8084 with replete levels of VitD and n = 15,133 with insufficient or deficient levels of VitD) from 19 studies were included in this analysis. Women with VitD < 20 ng/mL had a higher preeclampsia rate as compared to women with VitD ≥ 20 ng/mL (OR 1.35, 95% CI 1.10–1.66, I² = 57%, random-effect) (Figure 2). No publication bias was detected (Figure S2b, Egger's test: p = 0.415). Sensitivity analysis demonstrated the results were stable after excluding any one of the included studies (Figure S3b). There was a trend toward an increased risk of preeclampsia in women with VitD < 20 ng/mL in middle pregnancy but no significant difference in preeclampsia risk was seen in early pregnancy (early pregnay: OR 0.85, 95% CI 0.62–1.18, I² = 19%, fixed-effect; middle pregnancy: OR 1.59, 95% CI 0.87–2.92, I² = 61%, random-effect) (Figure 2a). The pooled data from studies with a case-control or cohort design demonstrated significantly increased preeclampsia rates in association with VitD < 20 ng/Ml, but it was not seen in pooled data from cross-sectional studies (case-control: OR 1.46, 95% CI 1.02–2.10, I² = 77%, random-effect; cohort: OR 1.24, 95% CI 1.02–1.51, I2 = 0%, fixed-effect; cross-sectional: OR 1.08, 95% CI 0.49–2.35, I² = 0%, fixed-effect) (Figure 2b).

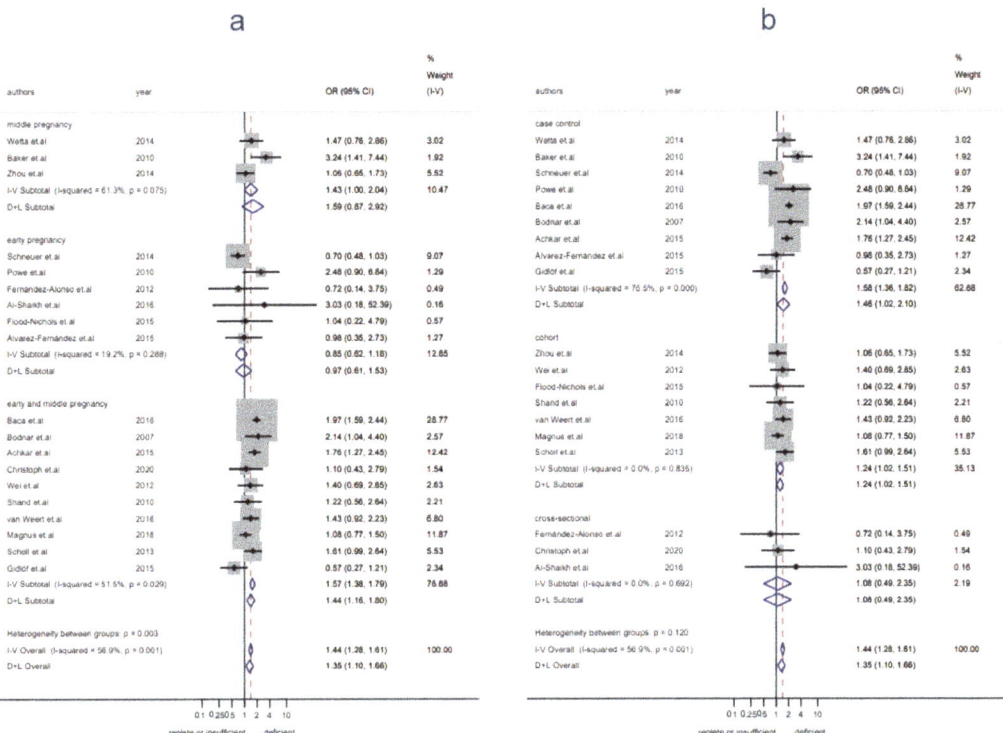

Figure 2. Studies evaluating replete vitamin D levels or insufficient versus deficient vitamin D levels. (**a**): Studies were stratified by gestational weeks (early, middle, and early and middle not specified); (**b**): studies were stratified by the study design.

3.4. Replete Levels of VitD (≥30 ng/mL) versus Insufficient Levels of VitD (20–30 ng/mL or 15–30 ng/mL)

A total of 11,091 pregnant women (n = 6856 with replete levels of VitD and n = 4235 with insufficient or deficient levels of VitD) from 11 studies were included in this analysis. Women with VitD insufficiency were more likely to develop preeclampsia as compared to women who were VitD replete (OR 1.44, 95% CI 1.24–1.66, I² = 23%, fixed-effect) (Figure 3). Publication bias was detected (Figure S2c, Egger's test: p = 0.005). Sensitivity analysis showed the results were stable after excluding any one of the included studies (Figure S3c). A slightly increased risk of preeclampsia was seen in women with insufficient VitD levels in early pregnancy, but it was not seen in middle pregnancy (early pregnancy: OR 1.40, 95% CI 1.00–1.96, I^2 = 22%, fixed-effect; middle pregnancy: OR 1.21, 95% CI 0.83–1.76, I^2 = 0%, fixed-effect) (Figure 3a). The pooled data from studies with a case-control design showed a significantly higher risk of preeclampsia in women with insufficient VitD levels, but it was not seen in pooled data from cohort studies or cross-sectional studies (case-control: OR 1.59, 95% CI 1.35–1.88, I2 = 0%, fixed-effect; cohort: OR 1.02, 95% CI 0.75–1.39, I^2 = 11%, fixed-effect; cross-sectional: OR 0.85, 95% CI 0.14–5.19) (Figure 3b).

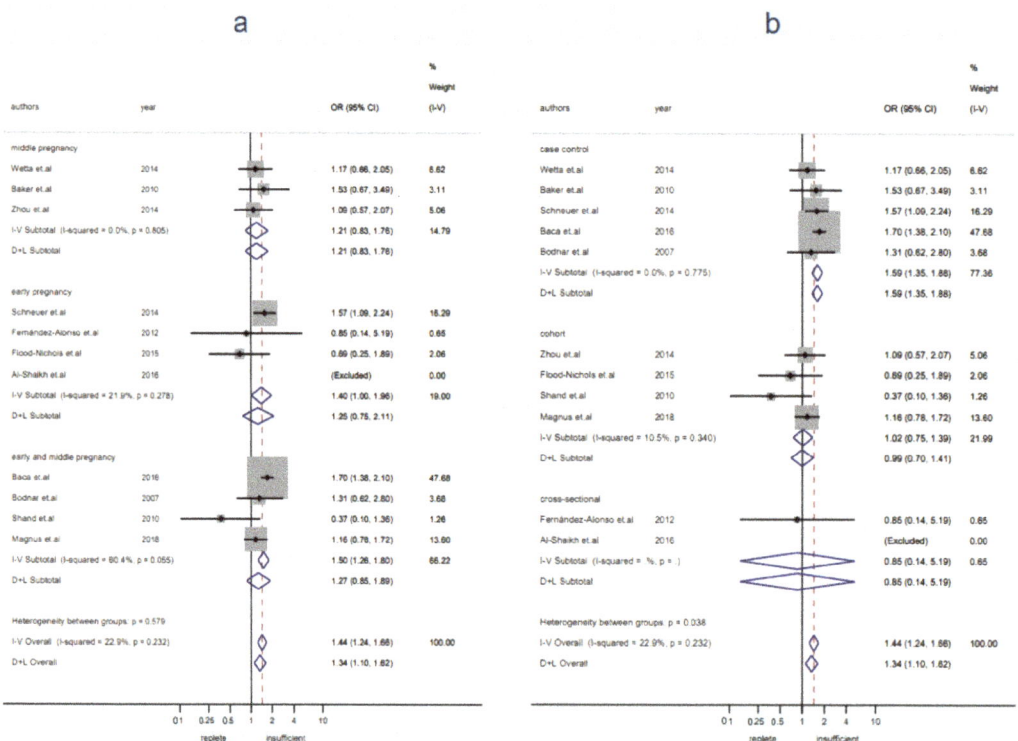

Figure 3. Studies evaluating replete vitamin D levels versus insufficient vitamin D levels. (**a**): Studies were stratified by gestational weeks (early, middle, and early and middle not specified); (**b**): studies were stratified by the study design.

3.5. Replete Levels of VitD (≥30 ng/mL) versus Deficient Levels of VitD (<20 ng/mL or <15 ng/mL)

A total of 8550 pregnant women (n = 4315 with replete levels of VitD and n = 4235 with deficient levels of VitD) from 11 studies were included in this analysis. Women with VitD deficiency were more likely to develop preeclampsia as compared to women with replete VitD levels (OR 1.50, 95% CI 1.05–2.14, I^2 = 64%, random-effect) (Figure 4). No publication bias was detected (Figure S2d, Egger's test: p = 0.188). Sensitivity analysis showed the results were stable after excluding any one of the included studies (Figure S3d). A slightly increased risk of preeclampsia was seen in women with deficient VitD levels in middle pregnancy, but it was not seen in early pregnancy (early pregnancy: OR 0.96, 95% CI 0.61–1.51, I^2 = 0%, fixed-effect; middle pregnancy: OR 1.78, 95% CI 0.93–3.41, I^2 = 54%, random-effect) (Figure 4a). The pooled data from studies with a case-control design showed a significantly higher risk of preeclampsia in women with VitD deficiency, but it was not seen in pooled data from cohort studies or cross-sectional studies (case-control: OR

1.99, 95% CI 1.24–3.18, I² = 71%, random-effect; cohort: OR 1.10, 95% CI 0.81–1.50, I2 = 0%, fixed-effect; cross-sectional: OR 0.71, 95% CI 0.14–3.62, I² = 0%, fixed-effect) (Figure 4b).

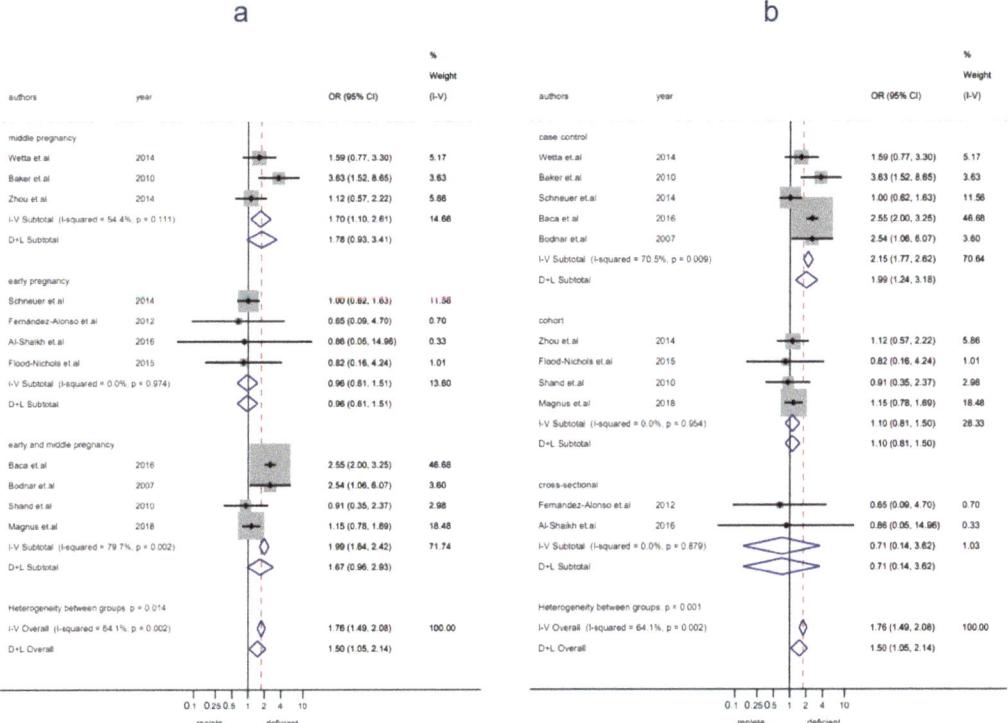

Figure 4. Studies evaluating replete vitamin D levels versus deficient vitamin D levels. (**a**): Studies were stratified by gestational weeks (early, middle, and early and middle not specified); (**b**): studies were stratified by the study design.

4. Discussion

Our study included data from 22 observational studies and demonstrated an association between VitD deficiency or insufficiency and pre-eclampsia risks in early to middle pregnancy.

The pathogenesis of preeclampsia remains incompletely understood. It is proposed that incomplete remodeling of spiral arteries of the uterus during placentation induces limited perfusion and hypoxia of the placenta, with subsequent release of antiangiogenic factors into the maternal circulation [49–51]. These antiangiogenic factors, including tyrosine kinase-1 and soluble endoglin, can lead to endothelial damage and the clinical features that define preeclampsia [52,53]. In addition, a large amount of proinflammatory cytokines (IL-1β, IL-6, and IL-8) are released from the neutrophils and monocytes in the decidua, leading to increased damage to the blood vessels [54,55]. A previous study demonstrated that increased VitD levels improved the invasion of the human extravillous trophoblast and thus proposed that VitD may exert a preventive effect on the development of preeclamptic disease [12]. Additionally, accumulating evidence have suggested that VitD plays a beneficial role in endothelial repair and angiogenesis [13–15] and that VitD deficiency is associated with the pathogenesis of cardiovascular diseases and arterial hypertension [16,17]. Therefore, VitD may have a role in augmenting endothelial repair and angiogenesis and controlling blood pressure in preeclampsia [18] and its immunomodulatory properties may also reduce the risk of preeclampsia development [13,19,20].

The association between VitD deficiency during pregnancy and preeclampsia has been much investigated. Previous systematic reviews of observational studies have demonstrated that women with VitD deficiency (at cutoff 20 ng/mL) were more likely to develop preeclampsia [27,28,56,57]. However, the gestation at which the blood was collected are not fully discussed in these systematic reviews. In this review, we focused on the association of VitD levels in early and middle pregnancy, and VitD supplementation at these points in pregnancy may provide an opportunity for disease prevention or modification. Our review also included several new studies and important studies that have been omitted in previous meta-analyses. Moreover, most previous reviews have compared VitD levels $\geq$ 20 ng/mL with VitD levels < 20 ng/mL, whereas our study compared VitD levels $\geq$ 30 ng/mL, <30 ng/mL, and <20 ng/mL. Our study demonstrates that VitD levels higher than 30 ng/mL are associated with reduced preeclampsia risk when compared with VitD levels < 30 ng/mL or <20 ng/mL, suggesting that women may benefit from the supplementation of VitD to a level of $\geq$30 ng/mL in early and middle pregnancy. This has been supported by previous observational studies and meta-analysis which demonstrated that VitD supplementation during pregnancy was related to a reduced rate of preeclampsia [58–62]. However, a systematic review of randomized trials found VitD supplementation did not significantly alter preeclampsia risk [63]. It should be noted that only three randomized trials with a total sample size of 654 were included in this systematic review [63], which may explain the inconsistency with other studies. A previous randomized trial suggested that VitD supplementation (4400 vs. 400 IU/d) in 10–18 weeks of pregnancy was not able to reduce preeclampsia risks [24]. However, VitD $\geq$ 30 ng/mL at the trial entry were related a reduced rate of preeclampsia [24]. It should be noted that only 74% pregnant women has a replete VitD levels in the 4400 IU/d group in late pregnancy [24], which may explain the nonsignificant difference of preeclampsia incidence for VitD supplementation in early or middle pregnancy. Future trials should further investigate whether VitD supplementation to the replete levels during pregnancy is associated with reduced preeclampsia.

Our review has several strengths. We limited the gestational age of blood collection to early and middle pregnancy. Additionally, we compared replete, insufficient, and deficient VitD status and found that women who were VitD replete had lower rates of preeclampsia than women with VitD insufficiency or deficiency. We also conducted sensitivity analysis and demonstrated that our results were robust after omitting any one of the included studies.

This systematic review also has several limitations. The available studies were heterogeneous in terms of gestational weeks, study design, methods of VitD measurement, and skin characteristics. Additionally, we included observational studies; therefore, there is the potential that unrecognized confounders may have impacted our results. Recognizing the limitations of studies included in meta-analyses, however, forms a basis for future studies with more optimal design and methods to define the role of VitD in preeclampsia. Future RCTs should consider initiating VitD supplementation in early or middle pregnancy or even before pregnancy in women with VitD insufficiency or deficiency.

In conclusion, our systematic review demonstrated that VitD insufficiency (20–30 ng/mL) or deficiency (<20 ng/mL) was associated with an increased risk of preeclampsia. This raises the possibility that VitD supplementation in early or middle pregnancy may represent a risk-modifying therapy.

Supplementary Materials: The following supporting information can be downloaded at: https://www.mdpi.com/article/10.3390/nu14050999/s1, Table S1: Search method for literature; Table S2: The Newcastle-Ottawa Scale (NOS) for assessing the quality of case-control studies; Table S3: The Newcastle-Ottawa Scale (NOS) for assessing the quality of cohort studies; Table S4: AHQR for assessing the quality of cross-sectional studies; Table S5: Vitamin D cutoff values and the calculated rate of preeclampsia in the included studies; Figure S1: Flowchart for study selection; Figure S2:

Funnel plot to assess publication bias. (a): Studies evaluating replete versus insufficient or deficient vitamin D levels; (b): Studies evaluating replete or insufficient versus deficient vitamin D levels; (c): Studies evaluating replete versus insufficient vitamin D levels; (d): Studies evaluating replete versus deficient vitamin D levels; Figure S3: Sensitivity analysis investigating the influence of a single study on the overall meta-analysis estimate. (a): Studies evaluating replete versus insufficient or deficient vitamin D levels; (b): Studies evaluating replete or insufficient versus deficient vitamin D levels; (c): Studies evaluating replete versus insufficient vitamin D levels; (d): Studies evaluating replete versus deficient vitamin D levels.

Author Contributions: Conceptualization, K.-L.H.; methodology, K.-L.H. and C.-X.Z.; software, K.-L.H., P.C. and C.-X.Z.; validation, K.-L.H., D.Z., S.H., P.C. and C.-X.Z.; formal analysis, K.-L.H.; investigation, K.-L.H. and C.-X.Z.; resources, K.-L.H. and C.-X.Z.; writing—original draft preparation, K.-L.H. and C.-X.Z.; writing—review and editing, K.-L.H. and S.H. All authors have read and agreed to the published version of the manuscript.

Funding: This study is supported by the National Key Research and Development Program of China (2018YFC1005003), The National Key Research and Development Program of China (2021YFC2700601), The National Natural Science Foundation of China (No. 81974224), the Key Research and Development Program of Zhejiang Province (2021C03098), the National Key Research and Development Program of China (2021YFC2700402). All these fundings have no role in study design, collection, analysis, and interpretation of data, writing of the report, and the decision to submit the article for publication.

Institutional Review Board Statement: Not applicable.

Informed Consent Statement: Not applicable.

Conflicts of Interest: The authors declare no conflict of interest.

References

1. Mol, B.W.J.; Roberts, C.T.; Thangaratinam, S.; Magee, L.A.; de Groot, C.J.M.; Hofmeyr, G.J. Pre-eclampsia. *Lancet* **2016**, *387*, 999–1011. [CrossRef]
2. Macedo, T.C.C.; Montagna, E.; Trevisan, C.M.; Zaia, V.; de Oliveira, R.; Barbosa, C.P.; Laganà, A.S.; Bianco, B. Prevalence of preeclampsia and eclampsia in adolescent pregnancy: A systematic review and meta-analysis of 291,247 adolescents worldwide since 1969. *Eur. J. Obstet. Gynecol. Reprod. Biol.* **2020**, *248*, 177–186. [CrossRef] [PubMed]
3. McDonald, S.D.; Malinowski, A.; Zhou, Q.; Yusuf, S.; Devereaux, P.J. Cardiovascular sequelae of preeclampsia/eclampsia: A systematic review and meta-analyses. *Am. Heart J.* **2008**, *156*, 918–930. [CrossRef] [PubMed]
4. McDonald, S.D.; Han, Z.; Walsh, M.W.; Gerstein, H.C.; Devereaux, P.J. Kidney disease after preeclampsia: A systematic review and meta-analysis. *Am. J. Kidney Dis.* **2010**, *55*, 1026–1039. [CrossRef] [PubMed]
5. Covella, B.; Vinturache, A.E.; Cabiddu, G.; Attini, R.; Gesualdo, L.; Versino, E.; Piccoli, G.B. A systematic review and meta-analysis indicates long-term risk of chronic and end-stage kidney disease after preeclampsia. *Kidney Int.* **2019**, *96*, 711–727. [CrossRef] [PubMed]
6. Javaid, M.K.; Crozier, S.R.; Harvey, N.C.; Gale, C.R.; Dennison, E.M.; Boucher, B.J.; Arden, N.K.; Godfrey, K.M.; Cooper, C. Maternal vitamin D status during pregnancy and childhood bone mass at age 9 years: A longitudinal study. *Lancet* **2006**, *367*, 36–43. [CrossRef]
7. Karras, S.N.; Anagnostis, P.; Annweiler, C.; Naughton, D.P.; Petroczi, A.; Bili, E.; Harizopoulou, V.; Tarlatzis, B.C.; Persinaki, A.; Papadopoulou, F.; et al. Maternal vitamin D status during pregnancy: The Mediterranean reality. *Eur. J. Clin. Nutr.* **2014**, *68*, 864–869. [CrossRef]
8. Hossein-nezhad, A.; Holick, M.F. Vitamin D for health: A global perspective. *Mayo. Clin. Proc.* **2013**, *88*, 720–755. [CrossRef]
9. Holick, M.F.; Binkley, N.C.; Bischoff-Ferrari, H.A.; Gordon, C.M.; Hanley, D.A.; Heaney, R.P.; Murad, M.H.; Weaver, C.M. Evaluation, treatment, and prevention of vitamin D deficiency: An Endocrine Society clinical practice guideline. *J. Clin. Endocrinol. Metab.* **2011**, *96*, 1911–1930. [CrossRef]
10. Kiely, M.E.; Wagner, C.L.; Roth, D.E. Vitamin D in pregnancy: Where we are and where we should go. *J. Steroid. Biochem. Mol. Biol.* **2020**, *201*, 105669. [CrossRef]
11. Wetta, L.A.; Biggio, J.R.; Cliver, S.; Abramovici, A.; Barnes, S.; Tita, A.T. Is midtrimester vitamin D status associated with spontaneous preterm birth and preeclampsia? *Am. J. Perinatol.* **2014**, *31*, 541–546. [PubMed]
12. Chan, S.Y.; Susarla, R.; Canovas, D.; Vasilopoulou, E.; Ohizua, O.; McCabe, C.J.; Hewison, M.; Kilby, M.D. Vitamin D promotes human extravillous trophoblast invasion in vitro. *Placenta* **2015**, *36*, 403–409. [CrossRef] [PubMed]
13. Poniedziałek-Czajkowska, E.; Mierzyński, R. Could Vitamin D Be Effective in Prevention of Preeclampsia? *Nutrients* **2021**, *13*, 3854. [CrossRef] [PubMed]

14. Schröder-Heurich, B.; von Hardenberg, S.; Brodowski, L.; Kipke, B.; Meyer, N.; Borns, K.; von Kaisenberg, C.S.; Brinkmann, H.; Claus, P.; von Versen-Höynck, F. Vitamin D improves endothelial barrier integrity and counteracts inflammatory effects on endothelial progenitor cells. *Faseb. J.* **2019**, *33*, 9142–9153. [CrossRef] [PubMed]
15. Brodowski, L.; Burlakov, J.; Myerski, A.C.; von Kaisenberg, C.S.; Grundmann, M.; Hubel, C.A.; von Versen-Höynck, F. Vitamin D prevents endothelial progenitor cell dysfunction induced by sera from women with preeclampsia or conditioned media from hypoxic placenta. *PLoS ONE* **2014**, *9*, e98527. [CrossRef] [PubMed]
16. Pilz, S.; Tomaschitz, A.; Ritz, E.; Pieber, T.R. Vitamin D status and arterial hypertension: A systematic review. *Nat. Rev. Cardiol.* **2009**, *6*, 621–630. [CrossRef] [PubMed]
17. Wimalawansa, S.J. Vitamin D and cardiovascular diseases: Causality. *J. Steroid Biochem. Mol. Biol.* **2018**, *175*, 29–43. [CrossRef]
18. Behjat Sasan, S.; Zandvakili, F.; Soufizadeh, N.; Baybordi, E. The Effects of Vitamin D Supplement on Prevention of Recurrence of Preeclampsia in Pregnant Women with a History of Preeclampsia. *Obstet. Gynecol. Int.* **2017**, *2017*, 8249264. [CrossRef]
19. Evans, K.N.; Bulmer, J.N.; Kilby, M.D.; Hewison, M. Vitamin D and placental-decidual function. *J. Soc. Gynecol. Investig.* **2004**, *11*, 263–271. [CrossRef]
20. Piccinni, M.P.; Scaletti, C.; Maggi, E.; Romagnani, S. Role of hormone-controlled Th1- and Th2-type cytokines in successful pregnancy. *J. Neuroimmunol.* **2000**, *109*, 30–33. [CrossRef]
21. Achkar, M.; Dodds, L.; Giguère, Y.; Forest, J.C.; Armson, B.A.; Woolcott, C.; Agellon, S.; Spencer, A.; Weiler, H.A. Vitamin D status in early pregnancy and risk of preeclampsia. *Am. J. Obstet. Gynecol.* **2015**, *212*, e511–e517. [CrossRef] [PubMed]
22. Baca, K.M.; Simhan, H.N.; Platt, R.W.; Bodnar, L.M. Low maternal 25-hydroxyvitamin D concentration increases the risk of severe and mild preeclampsia. *Ann. Epidemiol.* **2016**, *26*, 853–857.e1. [CrossRef] [PubMed]
23. Serrano, N.C.; Guío, E.; Quintero-Lesmes, D.C.; Becerra-Bayona, S.; Luna-Gonzalez, M.L.; Herrera, V.M.; Prada, C.E. Vitamin D deficiency and pre-eclampsia in Colombia: PREVitD study. *Pregnancy Hypertens* **2018**, *14*, 240–244. [CrossRef] [PubMed]
24. Mirzakhani, H.; Litonjua, A.A.; McElrath, T.F.; O'Connor, G.; Lee-Parritz, A.; Iverson, R.; Macones, G.; Strunk, R.C.; Bacharier, L.B.; Zeiger, R.; et al. Early pregnancy vitamin D status and risk of preeclampsia. *J. Clin. Investig.* **2016**, *126*, 4702–4715. [CrossRef] [PubMed]
25. Powe, C.E.; Seely, E.W.; Rana, S.; Bhan, I.; Ecker, J.; Karumanchi, S.A.; Thadhani, R. First trimester vitamin D, vitamin D binding protein, and subsequent preeclampsia. *Hypertension* **2010**, *56*, 758–763. [CrossRef] [PubMed]
26. Zhou, J.; Su, L.; Liu, M.; Liu, Y.; Cao, X.; Wang, Z.; Xiao, H. Associations between 25-hydroxyvitamin D levels and pregnancy outcomes: A prospective observational study in southern China. *Eur. J. Clin. Nutr.* **2014**, *68*, 925–930. [CrossRef]
27. Aguilar-Cordero, M.J.; Lasserrot-Cuadrado, A.; Mur-Villar, N.; León-Ríos, X.A.; Rivero-Blanco, T.; Pérez-Castillo, I.M. Vitamin D, preeclampsia and prematurity: A systematic review and meta-analysis of observational and interventional studies. *Midwifery* **2020**, *87*, 102707. [CrossRef]
28. Akbari, S.; Khodadadi, B.; Ahmadi, S.A.Y.; Abbaszadeh, S.; Shahsavar, F. Association of vitamin D level and vitamin D deficiency with risk of preeclampsia: A systematic review and updated meta-analysis. *Taiwan J. Obstet. Gynecol.* **2018**, *57*, 241–247. [CrossRef]
29. Serrano-Díaz, N.C.; Gamboa-Delgado, E.M.; Domínguez-Urrego, C.L.; Vesga-Varela, A.L.; Serrano-Gómez, S.E.; Quintero-Lesmes, D.C. Vitamin D and risk of preeclampsia: A systematic review and meta-analysis. *Biomedica* **2018**, *38* (Suppl. S1), 43–53. [CrossRef]
30. Wei, S.Q.; Qi, H.P.; Luo, Z.C.; Fraser, W.D. Maternal vitamin D status and adverse pregnancy outcomes: A systematic review and meta-analysis. *J. Matern. Fetal. Neonatal. Med.* **2013**, *26*, 889–899. [CrossRef]
31. Page, M.J.; McKenzie, J.E.; Bossuyt, P.M.; Boutron, I.; Hoffmann, T.C.; Mulrow, C.D.; Shamseer, L.; Tetzlaff, J.M.; Moher, D. Updating guidance for reporting systematic reviews: Development of the PRISMA 2020 statement. *J. Clin. Epidemiol.* **2021**, *134*, 103–112. [CrossRef] [PubMed]
32. Wells, G.; Shea, B.; O'Connell, D.; Peterson, J.; Welch, V.; Losos, M.; Tugwell, P. The Newcastle-Ottawa Scale (NOS) for Assessing the Quality of Nonrandomised Studies in Meta-Analyses. In Proceedings of the 3rd Symposium on Systematic Reviews: Beyond the Basics. Improving Quality and Impact, Oxford, UK, 3–5 July 2000. Available online: http://www.ohri.ca/programs/clinical_epidemiology/oxford.asp (accessed on 5 July 2000).
33. Baker, A.M.; Haeri, S.; Camargo, C.A., Jr.; Espinola, J.A.; Stuebe, A.M. A nested case-control study of midgestation vitamin D deficiency and risk of severe preeclampsia. *J. Clin. Endocrinol. Metab.* **2010**, *95*, 5105–5109. [CrossRef] [PubMed]
34. Schneuer, F.J.; Roberts, C.L.; Guilbert, C.; Simpson, J.M.; Algert, C.S.; Khambalia, A.Z.; Tasevski, V.; Ashton, A.W.; Morris, J.M.; Nassar, N. Effects of maternal serum 25-hydroxyvitamin D concentrations in the first trimester on subsequent pregnancy outcomes in an Australian population. *Am. J. Clin. Nutr.* **2014**, *99*, 287–295. [CrossRef]
35. Bodnar, L.M.; Catov, J.M.; Simhan, H.N.; Holick, M.F.; Powers, R.W.; Roberts, J.M. Maternal vitamin D deficiency increases the risk of preeclampsia. *J. Clin. Endocrinol. Metab.* **2007**, *92*, 3517–3522. [CrossRef] [PubMed]
36. Benachi, A.; Baptiste, A.; Taieb, J.; Tsatsaris, V.; Guibourdenche, J.; Senat, M.V.; Haidar, H.; Jani, J.; Guizani, M.; Jouannic, J.M.; et al. Relationship between vitamin D status in pregnancy and the risk for preeclampsia: A nested case-control study. *Clin. Nutr.* **2020**, *39*, 440–446. [CrossRef] [PubMed]
37. Fernández-Alonso, A.M.; Dionis-Sánchez, E.C.; Chedraui, P.; González-Salmerón, M.D.; Pérez-López, F.R. First-trimester maternal serum 25-hydroxyvitamin D_3 status and pregnancy outcome. *Int. J. Gynaecol. Obstet.* **2012**, *116*, 6–9. [CrossRef]
38. Christoph, P.; Challande, P.; Raio, L.; Surbek, D. High prevalence of severe vitamin D deficiency during the first trimester in pregnant women in Switzerland and its potential contributions to adverse outcomes in the pregnancy. *Swiss. Med. Wkly.* **2020**, *150*, w20238. [CrossRef]

39. Al-Shaikh, G.K.; Ibrahim, G.H.; Fayed, A.A.; Al-Mandeel, H. Impact of vitamin D deficiency on maternal and birth outcomes in the Saudi population: A cross-sectional study. *BMC Pregnancy Childbirth* **2016**, *16*, 119. [CrossRef]
40. Hemmingway, A.; Kenny, L.C.; Malvisi, L.; Kiely, M.E. Exploring the concept of functional vitamin D deficiency in pregnancy: Impact of the interaction between 25-hydroxyvitamin D and parathyroid hormone on perinatal outcomes. *Am. J. Clin. Nutr.* **2018**, *108*, 821–829. [CrossRef]
41. Wei, S.Q.; Audibert, F.; Hidiroglou, N.; Sarafin, K.; Julien, P.; Wu, Y.; Luo, Z.C.; Fraser, W.D. Longitudinal vitamin D status in pregnancy and the risk of pre-eclampsia. *Bjog* **2012**, *119*, 832–839. [CrossRef]
42. Flood-Nichols, S.K.; Tinnemore, D.; Huang, R.R.; Napolitano, P.G.; Ippolito, D.L. Vitamin D deficiency in early pregnancy. *PLoS ONE* **2015**, *10*, e0123763. [CrossRef] [PubMed]
43. Shand, A.W.; Nassar, N.; Von Dadelszen, P.; Innis, S.M.; Green, T.J. Maternal vitamin D status in pregnancy and adverse pregnancy outcomes in a group at high risk for pre-eclampsia. *Bjog* **2010**, *117*, 1593–1598. [CrossRef] [PubMed]
44. van Weert, B.; van den Berg, D.; Hrudey, E.J.; Oostvogels, A.; de Miranda, E.; Vrijkotte, T.G.M. Is first trimester vitamin D status in nulliparous women associated with pregnancy related hypertensive disorders? *Midwifery* **2016**, *34*, 117–122. [CrossRef] [PubMed]
45. Magnus, M.C.; Miliku, K.; Bauer, A.; Engel, S.M.; Felix, J.F.; Jaddoe, V.W.V.; Lawlor, D.A.; London, S.J.; Magnus, P.; McGinnis, R.; et al. Vitamin D and risk of pregnancy related hypertensive disorders: Mendelian randomisation study. *BMJ* **2018**, *361*, k2167. [CrossRef] [PubMed]
46. Scholl, T.O.; Chen, X.; Stein, T.P. Vitamin D, secondary hyperparathyroidism, and preeclampsia. *Am. J. Clin. Nutr.* **2013**, *98*, 787–793. [CrossRef]
47. Álvarez-Fernández, I.; Prieto, B.; Rodríguez, V.; Ruano, Y.; Escudero, A.I.; Álvarez, F.V. Role of vitamin D and sFlt-1/PlGF ratio in the development of early- and late-onset preeclampsia. *Clin. Chem. Lab. Med.* **2015**, *53*, 1033–1040. [CrossRef]
48. Gidlöf, S.; Silva, A.T.; Gustafsson, S.; Lindqvist, P.G. Vitamin D and the risk of preeclampsia–a nested case-control study. *Acta Obstet. Gynecol. Scand.* **2015**, *94*, 904–908. [CrossRef]
49. Kaufmann, P.; Black, S.; Huppertz, B. Endovascular trophoblast invasion: Implications for the pathogenesis of intrauterine growth retardation and preeclampsia. *Biol. Reprod.* **2003**, *69*, 1–7. [CrossRef]
50. Ishihara, N.; Matsuo, H.; Murakoshi, H.; Laoag-Fernandez, J.B.; Samoto, T.; Maruo, T. Increased apoptosis in the syncytiotrophoblast in human term placentas complicated by either preeclampsia or intrauterine growth retardation. *Am. J. Obstet. Gynecol.* **2002**, *186*, 158–166. [CrossRef]
51. Perez-Sepulveda, A.; Torres, M.J.; Khoury, M.; Illanes, S.E. Innate immune system and preeclampsia. *Front. Immunol.* **2014**, *5*, 244. [CrossRef]
52. Chaiworapongsa, T.; Chaemsaithong, P.; Yeo, L.; Romero, R. Pre-eclampsia part 1: Current understanding of its pathophysiology. *Nat. Rev. Nephrol.* **2014**, *10*, 466–480. [CrossRef] [PubMed]
53. Leaños-Miranda, A.; Navarro-Romero, C.S.; Sillas-Pardo, L.J.; Ramírez-Valenzuela, K.L.; Isordia-Salas, I.; Jiménez-Trejo, L.M. Soluble Endoglin As a Marker for Preeclampsia, Its Severity, and the Occurrence of Adverse Outcomes. *Hypertension* **2019**, *74*, 991–997. [CrossRef] [PubMed]
54. Borzychowski, A.M.; Sargent, I.L.; Redman, C.W. Inflammation and pre-eclampsia. *Semin. Fetal Neonatal Med.* **2006**, *11*, 309–316. [CrossRef] [PubMed]
55. Luppi, P.; Deloia, J.A. Monocytes of preeclamptic women spontaneously synthesize pro-inflammatory cytokines. *Clin. Immunol.* **2006**, *118*, 268–275. [CrossRef]
56. Hyppönen, E.; Cavadino, A.; Williams, D.; Fraser, A.; Vereczkey, A.; Fraser, W.D.; Bánhidy, F.; Lawlor, D.; Czeizel, A.E. Vitamin D and Pre-Eclampsia: Original Data, Systematic Review and Meta-Analysis. *Ann. Nutr. Metab.* **2013**, *63*, 331–340. [CrossRef]
57. Tabesh, M.; Salehi-Abargouei, A.; Tabesh, M.; Esmaillzadeh, A. Maternal vitamin D status and risk of pre-eclampsia: A systematic review and meta-analysis. *J. Clin. Endocrinol. Metab.* **2013**, *98*, 3165–3173. [CrossRef]
58. Fogacci, S.; Fogacci, F.; Banach, M.; Michos, E.D.; Hernandez, A.V.; Lip, G.Y.H.; Blaha, M.J.; Toth, P.P.; Borghi, C.; Cicero, A.F.G. Vitamin D supplementation and incident preeclampsia: A systematic review and meta-analysis of randomized clinical trials. *Clin. Nutr.* **2020**, *39*, 1742–1752. [CrossRef]
59. Fu, Z.M.; Ma, Z.Z.; Liu, G.J.; Wang, L.L.; Guo, Y. Vitamins supplementation affects the onset of preeclampsia. *J. Formos. Med. Assoc.* **2018**, *117*, 6–13. [CrossRef]
60. Khaing, W.; Vallibhakara, S.A.; Tantrakul, V.; Vallibhakara, O.; Rattanasiri, S.; McEvoy, M.; Attia, J.; Thakkinstian, A. Calcium and Vitamin D Supplementation for Prevention of Preeclampsia: A Systematic Review and Network Meta-Analysis. *Nutrients* **2017**, *9*, 1141. [CrossRef]
61. Oh, C.; Keats, E.C.; Bhutta, Z.A. Vitamin and Mineral Supplementation During Pregnancy on Maternal, Birth, Child Health and Development Outcomes in Low- and Middle-Income Countries: A Systematic Review and Meta-Analysis. *Nutrients* **2020**, *12*, 491. [CrossRef]
62. Palacios, C.; Kostiuk, L.K.; Peña-Rosas, J.P. Vitamin D supplementation for women during pregnancy. *Cochrane Database Syst. Rev.* **2019**, *7*, Cd008873. [CrossRef] [PubMed]
63. Pérez-López, F.R.; Pasupuleti, V.; Mezones-Holguin, E.; Benites-Zapata, V.A.; Thota, P.; Deshpande, A.; Hernandez, A.V. Effect of vitamin D supplementation during pregnancy on maternal and neonatal outcomes: A systematic review and meta-analysis of randomized controlled trials. *Fertil. Steril.* **2015**, *103*, 1278–1288.e4. [CrossRef] [PubMed]

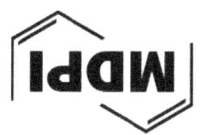

MDPI
St. Alban-Anlage 66
4052 Basel
Switzerland
Tel. +41 61 683 77 34
Fax +41 61 302 89 18
www.mdpi.com

Nutrients Editorial Office
E-mail: nutrients@mdpi.com
www.mdpi.com/journal/nutrients